Medical Wisdom
and Doctoring

Medical Wisdom and Doctoring

The Art of 21st Century Practice

Robert B. Taylor, M.D.

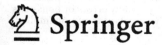 Springer

Robert B. Taylor
Department of Family Medicine
School of Medicine
Oregon Health and Sciences University
Portland, OR
USA
taylorr@ohsu.edu

ISBN 978-1-4419-5520-3   e-ISBN 978-1-4419-5521-0
DOI 10.1007/978-1-4419-5521-0
Springer New York Dordrecht Heidelberg London

Library of Congress Control Number: 2009942273

Printed on acid-free paper

Springer is part of Springer Science+Business Media (www.springer.com)

Knowledge and wisdom, far from being one,
Have oft-times no connection. Knowledge dwells
In heads replete with thoughts of other men;
Wisdom in minds attentive to their own.
Knowledge is proud that he has learned so much;
Wisdom is humble that he knows no more.
  From *The Task*, by British poet William Cowper (1731–1800)

Medicine can never abdicate the obligation to care for the patient
and to teach patient care.
  A quote from American medical educator and editor
  Maurice B . Strauss (1904–1974). From: Medicine
  1964;19:43.

To realize one's destiny is a person's only obligation.
  Advice from the man who calls himself king to the shepherd
  boy seeking his as-yet-unknown treasure and, ultimately, his
  Personal Legend, what he has always
  wanted to accomplish.

  Telling more about the *Personal Legend,* the man who calls
  himself a king continues:
…there is one great truth on this planet: whoever you are, or
whatever it is that you do, when you really want something, it's
because that desire originated in the soul of the universe. It's your
mission on earth.
  From *The Alchemist,* by Paulo Coelho, New York: HarperCollins;
  1993, page 22.

Preface

This book is about what we have learned in several millennia of medical practice and about the art of doctoring – using that wisdom in daily patient care. It is about the elderly woman with pneumonia you treated yesterday afternoon and the middle aged man with chest pain you saw this morning. It is about the child with croup, struggling for the next breath in the middle of the night, and about the medicines we use each day. It is about your community members who look to you for leadership and the medical student you are mentoring. It is also about you and me, as humble members of the most noble profession, and our families who support us and who worry about our well-being.

To fully appreciate the nobility of our calling, we physicians – indeed, all health professionals – need to know about current applications of our heritage from past generations of medical practitioners and scholars. These include how to think like both a professional clinician and an empathic human being; how to manage disease, illness and death; and how to care for our patients, their families, and ourselves and our families – in short, how to be a knowledgeable, wise and caring twenty first century physician.

As you read the pages that follow, you will discern three themes – as suggested by the introductory quotations. The first involves the legacy of medical knowledge and wisdom provided to us by our predecessors, and for which we should give thanks each day. Knowledge and wisdom, of course, are not quite the same. There is *medical knowledge*, the rapidly expanding treasury of objective data that helps us deliver evidence-based medical care, and there is *medical wisdom*, which is subjective, philosophical, and sometimes surprisingly intuitive. The second theme is the imperative of our service to others, the fundamental mission of medicine and doctoring. And the third is the physician's ongoing quest for self-actualization – in the words of Paulo Coelho, the seeking of one's personal legend, a journey that takes on special meaning for those would be healers.

In exploring the three themes, I have sought the time-honored advice of experienced healers and investigators – the wise physicians. A great deal of what follows might be considered "oral history," thoughts and tales seldom recorded in standard textbooks. Nevertheless, to make this the most scholarly work possible, I have attempted to support precepts and maxims with concrete examples derived from three sources: the current medical literature, anecdotes from the history of medicine, and the personal narratives of practicing physicians, including some of my own stories.

The book's title *Medical Wisdom and Doctoring: the Art of 21st Century Practice* was chosen to emphasize that the content is relevant to what physicians do today. You will read about some current diagnostic and therapeutic approaches, practical communication skills, pertinent ethical issues, and trends that just might foretell tomorrow's practice. In addition, there are chapters on caring for you, the physician, as well as for your family and your community – endeavors I consider essential to achieving your full potential as a physician.

Some items you will read describe the exploits of "great doctors" who have preceded us. These include Moses Maimonides, Ambroise Paré, John Snow, Francis Weld Peabody, the brothers Mayo and others. In addition, many of the topics presented have come from unsung medical heroes, the hardworking clinicians who, in their daily practice of medicine, have also been some of our most *wise physicians*, who have given us ideas and techniques that merit sharing with future generations. In the end, the selection of content is mine, based on four decades of experience in medical practice and teaching.

To continue with the "oral history" thought mentioned above, this book tells examples of medical lore passed from senior to junior clinician, from teacher to pupil, from mentor to mentee. Actually, we should hope that the precepts, methods, and wise words are being passed on, but such is not always the case. For both young and older physicians, the days are often too busy for reflective discourse and for "tales told around the campfire." What's more, with the proliferation of scientific knowledge, there seems to be scant time to share the *wisdom* of medicine. Hence, in some ways, what you will read in the coming pages represents what you may not have learned in medical school and residency, or what may sometimes be accorded low priority amid the demands of daily practice.

This book is written for physicians. Yet, the content is pertinent to all clinicians. For the medical student, resident in training and physician in early practice, nurse and physician assistant who provide patient care, the concepts presented can help avoid clinical misadventures and potentially painful experiential learning. Even if you have been in practice for two or three decades, this book is sure to present some approaches to healthcare you have not previously considered, and it will help satisfy your curiosity as to whether or not your daily practice of medicine is consistent with that of the *wise physicians*.

Of course, with time some advice needs to be tweaked a little to bring it up to date with twenty first century medicine. For example, in 1903, Sir William Osler advocated bedside teaching as a radical reform in teaching medical students.[1] Yet today, with short, focused hospital stays often measured in hours and with many alternative venues for patient care, teaching is more likely to occur in the physician's office, emergency department of the hospital, operating room, or even the patient's home or nursing home. For this reason, I have presented timeless maxims, supported by examples that relate to today's practice. Also, in the case of personal practice anecdotes, I have disguised names and circumstances to protect patient confidentiality, while trying not to lose the flavor of the stories.

I urge you to read *Medical Wisdom and Doctoring* for personal enrichment. You will find some quotes from Hippocrates and Pogo, Albert Schweitzer and Charles Barkley (yes, the basketball player Charles Barkley), Louis Pasteur and Little Orphan Annie. You will learn the success secrets of Applebee's Restaurants, the back-story of Joseph

Lister and Listerine, and the identity of the role model for Sherlock Holmes. Yet, for those who just must be learning something "useful," I have included some hard-core clinical pearls, such as the tip-off that can alert you when a patient may be developing herpes zoster ophthalmicus, the best way to test for diabetic peripheral neuropathy, what to consider when you encounter a unilateral right-sided varicocele, and the significance of pleuritic-type chest pain radiating to the left shoulder and relieved by leaning forward. I would be honored if some forward-thinking medical school professor designates this book as a required course text, but I have stopped short of providing details of how to diagnose and treat specific ailments.

The aphorism "Medicine is not only a science; it is also an art" is attributed to medieval physician Paracelsus (1493–1591)[2] and more than anything, this book is about the art of medicine. And so, what you hold in your hand is intended to be read on a quiet evening beside an open fire, on a long plane ride, or perhaps as something to ease the tedium of a night in the on-call room, because it presents concepts that should be savored when you have time for thoughtful reflection.

Now settle in and enjoy *Medical Wisdom and Doctoring*.

Portland, OR   Robert B. Taylor, MD

REFERENCES

1. Osler W. On the need of a radical reform in our methods of teaching senior students. *Med News* 1903;82:49-53.
2. Paracelsus. *Die grosse Wundarznei*. Quoted in Strauss MB. Familiar medical quotations. Boston: Little, Brown; 1968:295.

Contents

Contents

xi

About This Book

There are men and classes of men that stand above the common herd: the soldier, the sailor, and the shepherd not infrequently; the artist rarely; rarer still, the clergyman; the physician almost as a rule. He is the flower (such as it is) of our civilization; and when that stage of man is done with, and only to be marveled at in history, he will be thought to have shared as little as any in the defects of the period, and most notably exhibited the virtues of the race. Generosity he has, such as is possible to those who practice an art, never to those who drive a trade; discretion, tested by a hundred secrets; tact, tried in a thousand embarrassments; and what are more important, Herculean cheerfulness and courage. So that he brings air and cheer into the sick room, and often enough, though not so often as he wishes, brings healing.

Robert Louis Stevenson

Dedication to *Underwoods*. [1]

Shirley Iverson had health insurance, and with a new job at age 42, she was one of the lucky ones. Her chief problem was that she had recently moved to the city and had not yet established her "medical home." When she began having episodes of feeling weak and light-headed, she decided to seek help. Her quest began with a series of telephone calls to four medical offices, only to be told, "We are not taking any new patients," or "Our office is not on the panel for your insurance company." Eventually a large clinic offered her an appointment a week later, after verifying her insurance coverage. When she showed up for her appointment, she checked in at the front desk and then spent some time with the financial screener, who relieved her of thirty dollar co-pay. Next the medical assistant showed her to a room, asked her chief complaint, logged on to the electronic medical record, and instructed her to disrobe and to put on an examination gown. Another person in white – a nurse – came to take her vital signs and elicit details of the clinical history.

Finally, after all the telephone queries, day-of-visit encounters with four office employees, and a long wait sitting in a drafty exam gown, the door opened and the physician entered the room, shook her hand and sat down. "Hi, Ms. Iverson, I'm Doctor Johnson. It's great to meet you. Let's talk about what brings you in today." Somehow, the doctor's manner put her at ease, and Shirley sensed intuitively that she could relax and tell this physician her story.

In the twenty-first century, the process of accessing healthcare can seem like a visit to the headquarters of a large corporation, until, if you are fortunate, you get in the exam room with an experienced and empathic physician, and you recognize that this is a person whom you can trust with your health and your secrets. At least this is what should happen when patient and physician eventually get together. Actually it often does.

Shirley Iverson's story and the experiences of countless other persons seeking healthcare today provoke cognitive dissonance. Think about it: caring, trustworthy clinicians providing personalized care to individual patients in office exam rooms and at the hospital bedsides in what has become a Byzantine and impersonal healthcare enterprise directed by bottom-line administrators, corporate executives, and government officials. This is the world in which we live, and a paradox I wish I could remedy. In this book, I will, for the most part, ignore the current healthcare bureaucracy, a self-serving enterprise with remarkable inertia. Instead, I will pin my hopes on the most promising change agent, the seemingly anachronistic hero in this story – the wise and competent physician, diligently striving to care for each patient with the nobility that earned physicians the status we enjoy in society. The physician-hero, admittedly no longer the key decision-maker in healthcare politics and economics, just might hold the key to better healthcare for all in the future.

And so we seek to understand, and perhaps emulate, the wise physician-hero. In doing so, the coming chapters, like your life in medicine so far, will be a journey. I will be your guide, not because I claim to be wiser than you, the reader, or any of my colleagues, but because I have done the digging and sorting. I have conducted the literature searches, read the books and articles, and assembled a mountain of material, seasoned with a few stories from my own practice years, into the 15 chapters that follow.

In an effort to make this book scholarly as well as reflective, I have included numerous citations to the literature, using two reference styles. The first is a shorthand method, indicating the page numbers in the books found in the *Bibliography*, books describing events in medical history, practice methods, word origins, clinical aphorisms, and classic quotations. In addition, I have also used the traditional style of item-by-item, chapter-by-chapter citations in instances in which the reference source is used only once or twice in the book. I have included numerous citations of both types, in hopes that readers will want to learn more about the topics described.

Then there are the patient-centered stories, some related to me by colleagues, but most coming from my own encounters with patients. Because I will describe events from my professional experience by topic and not in any chronologic order, I will now give you a brief sketch of my life so far as a physician. I graduated from Temple Medical School in Philadelphia in 1961, spent the next 3 years in training, and completing my obligatory service time at the United States Public Health Service Hospital in Norfolk, Virginia. In 1964, accompanied by my wife and two young daughters, I left the USPHS and joined a four-doctor group in New Paltz, NY, a picturesque college town in the Hudson Valley of New York, some 90 miles north of New York City.

In 1968, I left the security of the medical group. In the nearby town of Gardiner, NY I built a 1,500 square foot medical office in what had been an old apple orchard. Here I was a "country doc" until 1978, when I left rural private practice to join the medical school faculty at Wake Forest University in Winston-Salem, NC, a life change sparked by my emerging interest in medical scholarship, chiefly in editing reference books for physicians.

After six years at Wake Forest University School of Medicine, in 1984 I accepted the chairmanship of the Department of

Family Medicine at Oregon Health & Science University in Portland, Oregon. I held this position until 1998, when I became professor/chairman emeritus, a position I hold now.

I tell the outline of my story, not as an exercise in literary narcissism, but as a framework to understand the anecdotes in the pages to come. My story, probably quite different from that of you, the reader, may help to show the diversity of our lives as persons and as professionals. Yet, as physicians we all recognize common milestones – the event of receiving an MD degree, the demanding years of training, the early years of practice, the career decisions we all face, and the life changes experienced as we grow older. These highlights of our lives, along with the stories our patients tell us, are the shared narrative of contemporary medical professionals.

There is more, of course, to the shared narrative of physicians, and that is the many chapters of exploits and service, of misbeliefs and missteps of the generations of healers that have gone before us. I think of this book as being about these events, and the lessons learned from them that influence what we do today.

All I ask is this: If this were a novel – let's say a thriller about a plot to blow up Washington, DC – I would ask you to suspend disbelief. But this is a book about becoming and being a wise physician. And so I urge you to dial down the filter of scientific skepticism that we all have, and seek personal enrichment in the pages that follow. I'll try not to disappoint. The coming chapters will discuss the art of clinical dialog, diagnostic skills, disease management, and caring for the patient rather than the disease. As examples of concepts presented, you will meet the young man declared prematurely dead (Chap. 7), the professor on the payroll of Big Pharma (Chap. 12), the doctor who said, "I don't know" once too often (Chap. 3), the patient who left his car to confront a rattlesnake deep in the Virginia's Dismal Swamp (Chap. 11), and the trichinosis that killed my Grandma's cat (Chap. 4).

Acknowledgments by an author are the humble recognition that no book, especially a retrospective work of this type, is a solo effort. I first thank my family: Anita D. Taylor, MA Ed, a true medical academician and a perceptive editor; our children Diana and Sharon; and our four grandchildren,

Francesca (Frankie), Elizabeth (Masha), Jack, and Anna (Annie). In addition, I want to acknowledge the contributions of many persons who, over the years, have shared their friendship, listening skills, stories and wisdom, some of which is reflected in the pages that follow. In no special order, these valued persons are: Robin Hull, Van Pine, Bob Bomengen, Jim Crowell, Ray and Nancy Friedman, Tom Deutsch, John Saultz, Bill Toffler, Scott Fields, Eric Walsh, Peter Goodwin, Coelleda O'Neil, Ben and Louise Jones, Marge Sosnik, Takashi Yamada, John Kendall, Joseph Van der Veer, and Alan Blum. In addition, I gratefully acknowledge the excellent work of my Springer editor, Katharine Cacace.

Now, it's time to begin. Whether you are a medical student seeking mature learning, or a seasoned practitioner wanting to become wiser than you are, the contents of this book can help. What you are about to read can not only assist you in making good patient care decisions, it can also help alert you to the potential for "unwise" choices in one's professional and personal life. So I invite you to join me as we explore the fascinating world of *Medical Wisdom and Doctoring*.

REFERENCES

1. Stevenson R L. Dedication. Underwoods, a collection of poems published in 1887.

I

Medical Wisdom in the Twenty-First Century

I knew a doctor who was honest, but gentle with his honesty, and was loving, but careful with his love, who was disciplined without being rigid, and right without the stain of arrogance, who was self-questioning without self-doubt, introspective and reflective and in the same moment, decisive, who was strong, hard, adamant, but all those things laced with tenderness and understanding, a doctor who worshipped his calling without worshipping himself, who was busy beyond belief, but who had time – time to smile, to chat, to touch the shoulder and take the hand, and who had time enough for Death as well as Life.

Michael A. LaCombe, MD[1]

This book is intended to help physicians achieve their full potential – to become wise physicians and to be able to apply wisdom in their daily practice – much like the doctor described above by LaCombe.

In this introductory chapter, I discuss some of the concepts imbedded in the title and elucidated in this book: These include the source of our current medical wisdom and methods of doctoring and the rationale behind my term *wise physician*; the art of medicine and service to humanity; aphorisms and precepts as vehicles to communicate medical wisdom; and the paradigmatic underpinnings of the twenty-first century practice.

TODAY'S MEDICAL WISDOM, OUR METHODS OF DOCTORING, AND WISE PHYSICIANS

What we offer patients in the office and hospital – today's doctoring – is the legacy of the generations of physicians and scientists who have preceded us. To borrow a metaphor

R.B. Taylor, *Medical Wisdom and Doctoring: The Art of 21st Century Practice*, DOI 10.1007/978-1-4419-5521-0_1,
© Springer Science+Business Media, LLC 2010

from English physicist Isaac Newton, we should think about those giants upon whose shoulders we stand. The following is a message by physician-educator Félix Martí-Ibáñez (1911–1972) to medical students at New York Medical College in the 1950s:

> You have chosen the most fascinating and dynamic profession there is, a profession with the highest potential for greatness, since the physician's daily work is wrapped up in the subtle web of history. Your labors are linked with those of your colleagues who preceded you in history, and those who are now working all over the world. It is this spiritual unity with our colleagues of all periods and all countries that has made medicine so universal and eternal. For this reason we must study and try to imitate the lives of the "Great Doctors" of history.
>
> Martí-Ibáñez 1961, p. 197.

Great Doctors

There are "Great Doctors"; there are "top doctors"; and there are *wise physicians*. This book is about the wise physicians – with insights into how they practice and live their lives, the precepts and maxims that they have bequeathed us, and the methods by which they heal, teach and inspire. But what is the relationship among the three groups? When discussing physicians of yesterday and today, do "great," "top," and "wise" mean the same thing?

In 2008, I wrote a book titled *White Coat Tales: Medicine's Heroes, Heritage and Misadventures*; the first chapter in the book told of the heroes, what Martí-Ibáñez calls the "Great Doctors" in history. Familiar names of the Great Doctors (and Scientists) include Imhotep, Hippocrates, Claudius Galen, Moses Maimonides, Andreas Vesalius, Thomas Sydenham, William Withering, Edward Jenner, Ignaz Semmelweis, John Snow, Joseph Lister, Robert Koch, Marie Curie, William Osler, and Sigmund Freud, all venerated for the medical advances and the knowledge they championed. I would consider many of them wise physicians but, in fact, we know their names today because each did something *memorable*. Not all, however, would be considered to have been wise in the truest sense of the word. Andreas Vesalius (1514–1564), whom Garrison (p. 218) asserts "alone made anatomy what it is today – a living, working science," became enraged when his work was criticized by colleagues, burned his manuscripts, turned his back on anatomic studies, and departed from Padua and went to Madrid, where he became a courtier, not a path that most of us today would encourage.

A few centuries later, German physician Robert Koch (1843–1910) discovered that tuberculosis is caused by the tubercle bacillus. The luster of this 1882 discovery was tarnished, however, when he later sought to market a secret remedy for tuberculosis, called ironically "tuberculin." The miracle drug was eventually found to be a glycerin preparation of tubercle bacilli, an embarrassing discovery prompting Koch and his new young wife to flee to Egypt, using funds he had received from the sale of his bogus remedy. (Porter, p. 441)

Lord Joseph Lister (1827–1912) is renowned for using carbolic acid (phenol) to help create a sterile surgical field in 1886, but his intellect was not matched by wisdom in his actions following the 1879 introduction of Listerine. Two entrepreneurs named Joseph Lawrence, himself a physician, and Jordan Wheat Lambert, concocted this proprietary remedy. In response to the unauthorized use of his name for a product marketed "to kill germs that cause bad breath," Lister "spent vast sums of money in unsuccessful efforts to suppress the term." (Dirckx, p. 82)

Marie Curie (1867–1934), who coined the term "radioactivity," carried glass tubes containing charmingly glowing radioactive isotopes in her pockets, eventually died of aplastic anemia, which we can logically assume was caused by exposure to "her" radium. (Taylor, p. 20)

Joseph Goldberger (1874–1929), known for demonstrating that pellagra is a niacin deficiency rather than a contagious disease, sought to prove his point by holding a "filth party," at which he, his wife, and several volunteers swallowed pellagra scabs, inhaled dried secretions, and injected themselves with blood taken from a pellagra victim. (Taylor, p. 23). His courage and tenacity earned him a place in the pantheon of Great Doctors, but today most would consider his actions foolhardy.

In fact, history is replete with the names of physicians and scientists who exhibited astounding vision, genius, and even serendipity, but not always great wisdom in their actions. And so, I submit that one seminal discovery, however ground-breaking, does not necessarily connote wisdom.

Top Doctors

Then there are the "top doctors," aka the "best doctors." What about the popular lists identifying "best" or "top" doctors? We Americans love the "best," and are fond of reading about the "best restaurants" and "best hotels." In magazines, we scan lists of the "best companies to work for," "best cities to live in," "best places to kiss," and even "best retirement communities." We admire the "best-dressed Hollywood stars." And part of our fascination with "the best" involves ranking America's physicians and hospitals. For example, the venerable American Association of Retired Persons (AARP) has published a list of top "out of town" hospitals for persons considering travel away from home for medical care. The list is based on ratings by physicians and, for example, it ranks the Mayo Clinic in Rochester, Minnesota as tops if you have a "mystery diagnosis."[2]

I was a "Top Family Doctor" nominee in 2009. With the notice came the opportunity to purchase a "Proclamation" wall plaque in a frame of finest imported mahogany hardwood (only $229) documenting my achievement. The selection criteria, I learned, include experience, training, professional associations, and board certification. In 2009, I was – at age 72 – no longer actively caring for my own panel of patients, and my nomination was probably based on the books I have written. It certainly wasn't because of my superior training – a single year of internship almost 50 years ago. I was undoubtedly a better physician 35 years ago, when I was in solo rural practice, but unknown outside my community. The "best" and "top" doctor lists in the newspapers and on the Internet are largely generated by nominations of fellow doctors, who, in turn are influenced by scientific papers published, national name recognition, even local publicity. A weakness of the system is lack of actual observation of the physician in practice. Few practicing physicians ever have their day-by-day care observed by colleagues.

In fact, when the local Portland, Oregon list of Top Docs was published in January, 2009 a respected local trauma surgeon wrote in response, "Here are my concerns about listing top trauma doctors: there is nothing scientifically valid about what is a 'top doc' in this survey – nothing about credentials, track record, publications, true peer reviews; any organization and/or group can nominate candidates and 'stuff' the ballot box, and that is in fact what is happening."[3]

It seems that Portland, Oregon is not alone is creating spurious lists. Writing about the *New York Magazine* 2006 "Best Doctors" list, Sepkowitz tells, "Half the selections are first-rate doctors, no doubt about it. Another 25% are people whom I don't know well (although I have my doubts), and 25% are certifiable duds – doctors who (hopefully) haven't seen a patient in years but have risen to the lofty realm of high society and semi-celebrityhood."[4]

And so, while many of "best" and "top" doctors are undoubtedly outstanding clinicians, a few probably aren't, and searching these lists – intended to identify those with superior training, knowledge and skills – may or may not lead you to the ideal doctor. My phrase *wise physician* has a somewhat different connotation.

Medical Wisdom and the Wise Physician

So what is medical wisdom, the *summum bonum* most of us physicians would like to possess? Let's start with what medical wisdom is not. It is not about a high intelligence quotient – IQ – and, in a sense, may be the antithesis. In Chap. 9, I will explain this further under the heading: "Don't aspire to be the smartest person in the room."

Just as medical wisdom is not the same as intellect, it is also not directly connected to science – the process of creating new knowledge based on measurable and verifiable facts. Discovering, for example, that depression is more common in migraineurs than in the so-called normal population is useful information, but not wisdom. Nor is medical wisdom the same as clinical intuition, the knack of finding answers to questions without conscious thought, a gift that defies quantification or explanation.

In my opinion, medical wisdom is the capacity to understand and practice medicine in a common-sense manner that is scientifically based, sensitive to patient needs, ethically grounded and professionally satisfying.

Based on this definition, the phrase *wise physician* describes those healers who provide excellent and up-to-date care for their patients while taking good care of their own families, their communities, and themselves. Most *wise physicians* do not get their names in history books, or even in the Sunday supplements. They practice exemplary medicine, doing their job thoughtfully and conscientiously, leaving a legacy of respect to be enjoyed by the next generation of aspiring healers.

To return to history, I believe the term wise physician describes Edward Jenner (1749–1823), who demonstrated the value of smallpox vaccination using material from a cowpox pustule in 1796, and yet who remained a country doctor throughout the balance of his practice life. Sir William Osler (1849–1919), who advocated patient-centered medicine, was also a wise physician and you will find his insightful sayings sprinkled throughout the pages to come. The brothers Mayo, surgeons whose famous clinic in Rochester, Minnesota is now the home of a prestigious medical school, were wise physicians, and some of the evidence is the treasury of aphorisms they have left us. (In the bibliography, see Willius: *Aphorisms of Dr. Charles Horace Mayo and Dr. William James Mayo*) And as you read on, *wise physician* describes the family physician in the tiny frontier town of Lakeview, Oregon, providing the full spectrum of health care for his patients, while contributing to his community and to the education of future doctors. It is about the doctor in the inner-city community health center, making life better in many ways for those who depend on the neighborhood clinic. It is about the retired physician who organizes a monthly "Senior Physicians' Seminar," with discussions of current ethical and philosophic topics in medicine. The book is about all of them, and is especially about their medical wisdom and their clinical skills, which they have all shared unselfishly (or are sharing today) with young persons aspiring to be tomorrow's next generation of "wise physicians."

I believe that we would all agree that our ideal physician would be intelligent, competent, diligent, humble, resourceful, trustworthy, and genuinely caring. He or she would be intelligent, but that is a baseline expectation for today's physicians; the medical school admissions process generally assures that those who are admitted have excellent grades and some modicum of interpersonal skills.

Competence, a core attribute of wise physicians, is different from intelligence. I have known physicians who had stunning intellects, but who lacked the common sense and attention to detail needed for the safe practice of medicine. Competent physicians exhibit sound medical knowledge and clinical skills. They approach diagnostic problems logically, advise rationally, and consult liberally.

The ideal doctor is diligent, actually a higher hurdle than native intelligence, because diligence takes energy, and calls for some level of compulsiveness. This means following up on laboratory tests and being up-to-date with every medication the patient is taking. As an example of diligence, when asked about taking work home heart surgeon Michael DeBakey replied, "Of course I take my work home with me. Any physician who doesn't should not be practicing medicine. There may be five or six open-heart operations scheduled the next day. All represent individual lives to me. I care about every patient; I worry about them. I think about all of them – their families and their hopes. I may be having dinner with you and talking about baseball, but my mind is with those patients. I wouldn't be a real physician if I didn't do that." (Manning and DeBakey, p. 8)

Humility is an attribute of the wise physician, who is always open to questioning an opinion or challenging dogma. Being humble helps avoid errors of arrogance, such as denying a young woman's request for a mammogram because you are sure her breast lump is too small to be significant. Just keep in mind that Murphy's Laws of Medicine, discussed in Chap. 11, can always trump your clinical acumen.

When I am ill, I want my physician to be resourceful, and not reliant on 5-year-old knowledge; thus, he or she will use the computer, check the literature, and call experts when needed. Trustworthiness is a physician attribute we can usually take for granted, and when a doctor seems to fail this expectation, as in the areas of truth-telling or maintaining confidentiality, the reason often lies in an ethical values conflict, not uncommon among persons with strong moral principles.

There is also the issue of caring for the patient, discussed in Chap. 2. For physicians evaluating other physicians, as in nominating colleagues for a "top-doc" list, this can be the most difficult attribute to assess, but it can be vitally important to the patient and family. Caring is sitting down and answering the patient's questions; caring is thinking about the meaning of a symptom or disease – back strain, for example – to the patient; caring is calling the family to report on progress of a hospitalized patient. This week, for example, my oldest granddaughter Francesca, who lives 600 miles away in Sun Valley, was in the hospital emergency room with gastroenteritis, dehydration and, as is sure to happen when a physician's family member is sick, some miscellaneous and slightly confusing other manifestations. The emergency physician, whom I have never met, called me – Grandpa Doctor in Portland – three times during the day to give me progress reports. In the end, Francesca responded to treatment and went home, and I greatly appreciated the extra effort of the physician to keep the parents and concerned grandfather informed of what was happening.

Under the general heading of caring, there is one more universal and more-or-less measurable attribute: The wise physicians are on the scene when their patients need them. They answer the phone when the patient is sick, make the hospital visits and even house calls, and they let their patients know, "I'll be there when you need me." And while providing the best possible care to their patients, they also safeguard their own health so they can "be there" when their patients need them.

One final trait that has always characterized the wise physicians is *passion*, which I hold is part of the definition of medical wisdom concerning personal satisfaction. Passion for excellence in patient care is what gets us out of bed in the morning and what lets us make the extra office or hospital call, sometimes even when we are tired and hungry. Passion is what keeps us learning decades after leaving medical school. Only the enormous energy that passion for medicine can bring will enable you to live up to diverse imperatives that will make you a wise physician.

ABOUT DOCTORING, THE ART OF MEDICINE AND SERVICE TO HUMANITY

What about doctoring and its personalized application, the art of medicine? As a little lexicographic background, "doctoring" is the past participle of the verb, "doctor," meaning to act as a doctor. This is bit of etymologic inconsistency, since "doctor" actually comes from the Latin *docere*, meaning "to teach," and does not denote healing at all. Nevertheless, doctoring is what we physicians do, and the art of medicine describes individuality, intuition, and sagacity that each physician brings to the work of doctoring each day.

The art of medicine has long been a favorite topic of doctors. Here, let's look at what some great minds have given us:

> The practice of medicine is an art, based on science.
> Sir William Osler, quoted in Bean and Bean, p. 123.

> It is our duty to remember at all times and anew that medicine is not only a science, but also the art of letting our own individuality interact with the individuality of the patient.
> German physician-philosopher Albert Schweitzer (1875–1965), quoted in Strauss, p. 361.

> You will see then that a distinction is drawn between the Art and the Science of Medicine. The Art in its Hippocratic sense has reference among other things to the practicing doctor's ability to inspire confidence in his patients and their relatives. This requires on his part an understanding of human nature, abounding unselfishness, unflagging sympathy, and observance of the Golden Rule.
> American neurosurgeon Harvey Cushing (1869–1939), quoted in Rapport and Wright, p. 507.

> Caring for the patient encompasses both the science and the art of medicine. The science of medicine embraces the entire stockpile of knowledge accumulated about man as a biologic

entity. The art of medicine consists of the skillful application of this knowledge to a particular person for the maintenance of health or amelioration of disease. Thus the meeting place of the science of medicine and the art of medicine is in the patient.

American cardiologist Herman L. Blumgart[5]

Now, let us take the next step: I believe that – with all the implied individuality, ability to inspire confidence, unselfishness, and skillful application of knowledge – the art of medicine, at its core, is nothing if not service to humanity.

Each fall, with the arrival of an incoming freshman class at our medical school, I am privileged to lead a small group seminar on "professionalism." The session comes a few days before the new students will receive their white coats and recite the *Declaration of Geneva*. At my session, we review the *Declaration of Geneva* as well as the original Oath of Hippocrates. Just for the record, the newer Declaration of Geneva, adopted by the General Assembly of the World Medical Association at Geneva in 1948 and subsequently revised several times, continues the same general theme of service and integrity as the oath attributed to Hippocrates.

In my opinion, the most powerful phrase in the Declaration of Geneva is found in the first lines: "At the time of being admitted as a member of the Medical profession, I solemnly pledge to consecrate my life to the service of humanity." Humanity is an expansive word, and this is a compelling statement, reasonably interpreted to mean that you and I will do our best to advance the welfare of humankind in general, and our patients, in particular. This pledge refers to the individual patient with diabetes sitting in your office, the nonagenarian with a stroke in the nursing home, the family of the child with cystic fibrosis, the children in a day care center threatened by an outbreak of rotavirus, and the residents of other lands who lack the health care benefits we take for granted. I tell my students that I hope they take this vow very seriously to serve humanity. If they do so, and make service to humanity the centerpiece of their professional lives, then they will, indeed, come to love the Art of Medicine.

Sometimes, the message of medicine as service to humanity takes a little time to sink in.

When I was in medical school, some among us called it "doctor school," as though we were attending a trade school and we were learning to become some sort of technicians. I am not sure we truly realized that, in the words of German pathologist Rudolph Virchow (1821–1902), "Medical instruction does not exist to provide individuals with an opportunity of learning how to make a living, but in order to make possible the protection of the health of the public." (Virchow, quoted in Brallier, p. 205) In spite of our youthful misconceptions and our middle-age strivings, sometimes sagacity develops with age. Speaking on the occasion of his 93rd birthday, American medical educator Eugene A. Stead, former chairman of the Department of Medicine at Duke University Medical Center, shared the following musing about his time as a student: "I was not particularly interested in providing service to all people. I never thought about that until my later years; I knew that the medical school wasn't that interested in that goal either. Now that I have grown older I realize how ignorant I was for most of my career, and I am a little ashamed of what a slow learner I was."[6]

It seems that, at some time during his professional life, Dr. Stead experienced the epiphanous realization that clinical science, medical knowledge, and doctoring are all about helping humans – typically, yet not necessarily always, one human at a time – achieve optimum health. May we all share his enlightenment.

ABOUT MEDICAL WISDOM EXPRESSED AS APHORISMS AND PRECEPTS

Creativity and new knowledge are expressed in many ways. Artists such as Rembrandt and Picasso used paint and canvas. Beethoven, Puccini, and other composers used notes, instruments, and sometimes voices to bring life to the music they created. Sculptors use stone, potters use clay, and weavers use fabric. Over the centuries, seasoned and thoughtful physicians have often packaged their insights as aphorisms and precepts – bite-sized kernels of experiential wisdom, often spiced with a metaphor or simile, or garnished with a twist of irony.

As the astute reader has surely deduced, I am a fan of medical sayings, which are the "meat and potatoes" of this book, with some axiomatic principles and friendly advice as philosophical condiments. Here is one of my favorite clinical aphorisms, courtesy of my favorite aphorist, Sir William Osler, having to do with the evaluation of abdominal pain:

> Adhesions are the refuge of the diagnostically destitute.
>   (Osler, quoted in Silverman, p. 103)

In these few simple words, Osler created the image of a befuddled physician, faced with a patient with unexplained abdominal pain, bereft of plausible etiologic notions, crouching behind a hedge of adhesions. Since I first heard this adage, it has stuck in my mind like a familiar refrain, and I have shared it with two generations of physicians in training.

Fascination with cunningly constructed, tightly packaged truths has long been a secret vice of doctors, perhaps because many physicians harbor a lingering desire to be writers. In fact, over the years, many physicians such as Sir Arthur Conan Doyle, Somerset Maugham, and Michael Crichton did so, trading clinical medicine for a life of creative writing.

Some might hold that physicians invented the aphorism, and there is some historical evidence, however debatable, to support such an assertion. Fowler states, without equivocation, "The word *aphorism*, meaning literally a definition or distinction, is of medical origin; it was first used of (SIC) the Aphorisms of Hippocrates, who begins his collection with one of the most famous of all famous sayings *Art is long; life is short*. The word has come to denote any short pithy statement containing a truth of general import." (Fowler, p. 31)

Bolstering the physician's claim to aphoristic rights, American medical educator Martin H. Fischer observed, "Since the time of Hippocrates, our father, the aphorism has been the literary vehicle of the doctor ... Laymen have stolen the trick from time to time, but the aphorism remains the undisputed contribution of the doctor to literature."[7]

As ancient example of succinctly stated wisdom, consider "First, do no harm," a precept we have all encountered. Even today, I recall one of my earliest medical school lectures, given by a surgeon. With the imperturbable self-possession that only a surgeon can portray, he strode to the blackboard and printed in large capital letters: *PRIMUM NON NOCERE!* No physician takes issue with this self-evident dictum, which dates to the time of Hippocrates, and in fact, even earlier to ancient Hindi medicine. (Taylor, 2008, p. 122) Hippocrates, who lived five centuries before Christ, gave us many clinical aphorisms that have stood the test of time. On example is the admonition, "In acute disease, it is not quite safe to prognosticate either death or recovery." (Strauss, p. 461)

This book is organized by precepts, maxims, and aphorisms, with the goal of making the messages relevant to today's practice of medicine.

ABOUT MEDICAL PARADIGMATIC CHANGE IN TWENTY-FIRST CENTURY PRACTICE

> Each generation has an obligation to remind succeeding ones about people, ideas and events that have gotten us to this point.
>
> American physician and educator John Geyman[8]

The practice of medicine we see today is not the medical practice of yesteryear, or even of yesterday. Things change, almost daily, and one of the goals of this book is to help present to younger doctors the philosophical insights, methodological changes, paradigmatic shifts that have led us to how we practice medicine today. For example, Hippocrates (ca 460–377 BCE) challenged the belief systems of his day by holding that disease comes from natural causes and not from intervention by some deity residing on Mount Olympus. Military physician Ambroise Paré (1517–1564) revolutionized wound care when, upon running short of boiling oil, he applied a cold solution of egg yolk, turpentine and oil of roses to battlefield injuries. Rudolph Virchow (1821–1902) pioneered the postulate that all life comes from life.

As recently as the early twentieth century, we could count on our fingers the available medications – digitalis, quinine, ergot, opium, salicylates, the ubiquitous purgatives, and a few others – that had any promise of benefit to patients. Writing in the New England Journal of Medicine in 1964, L. J. Henderson reflected, "Somewhere between 1910 and 1912, in this country, a random patient, with a random disease, consulting a doctor chosen at random had, for the first time in the history of mankind, a better than fifty-fifty chance of profiting from the encounter." (Strauss, p. 302) Why did Henderson specify those dates? The key innovation of that time was the introduction of arsphenamine, an arsenical derivative marketed as Salvarsan as a "magic bullet" to treat syphilis, a humble beginning for what would become the era of actually effective, disease-specific drugs. (Taylor 2008, p. 121)

The instruction of young physicians also changed, based on a study by Abraham Flexner (1866–1959), a previously unemployed former schoolmaster funded by the Carnegie Foundation for the Advancement of Teaching, who visited selected medical schools and subsequently prepared a report titled *Medical Education in the United States and Canada*. Before the Flexner report in 1910, medical education in the US was based on an apprenticeship model; today, science-based, specialty-oriented medical education prevails. (Taylor 2008, p. 22)

These advances and more – such as the introduction of ether anesthesia by William T. G. Morton in 1846, the development of the germ theory of disease by Louis Pasteur in the 1870s, and the discovery of the X-ray by Wilhelm Roentgen in 1895 – all had profound influence on medical practice. But changes were not limited to specific advances, nor did the evolution of medicine end at some date in the mid twentieth century.

Here, I describe some of the paradigmatic shifts that have occurred during my practice lifetime. I won't discuss the development of the Salk polio vaccine in 1952, the isolation of the human immunodeficiency virus (HIV) in 1983–1984, or the mapping of the human genome in 2005, as important as these all may be. Instead, I will focus on cultural shifts in medical education and practice, sea changes that have shaped how we currently decide who will be our doctors, the settings in which they will practice, how they relate to their patients, how they will think about themselves, and how they will earn their livings.

The Democratization of Medicine

In 1908, Henry Ford "democratized" the automobile, producing the first motorcar that was affordable by the average working American, fulfilling his goal, which was to "build a car for the great multitude."[9] In a somewhat analogous sense, we have witnessed the democratization of medicine. That is, medical knowledge is no longer the exclusive property of the chosen few – the physicians – and medical decision making is increasingly shared with patients and families. It was not always so. For example, in the Oath of Hippocrates, we find the line, "... I will impart a knowledge of the Art to my own sons, and those of my teachers, and to disciples bound by a stipulation and oath according to the law of medicine, *but none other*." (italics mine) In ancient times, medical knowledge was clearly intended for doctors only.

When we think about it, there is a direct link between medical knowledge and medical choices. In considering what happens when, let's say, a treatment decision must be made, the physician assumes the role of process leader even though the patient makes the ultimate decision. In this model, there are various types of leaders: dictatorial, autocratic, parental, facilitative, and others. Two or three generations ago the physician, the possessor of medical knowledge, typically assumed a parental leadership role. (Actually, because most physicians were male, a more precise descriptor would be "paternal.") What layperson could fathom the extravagant proliferation of cancer cells or the greasy accumulation of plaque in the walls of coronary arteries? In those days, when we were digesting the news that cigarettes just might cause cancer and had yet to learn about HIV and AIDS, it was therefore axiomatic that, "Doctor knows best."

The beginning of democratization may be dated to the social upheaval of the 1960s, when one of the tenets was to question authority, giving patients license to question their physician experts and to seek knowledge upon which to base their own health care decisions. Another step in the democratization of medical knowledge and decision making came with the proliferation of home medical guides, published by many medical experts and sources, including the venerable American Medical Association, whose *Family Medical Guide* is now in its fourth edition. The dike burst with the advent of the World Wide Web, bringing current medical information to everyone. Nor are we limited to PubMed and other professional sites. Today, patients (and physicians alike) search Google for answers to medical questions, and come to their physicians clutching printouts describing the latest medical advances.

With such data readily available to the informed patient, and with the current emphasis on "informed consent" influenced by the medico–legal climate of the day, it is only logical that medical decision making has become a shared enterprise, and the doctor's leadership style has morphed from parental to facilitative.

The Collectivization of Medicine

Early American medicine was largely an assortment of solo practitioners, working in small offices and occasionally in local hospitals, serving their communities. Today, the solo doctor is an endangered species, in part a casualty of the health maintenance (HMO) movement, described next. For example, today in my specialty of family medicine, 17.6% of physicians are in solo practice in contrast to 73% who report being in some sort of group practice arrangement.[10] The current trend is clearly toward fewer solo doctors and more large group practices.

The Commercialization of Medicine

The democratization of medicine can be considered a favorable trend, and the collectivization trend has been a mixed blessing, bringing economies of scale at the expense of autonomy, but I can find nothing to like about the progressive commercialization of medicine. I urge all to read

Chap. 1 of Paul Starr's book *The Social Transformation of American Medicine*, which begins: "The dream of reason did not take power into account." (Starr, p. 3) Writing in 1982, at the time when the health maintenance organizations (HMOs) and managed care were in their infancy, Starr wrote that, "The organizations that the profession once defeated or restricted have re-emerged as threats to its sovereignty. Again, the threats are of two related kinds – competition and control." (Starr, p. 27).

When I began private practice in 1964, my fellow physicians and I decided on our own fees; one generalist colleague, with a slightly ironic sense of humor, pegged his office call fee to the price of a postage stamp. When the price of a stamp went from 12 to 15 cents, the price of his usual office visit was increased from 12 to 15 dollars. In my office, I treated my patients, who paid me directly. If the patient had medical insurance, my staff filled in the form and returned it to the patient who would seek reimbursement for my fee. If a patient could not afford my fee, I would discount or waive the charge for the visit; that was how we provided care for the needy, and it worked. Of course, it was an honor to treat another physician or a member of a physician's family, and our colleagues received "professional courtesy."

Over the subsequent decades, we began sending our bills directly to insurance companies, and before long we contracted with them, offering discounts not available to our fee-paying patients. Then came HMOs, with which physicians made Faustian bargains that discounted our fees and that bundled us into "provider" panels. Our patients were now "covered lives." I still recall the setting and the disgust I felt when I first heard patients called "covered lives." Before long, we were part of HMOs offering managed care, and we sometimes found ourselves to be pawns in competing organizations.

As previously independent physicians became co-opted by HMOs and even hospital corporate systems, we began to lose a little of the luster of the professional – the knowledgeable, ethical, honorable, and humanitarian person – and we assumed the mantle of a vendor of services. As evidence, let me tell you about two personal experiences separated by almost four decades. In 1972, I wrote a health care guide for senior citizens. It was titled *Feeling Alive after 65*, parenthetically a title suggested by one of my older patients. My publisher arranged for me to be interviewed on a local radio station, but before doing so, I was required to obtain formal permission of my Ulster County Medical Society. I was, after all, going to discuss health issues and my book on the air, which might be considered a form of advertising – something ethical doctors did not do.

Now, I describe the contrast we encounter today. Last week on my car radio, I heard an advertisement for an imaging center, seeking patients who might need computed tomography or magnetic resonance imaging. Part of the recorded radio message was the testimonial of a local generalist physician, extolling the virtues of the imaging center and telling how happy her patients were when she referred them there. On my television I see cardiologists telling the advantages of getting care for one's cardiac disease at their proprietary "heart hospital;" and my Sunday newspaper has a large ad with the smiling face of an attractive plastic surgeon offering Botox and dermabrasion treatments.

The Computerization of Medicine

If the democratization of medicine has been generally good for humanity and the commercialization less so, the computerization of medicine may turn out to have been a mixed blessing. Time will tell.

Our current generation of freshly minted physicians has never known a world without computers, and the newest among them have never used a pen to write a progress note on a paper chart. Yes, the computer and subsequently the World Wide Web have represented "game-changing" technology. In medicine, the first beachhead was in billing, allowing doctors' offices to do accounting, and submit bills to insurers electronically. Then, there came word processing, allowing easier production of what were still paper documents. The Internet made finding up-to-date information much faster and easier than searching old journals, and, with some ambivalence, I discarded my Pendaflex folders full of old, tattered tear-sheets. In time, I began to communicate with colleagues by email, and it wasn't long until I received my first email query from a computer-savvy patient, someone in the university who had access to my email address. Then 3 years ago, our clinic made the major and painful transition to the electronic medical record (EMR). Now I read about mobile robots with camera/computer "heads" chug-chugging around hospital corridors, making "rounds" on hospital patients, while the physicians communicating with hospitalized patients via the robotic computer remain seated in their offices.

In addition to helping us manage information, computerization underlies much of the technology that makes medicine increasingly more subspecialized and sometimes mechanical, prompting Reynolds and Stone to write, "If I were a medical student or an intern, just getting ready to begin, I would be more worried about this aspect of my future than anything else. I would be apprehensive that my real job, caring for sick people, might soon be taken away, leaving me with the quite different occupation of looking after machines. I would be trying to figure out ways to keep this from happening." (Reynolds and Stone, p. 160)

All these advances, like it or not, set the stage for the e-medicine of tomorrow, and I will return to this discussion later in the book.

The Feminization of Medicine

Just in case you haven't been on a medical school campus recently, I can assure you that the face of medicine has changed. Until sometime in the latter half of the twentieth century, we assumed that physicians were men (with a few notable exceptions); today approximately half of medical students are women. The Association of American Medical Colleges (AAMC) provides annual statistics. For the 2007–2008 academic year, 49% of medical school applicants, 49% of enrolled medical students and 45% of residents and fellows were women.[11]

What might this mean for the future of medical practice? Here, we can only speculate and explore possibilities.

For example, with more female physicians, will we see more attention to the service and "caring" functions of medicine? Will we see an influence on the physician workforce? Until some space-age breakthrough allows men to bear children, female physicians choosing parenthood will take some time off work to be mothers. What will the portrait of medicine look like when most of the faces are women?

There will certainly be consequences resulting from the feminization of medicine, but no wise man would attempt to predict the future, especially regarding items related to gender.

The Politicization of Medicine

A generation from now we may look back to today and reflect that the politization of medicine was in its infancy as this book was written. Yes, there is Medicare and Medicaid, both begun in the 1960s. But fundamentally, medicine in the early twenty-first century is still largely a private-based enterprise, albeit dominated by large insurance and hospital enterprises.

Sadly, however, we have allowed some 40 million citizens to fall through the health insurance net, and health care costs have outstripped other items in the average person's budget, setting the stage for epic federal legislation sure to profoundly alter health care delivery in America.

Even states are getting in the game: From the state of Connecticut comes this report documenting the politicization of health policy. In 2006, the Infectious Diseases Society of America (IDSA) released updated clinical guidelines for the diagnosis and management of Lyme disease. In response, the Connecticut attorney general began an investigation, claiming a violation of state antitrust law. It seems that the IDSA allegedly violated Connecticut's antitrust law by recommending against the use of long-term antibiotics in the management of "chronic Lyme disease." Full details of this silly, yet chilling episode are found in a report by Kraemer and Gostin.[12]

However noble the cause, no legislative process can occur in a vacuum, and even today, the lobbyists, special interest groups, and the administration are all working to be sure that the inevitable legislation contains the wording they crave. For the house of medicine, the game is already in play.

The rising political tsunami and the other ideological and societal upheavals seen over the last half century have been truly transformative. Over our lifetimes, there will be even more new discoveries, new cultural trends, and new political initiatives. Happily, however, although medical knowledge and technical skills will change, medical wisdom is enduring, and that, in the end, is what this book is about.

WISE WORDS ABOUT MEDICAL WISDOM IN THE TWENTY-FIRST CENTURY

■ *Where there is love for humanity, there is also love for the art of medicine.* Attributed to Hippocrates. (Garrison, p. 16)

■ *Sciences may be learned by rote, but wisdom not.* English novelist and clergyman Laurence Sterne (1713–1768).
   This quote is from Sterne's *The Life and Opinions of Tristram Shandy, Gentleman,* a humorous novel first published in 1759.[13]

■ *Common sense in matters medical is rare, and is usually in inverse ratio to the degree of education.* Sir William Osler (Osler, p. 124)
   Give me the common sense doctor instead of the brilliant doctor any day.

■ *Medicine is an art, but it is an art which is always trying to become a science.* (Lindsay, p. 6.)
   I actually hope that medicine never fully succeeds in becoming a science, since much of our soul will be lost.

■ *Knowledge is a process of piling up facts; wisdom lies in their simplification.* American medical educator Martin H. Fischer (1879–1962) (Quoted in Strauss, p. 256)

■ *When knowledge is translated into proper action, we speak of it as wisdom.* American surgeon William J. Mayo (Mayo and Mayo, p. 60)
   This is an intriguing quote, perhaps reflecting the mentality of a surgeon, but I do not see wisdom as necessarily action-oriented.

▓ *The Compleat Physician is one who is capable in all three dimensions: he is a competent practitioner; he is compassionate; and he is an educated man.* American physician and humanist Edward D. Pellegrino. (Pellegrino, p. 157)

▓ *The good physician knows what to do in a clinical situation; the wise physician knows what not to do.* (Anon)
This aphorism reminds me of the surgical dictum: It takes years to learn when to operate, and even longer to learn when not to. Sometimes the wise thing is to do nothing for a while.

▓ *Statistical significance and clinical wisdom do not always agree.* (Anon)
And sometimes they are polar opposites. A friend who was a sociologist and pretty good with statistics told me, "I can demonstrate statistically that the amount of damage in a fire is directly related to the number of fire trucks on the scene."

▓ *Every doctor should be a student of the history of medicine. It teaches us that we are still works in progress.* American physician David Barton (Meador, No. 213)

▓ *We have lost something of the art of medicine in a headlong rush to embrace the science.* American public health physician Bill Kirkup[14]

REFERENCES

1. LaCombe MA. On professionalism. *Am J Med*. 1993;94(3):329.
2. AARP lists "top-ranked" US hospitals. Healthcare Finance News. Available at: http://www.healthcarefinancenews.com/news/aarp-lists-top-ranked-us-hospitals/; Accessed April 2, 2009.
3. Long WB. Top Docs (letter). *Portland Monthly*, Feb 2009; page 20.
4. Sepkowitz K. A few good doctors: don't look for them on a magazine top-10 list. Medical Examiner. Available at: Sepkowitz K. A few good doctors: http://www.slate.com/id/2143506/; Accessed March 14, 2009.
5. Blumgart HL. Caring for the patient. *N Engl J Med*. 1964;270(9):449–452.
6. Stead EA. Wisdom from a medical elder. *Can Med Assoc J*. 2004;171(2):1465–1466.

7. Fabing H, Marr R. *Fischerisms: being a sheaf of sundry and diverse utterances culled from the lectures of Martin H. Fischer, professor of physiology in the University of Cincinnati.* New York: Science Press; 1937.

8. Frey JJ. Five careers and eight airplanes: an oral history of John Geyman, MD. *Ann Fam Med.* 2007;5:368–370.

9. Boorstin DJ. *The Americans: the democratic experience.* New York: Vintage Books; 1974; 548.

10. Facts about Family Medicine. Available at: http://www.aafp.org/online/en/home/aboutus/specialty/facts/4.html/; Accessed April 1, 2009.

11. AAMC women in U.S. medicine: statistics and benchmarking report 2007-2008. Available at: http://www.aamc.org/members/wim/statistics/stats08/stats_report.pdf/; Accessed March 29, 2009.

12. Kraemer JD, Gostin LO. Science, politics, and values: the politicization of professional practice guidelines. *JAMA.* 2009; 301(6):665–667.

13. Sterne L. *The Life and Opinions of Tristram Shandy, Gentleman.* Book V. 1759 [chapter 32] London: Becket and DeHondt, publishers.

14. Kirkup B. Listen to the patient. *BMJ.* 2003;327(7411):401–403.

2

Caring for the Patient

I sought for happiness
Happiness I cannot see
I seek for richness of spirit
Richness eluded me
I looked for fulfillment
Fulfillment escaped me
But when I gave Medicine to my brethren
I found all three.

From an unknown source:
Quoted by Singapore physician C. H. Low.[1]

The title of this chapter has been shamelessly, yet respectfully, adapted from the title of a lecture given at Harvard Medical School in 1925, one of a series of late-afternoon sessions for medical students, and subsequently published in the Journal of the American Medical Association (JAMA) in 1927. The title of the lecture and the paper was simply "The Care of the Patient."[2] Peabody's lectures and writings were later collected and published in 1931, a project underwritten by his classmates from Harvard Medical School. In the preface to this volume, bacteriologist Hans Zinsser wrote of Peabody's collected works: "Their publication will serve to continue the influence of a voice that American medicine could ill afford to lose – one of clear-headedness, unsentimental idealism and the great wisdom of affectionate optimism."[3] I mentioned Dr. Peabody's work to one of our residents, who happens to be a graduate of Harvard Medical School; she replied that while in medical school, she was a member of the Francis Weld Peabody Society.

Peabody's lecture and subsequent article contain some of the most insightful descriptions of wise clinical practice

R.B. Taylor, *Medical Wisdom and Doctoring: The Art of*
21st Century Practice, DOI 10.1007/978-1-4419-5521-0_2,
© Springer Science+Business Media, LLC 2010

ever written. The thoughts expressed are as relevant today as they were some eight decades ago, and I still give photocopies of the article to medical students and residents whom I believe will appreciate the message. The theme of the work is summed up in the final three sentences: "The good physician knows his patients through and through, and his knowledge is bought dearly. Time, sympathy, and understanding must be lavishly dispensed, but the reward is to be found in that personal bond which forms the greatest satisfaction of the practice of medicine. One of the essential qualities of the clinician is interest in humanity, for the secret of the care of the patient is in caring for the patient."[2]

Peabody's "The Care of the Patient" has been quoted, reprinted, and photocopied countless times. Even today, it remains one of medicine's all-time most influential papers. The poignant back-story is that at the time of his lectures, Peabody was aware that he had incurable cancer, which caused his early death in 1927 at the age of 46.[4] I refer to Peabody's "The Care of the Patient" lecture at this point because, with great humility, I hope this chapter will reflect his message to readers.

FIRST, BE A HEALER

The dream of becoming a healer is why most of us became doctors in the first place. We wanted to take care of sick people. When I first considered attending medical school and being a physician, I am sure I was emulating the small town physicians who had treated my childhood injuries, removed my tonsils, and made home visits when I was too sick to get out of bed. In short, when I grew up I wanted to be a healer – just like them.

The *Oxford Handbook of Clinical Medicine* has a charming story, told as only the Brits can do, one that illustrates differences between caring for the patient and being a provider of health care services: A man cut his hand, and went to the home of his neighbor, a physician. The doctor was out for a short while, but his 3-year-old daughter asked the neighbor in, put her clean handkerchief on the laceration, which wasn't really very large, and had him sit in daddy's chair with his legs raised. "She stroked his head and patted his hand, and told him about her marigolds, and then about her frogs."

Then, Doctor Daddy returned home. "He quickly turned the neighbor into a patient, and then into a bleeding biohazard, and then dispatched him to Casualty (what we Yanks call the emergency room) for suturing." At the Casualty, he received "two desultory stitches" and care by a medical student who recommended a tetanus booster, to which – as it turned out – the patient was allergic.[5]

In this narrative, it is reasonable to ask: Who acted as a healer? Was it the physician, who over-reacted to a small cut that he probably could have managed with soap, water, one or two Steri-Strips, and reassurance? Was it the medical student, who placed two (probably unnecessary) sutures, and almost managed to transform a minor injury into an anaphylactic catastrophe? Or was it the 3-year-old girl, who used a clean dressing to help stop bleeding, placed the patient in the appropriate position to prevent syncope, and did her best to distract the injured man?

BE SURE TO CARE FOR THE PATIENT AS WELL AS THE DISEASE

British anatomist and politician Auckland Geddes (1879–1954) has observed: "So many come to the sickroom thinking themselves as men of science fighting disease and not as healers with a little knowledge helping nature to get a sick man well." (Brallier, page 148) Of course, there are moments for the physician to become the rational science-based warrior. Certainly the patient whom my resident and I saw last week with acute abdominal pain expected us to practice scientifically grounded, evidence-based medicine. And yet, when I am the patient, as all of us will be from time to time, I also value highly the clinician who takes the time to listen to my concerns and to explain what's going on with my body. In his 1925 lecture, Peabody advised, "There are moments, of course, in the cases of serious illness when you think solely of the disease and its treatment; but when the corner is turned and the immediate crisis is passed, you must give your attention to the patient."[2]

Caring for the patient is not always easy. Our current system of health care encourages disease-oriented thinking. There is National Institutes of Health (NIH) funding for biomedical research on diseases of the eye, heart, lung, blood and so forth, as well as on cancer, mental illness, and pretty much any disease that can muster a large army of advocates. There is, however, no national institute on the *care of the patient*. I recently received an invitation to attend a conference on how to deal with persons who did not respond to contacts from a diabetic registry, or cholesterol registry, or heart failure registry. The conference description discussed how a patient could be on three or four registries, a situation in which – was I such a patient – I would be annoyed to be so disassembled. Such disease-oriented registries, while valuable in collecting statistics, are not at the core of patient centered care.

And so, most patients are not keenly interested in Greek or Latin names of pathologic entities, disease registries, or silo-based guidelines that ignore all else. Nor are they enthralled by our fascinating hypotheses about disease causality. As Jung stated, "The patient is there to be treated and not to verify a theory."[6] After the hypothesizing diagnostic possibilities, naming the syndrome, cataloging the patient with others suffering like pathology, consulting the latest evidence, and all the rest of the impersonal acts that occur with disease diagnosis and treatment, the wise physician returns to the very personal business of caring for the patient.

RECOGNIZE THE DIFFERENCE BETWEEN DISEASE AND ILLNESS

Words matter, and physicians, as educated individuals, should strive to use words precisely. Thus, the time has come for me to differentiate between *disease* and *illness*. Clinicians sometimes use these words interchangeably, but they have quite different connotations, just as do leadership and management or house and home. The word *disease* refers to some biologic or mental abnormality such as, for example, lung cancer or schizophrenia. For physicians, a disease name might conjure up an image of the typical clinical presentation, the usual findings on imaging, the menu of therapeutic options and certain prognostic implications.

Illness, on the other hand, includes not only the disease, but also the patient's experience in regard to the disease, including pain or other type of suffering, its economic impact, and its influence on his or her life and that of the family and close friends. Thus, while disease tends to be somewhat concrete and generally identifiable in a few words, such as heart attack or asthma, illness is more comprehensive, involving the family, community, and the cultural and social context of the person who happens to have the disease. Thus an illness description of a 57-year-old male lung cancer patient might be a life-long smoker who is married, with two children, one of whom has Down syndrome and is dependent on the patient and his wife for care. Aware of the grim prognosis and the anticipated costs of medical treatment, the patient is worried – depressed might be a better descriptor – about not only his future, but also that of his wife and children.

TRY TO "FEEL" THE PATIENT'S EXPERIENCE OF THE ILLNESS

McWhinney describes an ideal clinical setting in which "the physician tries to enter the patient's world, to see the illness through the patient's eyes."[7] Today, such counsel seems self-evident, but seeking synergy with the patient was not always the case. Not too many decades ago, and certainly in Peabody's time, the prevailing model of medical care could best be described as paternalistic. In a highly imbalanced relationship, the physician prescribed and the patient complied. Think how the term "patient compliance" lingers in our clinical lexicon. The doctor, by virtue of his knowledge and skills, held the power and the patient's job was simply to follow "doctor's orders." Perhaps this explains why Peabody's ideas were noticed: He described a model of care not in favor at the time. In effect, he advocated that physicians change how they related to patients.

Today, the doctor–patient relationship is more balanced and physicians are encouraged to seek empathic understanding of their patients' illnesses. In fact, many clinicians do so, or at least they make the attempt.

Why the evolution in clinical practice, the transformation from a paternalistic to a collaborative relationship between patient and doctor? Here, I suggest several key influences: The first was the social upheaval of the 1960s, with the Viet Nam war, the civil rights movement, and a general distrust of experts – which, to some degree, came to include physicians as not-necessarily-trustworthy experts. This era also saw the rise of primary care, promising to reunite a fragmented health care system and return it to the people. Primary care, notably family practice, did not emerge in response to host of new technologic wonders, but as a social movement consistent with the times.

Another paradigm-changing influence was the development of the World Wide Web, opening the libraries of once-arcane medical knowledge to anyone with access to the Internet. The result of the social changes in America, the influence of physicians committed to relationship-based, personal care, and search engines allowing easy access to medical information has been the democratization of health care, with doctors seeking patients' opinions about their illness and the care decisions being made.

THINK ABOUT THE IMPACT OF ILLNESS ON THE PATIENT

"Feeling" the experience of the illness calls for considering how being sick is upsetting the patient's world. Part of the clinical skills exhibited by wise physicians is managing both the disease and the mischief the disease is causing in the patient's life.

When a disease is present, there is always an impact, even if not mentioned by the patient or parent, and regardless of whether or not the physician thinks of them at all. Consider, for example, a patient seen on Wednesday last week. Joey is a 17-year-old boy, brought to the office by his mother because of a severe sore throat, cough, and fever. Now, for a family physician, this is about as routine as it gets. Yet, there is an impact. For example, Joey will miss an important school exam on Thursday, and probably won't be well enough to play in the school basketball game on Friday evening. Missing the exam may lower his end-of-the-year class standing just a bit, and missing the basketball game may hurt his chances of getting a needed college scholarship.

The disruption of a minor, self-limited illness pales in comparison to what happens when a person has a chronic, progressive disease. In this setting, I think of Martha, who has chronic obstructive pulmonary disease (COPD), now retired following a two decades of working in a smoky barroom. Her COPD has led to physical inactivity and compensatory over-eating, bringing her weight to 236 pounds, in turn contributing to her type 2 diabetes mellitus. Thus, at age 58, Martha cannot climb more than one flight of stairs. She cannot go for walks with her two sisters. She isn't comfortable flying to visit her grandchildren who live across the country. And she can't visit her old friends in the smoke-filled tavern.

Schillerstrom et al looked at the impact of various medical illnesses on the executive function, which the authors define as "one's ability to plan, initiate, sequence, monitor, and inhibit goal-directed behaviors."[8] We all know that the executive function can be adversely affected by dementia, including Alzheimer disease. The authors, however, also found that the executive impairment can occur with a variety of chronic medical diseases, including COPD, diabetes mellitus, and hypertension. In some settings, the executive impairment may be inapparent to the patient and the physician, and is first suspected by the family. Other times, the patient is well aware of cognitive decline.

Here is an example of how executive function impairment may be first suspected by the patient and family who, by limiting social interactions, may both unwittingly contribute to progressive cognitive impairment. When I lived in the small town of New Paltz, New York in the 1960s and 1970s, I was both physician and friend of the boxer Floyd Patterson, one of the finest persons ever to become a sports legend. Floyd was a bright individual who helped scores of young men learn the sport and who championed boxing safety, including the use of thumb-less gloves and headgears.

Sadly I learned later, two decades after I had moved away, that Floyd had, like other aging pugilists such as Joe Lewis, Jerry Quarry, Ingemar Johansson, and Muhammad Ali, suffered the long-term effects of too many blows to the head. Recently, I read an excellent biography of Patterson, written by Alan Levy.[9] Levy tells how, at a boxing commission meeting in 1998, Patterson could not recall the names of fellow commissioners. "He resigned from the commission the very next day. He knew what was occurring. It had already begun, but he and his friends had kept it quiet...Mrs. Patterson first emphatically denied rumors that her husband often appeared lost and confused." The author goes on to tell how he went "into relative seclusion" in his rural home in New Paltz, how by 2000, he could not recall his wife's name and how, "shut away," he died on May 11, 2006 at age 71. Patterson's relative seclusion and being shut away (Levy's words) avoided embarrassment to this proud man, but the paucity of human contact may just have accelerated the mental decline.

CONSIDER HOW THE INDIVIDUAL PATIENT'S ILLNESS AFFECTS THE FAMILY

Let us return to 17-year-old Joey, described above, and his mother. Joey's mother is a single mom, supporting herself and young son as a receptionist in a local real estate office. In order to drive her son to see the physician today, she lost half a day of work, income she needs to help with the monthly rent. There will be a co-pay for the doctor visit, even though she is lucky enough to have some health insurance. Then, the mother will also have to pay for Joey's prescription.

When a patient is ill, the rest the family also suffers a disruption of their routine and a threat to their sense of invulnerability. The more serious or the more chronic the illness, the greater the perturbations. Think of the effect of Floyd Patterson's progressive dementia on his wife and children.

To consider another example, being the parent of a diabetic teenager means that there must be daily vigilance regarding nutrition, frequent visits to the physician, doctor bills related to the disease, and unanticipated trips to the hospital when things go wrong. Occasionally, the patient may seem to use the disease to exert influence in the home and to manipulate other family members. Eventually, siblings may come to resent the diabetic family member, and then they may feel guilty about their feelings of resentment. Parents worry that another of their children might develop the disease. And all the while, they just wish and pray that it would all go away.

Hence, for the physician, the diabetic teenager means insulin dosage adjustments and diet advice. For the family, the illness means emotional stress, difficulty when making family plans, costs other families don't face, household power struggles, and the ongoing fear of diabetic complications.

For parents of a child with chronic illness, the news is not at all grim, however. In a 7-year study of 191 children with cancer, Lansky et al found a person-year divorce rate of only 1.19%, lower than the 2.03% person-year rate among comparable married couples with children. Although the study confirmed the stress faced by the families of children with cancer, the higher divorce rate that might have intuitively been expected was not found.[10]

SOMETIMES, THE KEY TO UNDERSTANDING THE CLINICAL PROBLEM LIES IN THE MEANING OF THE SYMPTOM TO THE PATIENT

Another part of feeling the patient's experience of the illness is understanding the significance of various disease manifestations to the individual. We sometimes get a hint of the meaning of symptoms when we ask patients what they think might be causing the illness. Sometimes the query is more direct: "What does your pain (or other symptom) mean to you?" The patient with low back pain may be worried about cancer, because that is just how his uncle's prostate cancer revealed itself not long before he died. A young woman with worsening Crohn disease may be most worried about losing her job. In another setting, the meaning of a clinical manifestation may be the fear of imperiling important relationships, as in the setting of a college student who has just received a diagnosis of genital herpes. A heart failure patient's chief concern could be that she may not live to see her granddaughter graduate from college next year.

Here is a useful question for a patient with chronic or serious disease: "How would your life be different if you did not have this disease?" Then, be silent and allow the patient to answer.

PART OF CARING FOR THE PATIENT IS "LAYING HANDS" ON THE PATIENT

Here is another lesson I learned from a patient early in my practice years. My patient, Mr. Roma, was an elderly Italian–American, and English was clearly his second language. Every few months, he would come to the office accompanied by his wife, for follow-up of his hypertension and type 2 diabetes mellitus. On the day of my "lesson," my schedule was especially busy. Fortunately, I thought, Mr. Roma was doing well. His weight was stable. The nurse reported a capillary blood glucose of 86. Excellent! The blood pressure reading, also recorded by the nurse, was 130/82. Great! Mr. and Mrs. Roma and I chatted a little about his diet and his medication, which required no adjustment, and I instructed him to return in 3 months. I was ready to move on to my next patient.

"Wait a minute, Doctor! You haven't examined me. That is what I pay you for," he said.

Of course, he was right. I had not visualized his eye grounds, listened to his heart or checked his feet – all good things to do when caring for a diabetic patient. I had examined these areas recently, just not today. This was not good enough for Mr. Roma. He had come for a "check-up," and that meant an examination.

Appropriately chastised, I personally repeated his blood pressure determination and performed a screening physical examination. And today, I advise student and residents to perform some sort of physical examination – to "lay hands" – on every patient they see, even if it is only taking the blood pressure myself and checking the pulse.

PROCEED CAUTIOUSLY WHEN A PATIENT CRITICIZES HIS OR HER LAST PHYSICIAN

Before long, this same individual might be criticizing you to the next physician – or perhaps to an attorney. The patient's grievance may be quite legitimate, or may be evidence of a blaming mindset. Always remember that there is another version of the story, one that you may never hear.

DIFFICULT PATIENTS EXIST; SO DO "DIFFICULT DOCTORS"

They appear to whine, they blame, they question every-thing, and they seldom seem to respond to our best therapy. According to Jackson and Kroenke, up to 15% of patient–physician encounters may be labeled as "difficult" by the physicians involved. Some common predictors are anxiety and depression, multiple somatic complaints, and exception-ally severe symptoms.[11] And other patients just seem deter-mined to resist our most diligent efforts to heal.

In the medical literature, the accepted phrase is "difficult patient," a label I really don't like. These persons are gener-ally not "difficult" so much as they have a different worldview than their physicians, but I will use the term here because that is the phrase commonly used today. The difficult patient is irritating and frustrating, and most physicians would not be upset to see these individuals change doctors.

Who might the physician perceive as a "difficult" patient? If you will excuse the psychological jargon in the titles, I will describe some types of difficult patients under headings used in the report of a study by Mas and colleagues.[12]

- *Dependent clinger*: This type was the most common difficult patient in the study cited. These patients are often seen as "frequent fliers" in the medical office. They call often and become well known to the staff members, who come to consider them annoying, at best. They also have numerous office visits, many not really necessitated by their illnesses, although dependent clingers tend to have a long and colorful medical problem lists. One feature tends to be common among this group: They offer new symptoms late in the visit, often with their hand on the doorknob. "Oh, doctor, I forgot to tell you about the chest pain I had last night."
- *Entitled demander*: "I'm sick and I need to see the doctor this afternoon, but I can't leave work until 5 PM." Or "My car is in the shop for repair, and so can the doctor make a house call?" Or "I don't care if the doctor is with a patient; I need to speak with her now." This person's parents never told him to be sensitive to the needs of others. He – or she – has an illness of some kind, and that confers entitlement to

what he wants when he wants it. An interesting variant of the entitled demander is the VIP or celebrity patient, who requires special attention throughout the course of an illness. Although many such persons are actually humble and respectful of the medical team, the situation itself creates a sense of undeserved advantage.

- *Manipulative help-rejecter*: I once had a patient who had fallen from a ladder while working. He suffered a back injury – a worker's compensation case. Five years after the injury, he continued to visit my office frequently, requesting physical therapy, muscle relaxants, and a lot of attention. He continued to nurture his pain and his worker's compensation case, and of course he continued to be totally disabled for work.

- *Self-destructive denier*: Oscar Yates, a 76-year-old widower who lived alone, seemed to enjoy rejecting my best stop-smoking efforts: "Yes, I smoke cigarettes. I know they are bad for me, but smoking is what I enjoy most in life, and I don't plan to quit." This sort of attitude can – metaphorically, of course – drive a physician crazy. Alcoholics and drug seekers are other examples of self-destructive deniers. Teen-age risk-takers also fit into this group. As an aside, Oscar eventually stopped smoking, all on his own, explaining that finally he became ready to quit.

- *Somatizer:* The word comes from the Greek *soma*, meaning body. For these persons, everyday stress seems to affect some part of their bodies, resulting in headaches, fatigue, abdominal pain, backache and so forth. Of course, no amount of explanation relieves the symptoms of the somatizer, who generally lacks insight into the mind–body connection.

- *Emotive seducer*: This patient coaxes the physician into a web of involvement, generally concerning crises in her – or his – life. In my experience, most of the emotive seducers are women. Terrible things happen in their lives, over and over, prompting visits to the physician for comfort and solace. Wise physicians soon learn to be quite wary of the emotive seducer.

If faced with a "difficult patient," ask first if there is something you just don't understand yet. Consider that occasionally the core problem may have a legitimate medical label: For example, quite often patients with borderline personality disorder are dismissed as "difficult patients."[13] These individuals and others like the patient with multiple interrelated problems may really be "heartsink" patients (See chapter 7), rather than "difficult" patients.

Of course, the patient is only half of the "difficult" patient–physician dyad. The other person in the dysfunctional relationship is the physician. Sad to say, some physicians can be dogmatic, defensive, or arrogant; others are harried and tired. In a revealing study, Krebs et al wondered if there are identifiable traits of physicians who are likely to express frustration with patients, tending to label them as difficult. In a survey of 1,391 physicians, the authors found that physicians tending to express irritation with patients had certain characteristics. These physicians tended to be younger, to work long hours, to have more than their share of patients with psychosocial problems or substance abuse, and to practice in a medical subspecialty. The physicians who felt annoyance with patients also were likely to suffer anxiety, stress, and depression.[14]

Wise physicians do their best to approach the difficult patient encounter with equanimity, and attempt to view such interactions analytically. Think of the interaction in the model proposed by in a qualitative study by Elder et al. "Difficult encounters occurred when these patient behaviors and medical problems clashed with physicians' personal and practice traits."[15]

Here is a suggested viewpoint: As a physician, try to feel honored that you have a few "difficult patients." That they stick with you is a tribute to your ability to exhibit patience and to your personal optimism. And the next time things seem to be exasperating, try this approach: "This visit isn't going well. Can we start over at the beginning?"

SOME PATIENTS WILL ALSO BE YOUR FRIENDS

I have heard a few medical students remark: "I would never treat a friend." To this aspiring physician I would say, "Then you should plan never to practice in a small town." As a family doctor for 14 years in a small town setting, I can't say I knew everyone in town, but I think that most people in town knew who I was – The Doctor. What's more, many of my friends were also my patients. (I must confess that I took some pride in their faith in my abilities.) I treated their sore throats and their fractures, I diagnosed their diabetes and cancers, and I did my best to be there when they needed me. I did not consider it unusual to see a person at a social event Saturday evening and then examine him or her in the office on Monday. That is what small town doctors do.

Occasionally a patient would remark that, in the office setting, I seemed more "formal." When I was in small-town practice I didn't wear a white coat, perhaps because I feared it might frighten the children who visited my office. The white coat came later when I became an "academic physician." The perceived formality, instead, was my *persona* as a physician. Figuratively, I put on my "doctor hat," and assumed the physician role.

In his book on *Doctoring*, Eric Cassell writes about the friend as patient: "A patient as a patient is not a friend even if the patient is a friend. A friend who is a patient is a patient while a patient and a friend in other settings. (This may be a difficult distinction to maintain on occasion. When I see my friends who are also patients in personal settings, I literally cannot remember intimate medical details about them.)"[16]

Actually, although I greatly respect Eric Cassell and his work, I must wonder about the parenthetical comments. When I have a patient who is also a friend, and I see the friend at the grocery store or on the street, I really don't have amnesia for the medical details. In fact, I often pay special attention to the patient-friend in these settings, wondering about behavior that may influence the disease and how the disease might be influencing his or her life at that moment. For example, if treating a patient-friend with a weight or cholesterol problem, I will quietly sneak a glance at the foods in the shopping cart or portions consumed at a dinner. If treating my patient-friend for an injury or back strain, I will watch how he moves his body even if I happen to be observing him outside the office setting.

All of us who have practiced in small towns know that, if you exclude your patients from your circle of friends, you may be quite lonely. I have always had friends, and even a few physician colleagues as patients. Or, from another perspective, my wife and I have ended up as friends with persons who began as patients. We, as physicians, just need to remember which hat we are wearing when – the friend hat or the doctor hat. It is really not difficult.

SOME OF YOUR MOST IMPORTANT LESSONS WILL BE LEARNED FROM PATIENTS

In my very first week of private practice, when I was the new doctor in the small group, I was assigned to take care of emergency patients. One of these was an 11-year-old girl with a laceration on her arm. Clearly, she needed a few sutures. I instructed the nurse to prep the wound and open a suture set while I went to see the next patient. A few minutes later, there was a ruckus in the hall – a hysterical girl and an angry mother. I exited the exam room to be greeted by the mother's wrath: "Doctor, I know you're young and new to town. And you have some lessons to learn. Don't ever set out needles and thread and scissors and then leave the room for a child to stare at and wait for you. I'm not surprised my daughter panicked!" As reader, you may or may not agree with the mother's stance, but for me it was a lifelong professional lesson: Don't set out an open suture set for an adolescent to ponder. And, with children, if you describe a procedure that may cause pain, such as an injection, get it done fast.

In medical history, there are numerous examples in which lessons learned from patients have advanced medical science. In the late eighteenth century, English physician and amateur botanist William Withering (1741–1799) learned from a village woman – some say a gypsy – that a tea she brewed from a secret recipe could cure dropsy (heart failure). After convincing the woman to share her recipe with him, Withering concluded that the active ingredient was the foxglove plant. The doctor began to use foxglove tea to treat heart failure patients in his practice, and subsequently described the success of this method in a paper published in 1785 titled "An Account of the Foxglove and Some of Its Medical Uses." (Taylor, page 15)

A few years later, a physician in the village of Berkley in Gloustershire, England wondered about the boasts of local milkmaids: "I won't get the smallpox; I've had the cowpox." In 1796, the physician, Edward Jenner (1749–1823), conducted a human experiment by inoculating a local boy with material from a cowpox pustule. Only mild disease developed, and when later Jenner exposed the boy to variolar material, no sickness occurred. Jenner, like Withering, reported his results, thus assuring a place in medical history – thanks to lessons learned from village milkmaids in his practice. (Gordon, page 65)

Although the advance should be attributed to a caregiver rather than to the actual patients – newborn infants – a chance observation led to the phototherapy technique used today to treat elevated and potentially toxic bilirubin levels in newborns. A nursery attendant, Sister J. Ward, noticed that jaundiced babies lost their yellow hue faster when exposed to sunlight, and so she clustered them near the nursery window.[17] Today, light therapy is commonly used to treat neonatal hyperbilirubinemia.

In a somewhat similar vein, the observation of mothers of children with cystic fibrosis that their children tasted salty when kissed led to the finding of a high salt content in the sweat of affected children, and eventually to a sweat test used to help diagnose the disease. (Collins, page 112)

On a more humble note, some of my patients have taught me the dignity of the human spirit, accepting with equanimity various types of chronic illness, disability, loss of family members, and even terminal disease.

DON'T DISMISS LIGHTLY A PATIENT'S RESEARCH ON THE INTERNET AND IN MAGAZINES AND NEWSPAPERS

For example, over the years, patients have told me about new remedies, which are sometimes discussed in the media before they are announced to the medical world. Years ago, my first knowledge about using antibiotics to treat peptic ulcer disease came from a patient, a stockbroker who had read an early report in the *Wall Street Journal*. Patients have told me about herbal remedies outside my traditional therapeutic armamentarium, agencies where my other patients can obtain needed social services, and the locations of helpful web sites I would have never found otherwise.

GIVE THE PATIENT THE BEST DIAGNOSIS POSSIBLE AT THE TIME

You help the patient in many ways when you give the disease a name. By telling the patient with pelvic pain that she has endometriosis, you are also saying that she does not have ovarian cancer, which might be just what she was worried about. A specific diagnosis, such as Achilles tendinitis or gallstones, gives the patient something to look up on the Internet. Even if the exact nature of the disease is still unclear, it helps to offer a general, descriptive diagnosis, such as "allergic rash," "probable viral infection," or "irritation of the stomach lining." At the end of a visit, there may be a cluster of family members in the waiting room waiting to ask, "What did the doctor say is wrong with you?" A reply from the patient, "The doctor doesn't really know," is not a satisfying answer.

Lipkin relates what happened to him on one occasion when he and the patient sought a diagnosis: "There are those who respect the frank statement, 'I'm not sure what's wrong but I will try to find out.' But once, after I had made such a remark, a highly intelligent but anxious woman replied angrily, 'Don't tell me you don't know! When my brother asked my father how many tiles there were on the room of the cathedral, he told him 174,692. My brother was satisfied. I don't care what you tell me. Just tell me something definite!'" (Lipkin, page 167)

SOMETIMES IT'S APPROPRIATE TO USE HUMOR IN THE EXAM ROOM

Sometimes! Describing his personal health problems, Norman Cousins has popularized the therapeutic value of humor.[18] What is the role of humor in the clinical encounter? What is and is not appropriate? When suitable to the context, humor can relieve anxiety and help to humanize the physician.

But what is proper can be a tricky issue, chiefly because of the vulnerability of the patient in any medical setting.

Patients seem to be keenly aware when the physician uses humor. In a study of 250 consecutive encounters in 15 practices, Granek–Catarivas et al found that almost 60 per cent of patients reported that the doctor had used some humor during the visit, while only 38% of these physicians reported using humor. The authors concluded, "Patients seem to be more sensitized to humor than physicians, probably because of their high stress level during medical encounters."[19]

Probably safest is patient-generated playful humor. During my medical school years, a group of us were examining an elderly lady with a loud murmur. When the blood flow in the heart is disturbed by a faulty valve, there is often turbulence that can be palpated through the chest wall. For historical reasons I have never quite understood, this phenomenon is called a "thrill." One day, we earnest trainees in our short white coats surrounded the hospital bed and as instructed by our attending physician, one by one, we ceremoniously pressed our examining hands on the lady's chest. Then, it was the turn of one slightly anxious young male student. As he finished his exam, the instructor asked him, "Did you feel a thrill?" At this point, the patient chimed in, "Sonny, if I were 50 years younger, you would have." Slightly raunchy, but no harm done, and the until-then passive patient clearly had assumed control of the situation.

Then, there is physician-generated situational humor. In another setting, a physician was doing a rectal and prostate exam on a male patient, who turned his head and remarked, "Doc, I hate this part of the examination." To this the physician replied, "Yes, and it's not the highlight of my day either." This remark is a little risky, but probably okay if it helps relieve the distress of an uncomfortable examination.

Most dangerous are physician-generated attempts at humor that might be interpreted as being at the patient's expense. An elderly man was undergoing prostate surgery likely to result in loss of any sexual function he might have had. When he asked his surgeon about possible effects of the surgery, the reply began, "Well, to begin, you will have to stop chasing the young girls." This seems crass and even somewhat cruel. It was clinical humor gone wrong.

The bottom line is this: Use humor in the clinical setting if it is not at the patient's expense and if it might brighten the patient's day a little. Keep in mind the power of the physician's words to hurt as well as to heal. Before making what seems a hilariously witty remark, the wise physician will reflect for a moment. If the little inner voice questions the appropriateness of the comment, then it is probably best left unsaid.

DURING THE MEDICAL ENCOUNTER, ASK THE PATIENT TO TELL ABOUT SOMETHING NONMEDICAL

How's your mom? Have you had time for some golf lately? How's your dog? What did you think of the football game on Saturday? Part of caring for patients is getting to know them as persons. This brings us to chatting.

Chatting is the art of making small talk, something else they never taught us in medical school. Yet, making small talk can have a significant influence on what patients think of us and our services. Gross et al assessed patient satisfaction in 2,315 patient–physician encounters. Two of their findings are pertinent here. First of all, they found that the longer the duration of the visit, the greater the patient's satisfaction was likely to be. And second, patient satisfaction was enhanced when the physician spent a little time chatting about nonmedical topics.[20] Delving a little into the patient's life doesn't take very long, it helps enrich the patient's life story and, who knows, you may just learn something that will prove clinically useful.

OCCASIONALLY SHARE A LITTLE ABOUT YOURSELF

One facet of nonmedical chatting can be revealing a bit about you to the patient. This can be telling about your recent trip, your grandchildren, or even your personal adventures in patienthood. When advising a flu shot, you might include, "I had mine last week." If you had successful surgery in the past, why not mention this when recommending surgery to a patient?

The patient who has lost a family member to death might be comforted by hearing something like, "I understand. My father died a few years ago, and it was a very hard time for me."

Beach et al found that in 1,265 clinical encounters, physician self-disclosure occurred in 15.4 per cent of instances. The authors grouped the disclosures into several categories: The most common disclosure involved reassurance, followed by counseling, rapport building, casual comments, intimate comments (such as "I cried a lot with my divorce, too".), and extended narratives generally unrelated to the patient's condition.[21]

AVOID LETTING THE PATIENT BELIEVE THAT YOU ARE INFALLIBLE

Sharing personal information with patients has one more benefit – it helps to humanize the "god-like" image of the physician. It is good for patients to feel confidence in their physicians, but the sense of confidence should stop short of omniscience with a hint of deification. A patient considering you to know everything and to be immune to error is dangerous for both of you. When this occurs, the patient ceases to question, and problems may not be mentioned. "After all, the doctor knows what he is doing." The risk to the doctor is the patient's disillusionment when things go wrong.

Here, I will wonder in print if the potential to be considered omniscient, omnipotent and infallible doesn't apply especially to surgeons, and within the surgical realm, to neurosurgeons and cardiothoracic surgeons, in particular. I believe that surgeons tend to have immense confidence in their abilities that lets them do their daily work; it takes a certain bravado to cut into the thorax or skull of another person. And perhaps, from time to time, the surgeon's self-assurance is unconsciously communicated to patients, possibly resulting in expectations of perfection. That surgical outcomes are sometimes less than perfect, and short of patients' occasionally inflated expectations, is reflected in the high malpractice liability insurance premiums paid by surgeons and in the occasional huge court award.

SOMETIMES COMFORT IS ALL YOU HAVE TO OFFER

"To cure sometimes, to relieve often, to comfort always – this is our work. This is the first and great commandment." Often attributed to Hippocrates, the first part of the quote is inscribed on the statue of Dr. Edward Livingston Trudeau (1848–1915) commemorating his tuberculosis sanitarium at Saranac Lake, New York. (Strauss, page 410.) Here, I will share a personal insight: In my career I have been both a primary care physician and an administrator – specifically, the chairman of a large medical school department. After a year of so in my administrative role I had what I considered a brilliant revelation, which is: Many of the persons coming to me – their chairman – with job problems didn't really expect me to fix them. They knew the limits of power of my office. What they wanted me to do was *listen*. Now, this can be very difficult for us physicians, who are biased toward action, toward identifying the problem, and finding a remedy. But in this work setting, the employee sometimes exhibited greater wisdom – looking for empathic comfort rather than an action-based response.

My next epiphany was that this administrative lesson had relevance in my clinical practice. In many situations, especially when chronic or terminal disease is involved, the patients and families know we can't offer cure; what they want us to do is to listen and understand. The best physicians do their best to be optimistic, even in the direst situations, and often the physician's hopefulness is the best medicine available.

ACCEPT HOW PATIENTS WILL JUDGE YOU

We have all been judged – evaluated – since the day we entered kindergarten and medical schools have raised evaluation to an art form. Being evaluated does not end upon receiving the MD degree, and perhaps the process becomes even intensified. There are specialty certification examinations, state licensing boards, and more, but here I focus on evaluation by patients. Every patient evaluates the doctor on each visit, and will probably not be shy about sharing conclusions with family and friends. How do patients evaluate their physicians?

Hurst writes, "In the final analysis, patients trust doctors to do the right thing. The right thing, of course, is for doctors to act scientifically when they can, but most patients are willing to leave the science to the physician. The patient's judgment about the physician is commonly based largely on how the physician handles the patient's general response to the illness. Patients may even recognize and appreciate the vow their doctors have made to obtain the best possible medical care for them despite the numerous obstacles that are commonly placed in the doctor's way."[22] Wise physicians know that patient judgments include intangibles such as punctuality, willingness to listen, perceived truthfulness, optimistic hopefulness, respect for the patient as a person, and even a willingness to disclose a little about themselves.

BEWARE THE POTENTIAL FOR CARING GONE WRONG

Adler writes about sociophysiology, what happens when persons in a bonded dyadic relationship exhibit a correlation of autonomic activity indicators. When this happens in a caring relationship, there is a reduction in the secretion of stress hormones, shifting the neuroendocrine system toward homeostasis.[23] To me, part of what Adler seems to be describing is what happens when two persons – in our case, patient and physician – begin to think as one, almost as if they shared one nervous system. When this occurs, critical thinking may suffer and clinical judgment can be suspended, a pathologic state endangering the quality of health care received.

One example of pathology in the patient–physician relationship is the *disease denial and rationalization syndrome*.[24] In this setting, both patient and physician enter into an unspoken pact to ignore the need for action in the clinical setting. Here is what happens: Mrs. Pella, age 66, has been Doctor Resnick's patient for almost 15 years. She sees him every 2 or 3 months for her various ailments, which include obesity with a body weight a little over 200 pounds, type 2 diabetes and hypertension. Her high blood pressure has never been under good control and at each visit Mrs. Pella and Doctor Resnick have more-or-less the same conversation. The script goes like this:

"Mrs. Pella, your blood pressure today is 164/96. I know that you are taking your diuretic every day, but I think we need to add another medicine to bring down your blood pressure. Also you need to lose weight."

"Doctor, I understand what you're saying. I've been under some stress, with my son, you know. Let me work on my weight until next time. I am sure I can take off a few pounds, and then let's see if this lowers my blood pressure."

"Okay, I'll see you in 2 months. Be sure to keep taking your diuretic and don't forget to lose some weight."

Of course, Mrs. Pella's weight stays stubbornly at the 200+ level, needed adjustments in antihypertensive medication are not made, and the blood pressure doesn't budge.

Visit after visit, year after year, Mrs. Pella and Doctor Resnick repeat the same script, almost as if they were actors in a play. Together they are denying the significance of her persistent hypertension and rationalizing the need for additional therapy. Dr. Resnick truly cares about Mrs. Pella and both feel that they have an excellent patient–physician relationship. And, in a patient-satisfaction sense, they do, except that their association has entered a pathologic zone – a caring relationship gone wrong – manifested as the disease denial and rationalization syndrome.

BE THERE FOR THE PATIENT

Whatever else the physician does, he or she must show up when needed. When a patient has a broken bone, a stroke, or a severe infection, the patient's physician – or else a surrogate covering for the personal physician – must be available. In my upstate New York practice, I lived eighteen miles of backcountry road from the hospital where my patients were admitted. One Sunday morning in January, I had a single hospitalized patient, Mrs. Martinez, a very elderly woman I was treating for heart failure. She had made good progress and was medically stable. Overnight there had been a foot of snow. What should I do? Dutifully, I braved the elements, made the trip to the hospital, examined my patient, adjusted the medication just a little, and then drove home on the snowy roads. When I arrived home I called Mrs. Martinez's daughter and reported on progress. I still recall her response: "Dr. Taylor, I just knew you would get to the hospital to see mom. We have such faith in you!" Somehow, her words made the winter trip more than worthwhile.

Writing for family doctors, but articulating a message pertinent to all physicians, Phillips and Haynes have provided me with one of my favorite quotations: "You can pretend to know, you can pretend to care, but you cannot pretend to be there." The authors go on to explain, "It is by being there for patients that family physicians provide the things patients seek: touch, trust, understanding, comfort, and healing."[25]

WISE WORDS ABOUT CARING FOR THE PATIENT

▓ *[In the case of] one whom you find who falls ill only on rare occasions, do not change any of his habits in his entire regimen.* Medieval Jewish rabbi and physician, Moses Maimonides (1135–1204). (Maimonides, page 51)

This reminds me a little of baseball players who won't change their sox as long as they are on a winning streak.

▓ *A cheerful face is nearly as good for an invalid as healthy weather.* American statesman Benjamin Franklin (1706–1790) (Quoted in Strauss, page 375.)

One of America's most inspired aphorists, Franklin suffered recurrent disabling attacks of gout, one of which prompted him to demur as lead author of the United States Declaration of Independence, ceding the opportunity to Thomas Jefferson. (Taylor 2008, page 189.) With recurrent gouty pain, Franklin must have highly valued cheerful faces about him.

▓ *The physician must generalize the disease, and individualize the patient.* German physician Christoph Wilheim Hufeland (1762–1836). (Quoted in Brallier, page 207).

We should all remember this aphorism when applying consensus-based clinical guidelines to individual patients.

For example, guidelines for prostate cancer screening or breast cancer therapy must always be tempered by the clinical context and the patient's preferences.

▨ *In spite of all our advances in medical knowledge, it is still true that it is more important to know what sort of patient has a disease than what sort of disease a patient has.* American physician and author James J. Walsh (1865–1942).[26]

▨ *A physician is obligated to consider more than a diseased organ, even more than the whole man—he must view the man in his world.* Harvey Cushing (1869–1939) (Quoted in Brallier, page 232.)

Cushing presents a good example of the distinction between disease and illness.

▨ *There are some patients whom we cannot help; there are none whom we cannot harm.* Arthur L. Bloomfield (1888–1962). (Quoted in Strauss, page 637).

We physicians should consider this aphorism whenever we write a prescription, especially for a drug with which we are newly acquainted.

▨ *Empathy is the physician's only panacea.* (Meador, No. 185.)

▨ *No matter how knowledgeable and skillful the physician, the healing process starts with a smile.* (Meador, No. 16)

Why not? A cheerful greeting adds no minutes to the length of the encounter, and it certainly makes the patient feel better.

▨ *Regardless of advances made, effective treatment will continue to depend on knowing the patient and his environment.* (Reveno, page 105)

▨ *Every patient invites the doctor to combine the role of the priest, the philosopher, the poet, and the scholar.* American essayist and editor Anatole Broyard (1920–1990) (From Broyard's essay "Doctor, talk to me." In: Reynolds and Stone, page 180)

Such a ponderous job description is one more reason why we, as a society, should encourage the best and the brightest to become our healers.

■ *But of course, without* sostradanya *(compassion) no man is a doctor. A doctor must give a part of his heart to his patient.*[27] This metaphoric saying, quoted by Crawshaw, is attributed to "an elderly Russian physician" who was undoubtedly the type of doctor Francis Weld Peabody would have admired.

REFERENCES

1. Low CH. Reflection for young doctors and doctors of tomorrow. *Singapore Med J.* 1998;39(12):535–536.
2. Peabody FW. The care of the patient. *JAMA.* 1927;88(12):877–882.
3. Zinsser H. Introduction. In: Peabody FW, ed. *Doctor and Patient.* New York: Macmillan; 1930:11.
4. Tishler PV. The care of the patient: a living testimony to Francis Weld Peabody. *Pharos; Alpha Omega Alpha Honor Med Soc.* 1992;55(3):32–36.
5. Longmore JM, Rajagopalan SR, Wilkinson I. *Oxford Handbook of Clinical Medicine.* London: Oxford University Press; 2006:2.
6. Jung C. Psychological reflections. In: Jacobi J, ed. *Bollingen Series 21.* Princeton: Princeton University Press; 1970:84.
7. McWhinney I. The need for a transformed clinical method. In: Stewart M, Roger D, eds. *Communicating with Medical Patients.* London: Sage; 1989.
8. Schillerstrom JE, Horton MS, Royall DR. The impact of medical illness on executive function. *Psychosomatics.* 2005;46(6): 508–516.
9. Levy AH. *Floyd Patterson: A Boxer and a Gentleman.* Jefferson, NC: McFarland; 2008:263–264.
10. Lansky SB, Cairns NU, Hassanein R, Wehr J, Lowman JT. Childhood cancer: parental discord and divorce. *Pediatrics.* 1978;62(2):184–188.
11. Jackson JL, Kroenke K. Difficult patient encounters in the ambulatory clinic: clinical predictors and outcomes. *Arch Intern Med.* 1999;159:1069–1075.
12. Mas GX, Cruz DJM, Fañanás LN, et al. Difficult patients in primary care: a quantitative and qualitative study. *Aten Primaria.* 2003;31(4):214–219.
13. Sansone RA, Benjamin A. Borderline personality: somatic presentations in the primary care setting. *Primary Care Reports.* 2007;13(3):1–11.
14. Garrett KEE, JM KTR. The difficult doctor? Characteristics of physicians who report frustration with patients: an analysis of survey data. *BMC Health Serv Res.* 2006;6(6):128–132.

15. Elder N, Ricer R, Tobias B. How respected family physicians manage difficult patient encounters. *J Am Board Fam Med.* 2006;19(6):533–541.

16. Cassell EJ. *Doctoring: The Nature of Primary Care.* New York: Oxford; 1997:109.

17. McDonagh AF. Phototherapy: from ancient Egypt to the new millennium. *J Perinatol.* 2001;21:S7–S12.

18. Cousins N. *Anatomy of an Illness as Perceived by the Patient.* New York: Bantam; 2005.

19. Granek-Catarivas M, Goldstein-Ferber S, Azuri Y, Kahan E. Use of humor in primary care; different perceptions among patients and physicians. *Postgrad Med J.* 2005;81(952):126–130.

20. Gross DA, Zyzanski SJ, Borawski EA, Cebul RD, Stange KC. Patient satisfaction with time spent with their physicians. *J Fam Pract.* 1998;47(2):133–137.

21. Beach MC, Roter D, Larson S, Levinson W, Ford DE, Frankel R. What do physicians tell patients about themselves? A qualitative analysis of physician self-disclosure. *J Gen Intern Med.* 2004;19(9):984–989.

22. Hurst JW. What do good doctors try to do? *Arch Intern Med.* 2003;163:2681–2686.

23. Adler HM. The sociopathology of caring in the doctor-patient relationship. *J Gen Intern Med.* 2003;18(4):317–322.

24. Hentschel U, Smith G, Draguns JG. *Defense Mechanisms: Theoretical, Research and Clinical Perspectives.* New York: Elsevier; 2004:489.

25. Phillips WR, Haynes DG. The domain of family practice: scope, role and function. *Fam Med.* 2001;33(4):273–277.

26. Quoted in: Medical epigrams. *Bull Hong Kong Chinese Med Assn.* 1948; 1(1): 42–43.

27. Crawshaw R. Humanitarianism in medicine. In: Smith MED, ed. *Living with Medicine: A Family Guide.* Washington DC: American Psychiatric Association Auxiliary; 1987.

3

Clinical Dialogue and Communication

You nearly always get more useful information using a chair than a stethoscope.

Meador, rule no. 141

We spend much of our waking time communicating with others, by speaking, writing, and through "body language." Communication is a little like sex. It is a normal function and most of us think we are good at it and some are, but many aren't. Superior clinical communication is a learned skill. Speaking with patients, families, and colleagues calls for a studied blend of selective curiosity, quiet intensity, and the ability to attend to what is *not* being said.

The process of clinical care is about helping patients manage their "stories."

Assuring that a patient's story is well told is a key responsibility of the physician, and for this reason, I chafe when a patient is called a "poor historian." We, the physicians, with some degree of formal training in how to communicate effectively, are the *historians*. The process of eliciting the patient's story was well captured by Berger as he described British general practitioner Dr. Sassall, doctoring in rural England in the 1960s:

> It is as though when he talks or listens to a patient, he is also touching them with his hands so as to be less likely to misunderstand; and it is as though, when he is physically examining a patient, they were also conversing.[1]

To orchestrate the storytelling, the physician needs highly tuned facilitative and listening abilities. Clinical dialogue is much more than data collection, and is much more than, "Just the facts, m'am." It is helping the patient tell a part of his

R.B. Taylor, *Medical Wisdom and Doctoring: The Art of 21st Century Practice*, DOI 10.1007/978-1-4419-5521-0_3,
© Springer Science+Business Media, LLC 2010

or her life narrative, and the clinical process is sometimes called "narrative-based medicine."[2]

As if to highlight the internationality of medical wisdom, Saito, writing in a Japanese medical publication, has proposed a framework to define narrative-based medicine.[3] The author proposes that narrative-based medicine has four defining features:

1. The illness is viewed as an evolving chapter within the larger story of the patient's life and "life-world."
2. The patient is acknowledged as both the narrator and subject of the story.
3. Medical hypotheses, theories and pathophysiologies are regarded as socially constructed narratives, and more than one can coexist at any time.
4. New stories may emerge from the patient–clinician dialogue and these new stories may have therapeutic impact.

From Launer, Saito and others, we learn that narrative is not peripheral to the clinical encounter; in fact, it is the bedrock of what happens between patient and physician. Metaphorically, the patient comes to the physician offering the complaint and wish: "My story is broken and I hope that you can help me fix it." In practice, I have heard this concretely expressed as: "My back has been hurting for weeks; I can't work and I am afraid I will lose my job." And "I have been having nausea and stomach pain for months, ever since my son got in trouble with the police." Of course, sometimes the patient is not forthcoming with the fears and concerns about work and family problems; the astute clinician has to ferret out these important facts as the story unfolds.

Charon refers to *narrative competence*, that is, the ability to acknowledge, absorb, interpret, and act on stories and the plight of others. The author holds that this "ability is required for the effective practice of medicine."[4] That communication skill, aka narrative competence, is important is underscored by the study by Tamblyn et al, highlighting what can happen when communication skills are lacking. These investigators looked at 3,424 physicians taking the Medical Council of Canada clinical skills examination between 1993 and 1996, and followed them through their first two to 12 years of practice. The found that poorer scores "in patient–physician communication and clinical decision making on [the] national licensing examination predicted complaints to medical regulatory authorities."[5]

In an editorial commenting on the 2007 Tamblyn et al study, Makoul and Curry tell, "In a diverse set of studies since [the late 1960s], effective communication has been linked with increases in patient and physician satisfaction, better adherence to treatment plans, more appropriate medical decisions, better health outcomes, and fewer malpractice claims."[6] Any process with so many potential benefits to both patient and physician surely merits diligent study and practice.

The "setting" of this chapter is the clinical interview, which Cassell terms the physician's "first and most basic clinical skill." (Cassell, page 148) The clinical interview may occur in one of a number of venues: the physician's office, emergency room, hospital bedside, nursing home, the patient's home, and more. No matter where the exchange occurs, the clinical maxims are the same. The concepts discussed below tell some specifics of how wise clinicians conduct the clinical interview. I start at the beginning of the encounter, what happens after you enter the room – greeting the patient.

ALWAYS GREET THE PATIENT BY NAME

A person's name is very important to him or her. Use it from time to time during the clinical interview, beginning with the moment when you first encounter the patient: "Mr. Jones, good morning. I'm Doctor Taylor." Or if this is a long-standing patient who is also a friend: "Good morning, Mary. Good to see you again."

Whether to use patient's first or last name is clearly a situational decision. Although generally not an issue with younger persons, the too-familiar use of a mature patient's first name can cause offence. I am in my 70s and yes, from time to time I am a patient in the office of a doctor or dentist. I confess that I feel a little disrespected when a nurse who is just a few years older than my granddaughter opens the door to the exam area, looks at the medical record and, in loud voice, summons "Robert." I caution students that saying Mr. Jones and Mrs. Smith will never offend. Move to a first-name basis when invited by the patient to do so.

While I am on my "addressing the patient with respect" soapbox, let's think for a moment about the risks of using first names when the doctor or nurse does not know the patient well. I have a friend named Harold Evan McKnight. (OK, I have changed the name a little.) All his family and friends call him Evan, not Harold. And my friend Evan tells me that when he receives a telephone call asking to speak to "Harold," he knows it is not from someone he knows well. He calls the name "Harold" his nuisance-call detector.

SIT WHEN TAKING A MEDICAL HISTORY

In both office and hospital, you will seem to be much less rushed if you sit while conversing with the patient, even if you are under time pressure. Don't appear to the patient to be a doctor who seems to make a brief guest appearance and then speeds off to something important. Groopman calls this physician on roller skates the "18-second doctor."[7] Then, there is the tale of the hospitalist who makes rounds on his charges at 2 a.m., explaining that seeing his patients at that hour goes much faster than when they are fully awake.

A good research study would be to sit while speaking with 100 patients and then stand while speaking with another 100 patients. Then, ask each to estimate the time of the doctor–patient encounter. My hypothesis is that the patients interviewed while you both were seated will guess the time to be significantly longer than the patients interviewed while the physician stood. As part of the study, I would also note the time expended in the visits. My hypothesis is that the actual length of the visit, measured in minutes and seconds, will be no different whether the physician stands or sits during the clinical interview.

BE SURE THE PATIENT KNOWS YOUR NAME AND YOUR ROLE IN HIS OR HER CARE

Identifying yourself is more important today than ever. Even in a restaurant of modest pretensions, I am likely to be greeted with, "Hi. I'm Karen and I will be your server tonight." In a health care setting, we should aim even higher. Knowing the health professional's name and role was scant problem when patients received care from their personal physicians, and when hospital physicians wore white coats or perhaps business suits, and nurses wore crisp white uniforms and caps. Today, patients are faced with a huge cast of health care professionals and students, many of whom wear outfits that don't tell their respective roles and who display name tags with tiny, unreadable print. Help the patient – and family members – avoid confusion by clearly stating who you are and why you may be important in the patient's care.

Introducing yourself, shaking hands with the patient, sitting down to talk, and explaining your role in the health care pantheon are all part of what Kahn calls *etiquette-based medicine*.[8] What Kahn advocates is a service oriented mentality based on respect for the patient and family, and that is evident in all phases of the medical encounter. In Chap. 7, I will tell some ways we clinicians can learn from the service experts. In the meantime, the following are some more ways to practice etiquette-based medicine.

MAKE EYE CONTACT APPROPRIATE FOR THE CLINICAL SITUATION

Making proper eye contact is a key skill in clinical communication. Any thoughtful medical student will advise making eye contact with the patient. But here I wish to temper this advice. First of all, not all eye contact is good. Here is a suggestion: When you are engaged in conversation with a friend, note the eye contact you both make. You will find that you maintain eye contact only about 5 seconds or so at a time. Then, you look at something or someone else for a while before reestablishing eye to eye contact. Any longer than 5–8 seconds of eye contact is staring – a little strange, at best, and intimidating to many persons.

On the other hand, recognize if the patient and you are not making eye contact at all. Reluctance to make eye contact at all is a note-worthy physical finding that needs to be explained. Who is not making eye contact? Is it you, already composing your note on the computer? Or is it the patient, who may be manifesting depression, anxiety, fear, shame or anger? Could a lack of eye contact at a key point in the interview – such as when discussing an illegal act or sexual encounter – indicate that the patient is being less than truthful? Or perhaps the lack of eye contact is nothing more than a cultural norm. In some societies, direct eye contact is considered rude, intimidating, and a sign of disrespect.

RECOGNIZE THE POWER IMPLICATIONS OF RELATIVE EYE LEVELS

Be sure not to hover over the patient – standing when the patient is sitting, or even sitting on a chair that is higher than the patient's. I once witnessed an oral examination in a medical school in Italy. Visualize the scene: The site was the floor of a tiered lecture hall, with a number of students watching the proceedings. On the floor of the amphitheater was a rectangular table. At the middle of one side of the table, the professor sat in a high-backed armchair. At each end of the table were two assistant professors seated on ordinary side chairs. Across from the table sat the hapless student examinee, seated on a low stool that placed his eye level far below that of the professors. I never forgot that height-based exercise of power.

DECIDE UPON YOUR DEFAULT OPENING QUESTION THAT BEGINS THE CLINICAL INTERVIEW

I like beginning the clinical interview with the phrase: "What brings you in today?" Yes, occasionally the answer is "the city bus," but generally this open-ended query prompts the patient to state the chief complaint clearly. There are advocates for the phrase, "How are you feeling?" I abandoned this question after a series of unhelpful responses, such as "bad" and "really sick." "What seems to be the trouble?" may prompt the frequent reply, "That's what I'm here to find out." Also, "What can I do for you today?" gets me far too many "Take my pain away" responses. In the end, you will decide on your default opening gambit.

OPEN-ENDED QUESTIONS YIELD THE BEST INFORMATION

I have young grandchildren, four of them, and I find I learn the most when I use the phrase, "Tell me about. . ." This is a good approach with patients. For example: In the setting of a patient with chest pain, asking, "Does the pain feel like pressure?" is subtly coaching the patient. Much better is, "Tell me about the nature of your pain."

Now, you may think this is somehow just logical and natural. Well, using open-ended questions in the medical interview may be logical, but it is not necessarily natural.

When we feel rushed, we tend to revert to yes–no questions, unconsciously hoping to shave a few minutes off the time of the visit. Also, the electronic medical record prompts us to ask focused questions and seems to want to make us all *Quiz-Docs*.

What is a Quiz-Doc? In his 82nd year, Dr. Seuss reflected on his experiences with doctors[9]: He coined the term *Quiz-Docs*, described, in the distinctive Dr. Seuss cadence, as those who "start questioning, asking point blank, how your various parts are faring."

INJECT A LITTLE IMPROVISATION INTO THE MEDICAL INTERVIEW

Our medical students sometimes emerge from their internal medicine rotation convinced that the clinical interview consists of filling the blanks, eliciting answers to questions found in their H & P outline. You remember this outline: Chief complaint, history of the present illness, past medical history, social history, and so forth. As important as all these elements may be, the richest historical narratives rely on the physician's unscripted ability to improvise – to respond to cues provided during the dialogue with the patient.

Haidet likens the unscripted communication in the clinical interview to the improvisation found in jazz music, which he describes as "the primary vehicle that jazz players use to relate and communicate musically with one another." Such a person-centered notion is the antithesis of the classic H & P template, and admittedly takes a lot of experience and even some measure of self-confidence. The outcome – thinking of clinical dialog as a composition and following the meandering themes that emerge – can yield a much richer record of the patient's problems.[10]

THE MOST EXPERIENCED CLINICIANS WILL MAKE NO CLEAR DISTINCTION BETWEEN TAKING A HISTORY AND PERFORMING A PHYSICAL EXAMINATION

While taking a medical history, wise physicians assess the patient's attentiveness, affect, and apparent level of anxiety, skin quality and tone, and general appearance of good health or poor. Subsequently, the time of the physical examination is an opportunity to clarify issues raised or to explore new pages in the medical history. In fact, continuing the elicitation of the patient's narrative can be a useful distraction during the examination. Only inexperienced clinicians remain mute during the physical exam, a behavior which represents both time and opportunity wasted, but which might alarm the patient being examined; that is, is the doctor finding something worrisome?

IF THE PRESENTING COMPLAINT SEEMS A LITTLE VAGUE, CONSIDER IF IT MIGHT BE A "TICKET OF ADMISSION"

Have you ever entered an exam room to discover, sometimes after more than a few minutes have passed, that the patient's actual reason for seeking care is not what was reported to the nurse, or even to you at the beginning of the interview? For me, one memorable case was a young woman who visited my office several times complaining of vague abdominal pain. Repeated physical examinations, various tests, and imaging failed to reveal any biologic abnormality. However, as she told her story, a picture emerged. She was a young mother with three children under the age of seven. Her husband was an auto mechanic who worked long hours. After work, he relaxed by playing softball with his buddies, and then stopped off for a few beers. This happened most nights, leaving my patient alone to feed the children, bathe them and get them to bed. She reported that her pain was usually worse in the evening and, in fact, she had considerable insight into its origin – the fact that she was a lonely "softball widow."

Despite her insight, she had offered the chief complaint of abdominal pain. It would be the rare patient who would begin a clinical encounter by saying: "Doctor, I'm here because I'm frustrated, lonely, and angry about my husband out with the guys every evening, while I am stuck home by myself with the kids." Thus, "abdominal pain" became her *ticket of admission* to medical care. What the softball widow really wanted, of course, was a chance to tell about her distress and a sympathetic ear to listen, even though she probably would have had difficulty describing what she really needed from the physician.

Patients can use the ticket of admission in various settings, which include: embarrassment about the nature of the problem, fear of appearing silly in the doctor's eyes, concern about the meaning of a symptom, and worries about loss of function or even death.

LEARN THE SKILL OF ACTIVE LISTENING

Be wholly present for the patient, with no interruptions – except, perhaps, in the setting of a life-threatening emergency calling for action first. In the usual clinical interview, pay attention to the patient's posture and to yours. Then, tune in to the narrative being told. Counselors use the term *listening with the third ear* – a metaphor attributed to psychoanalyst Theodore Reik.[11] To me this means not only hearing words and phrases, but being sensitive to how things are said, what is unsaid, and the patient's demeanor and body language. Consider if there is a subtext to the narrative, a pathway that should be explored. For example, if symptom such as vague chest pains began 6 weeks ago, what was going on at that time? And does the patient's posture seem to change when answering the question? Does he or she break eye contact, look away, or seem to become a little tense?

Sometimes, your third ear will sense that something is not being said. It may be an omission in the narrative of a key family member, or a past illness, or an important life event. Spanish cellist Pablo Casals once remarked, "The most important thing in music is what is not in the notes." Remember that the most important revelation in the clinical history may not be expressed in words.

PAY ATTENTION TO THE PATIENT; HE OR SHE IS TELLING YOU THE DIAGNOSIS

The adage of listening to the patient is attributed to Sir William Osler (1849–1919).The concept was stated a little differently by British and U.S. neurologist Oliver Sacks (b. 1933), author of the book *Awakenings*, who wrote: "There is only one cardinal rule: Always listen to the patient," (Quoted in Brallier, page 211) We should all be happy that, like the zebra metaphor (see Chap. 4), the "listening" aphorism has become part of the lore of medical education.

You, the clinician, and the patient share a goal – to arrive at an accurate diagnosis that allows effective therapy. In achieving this role, your best consultant is the patient. Writing in the Singapore Medical Journal, Low provides us with an illustrative tale: "I remember as a young doctor a child was admitted for loss of appetite, vomiting and dehydration. For many days, he was investigated extensively, and only after 7 days was a barium swallow ordered which revealed a 'seed' obstructing the esophagus. Everyone had not listened carefully to the child and had overlooked the story of 'accidentally swallowing a large seed' which started all the symptoms."[12]

LISTEN MORE THAN YOU TALK

US President Lyndon Johnson (1908–1973) once said: "You aren't learning anything when you're talking." The best clinicians talk much less than half the time.

One day in the office, I met with two parents who wanted me to "talk to" their 15-year-old daughter about some behavioral issues. It seems that she was becoming distant, acting rudely to parents and teachers, and engaging in some risky behavior. "I'm not sure that I should talk to your daughter," I replied, "but I will be happy to listen to her." Today decades later, I recall what happened with surprising clarity. Now remember that I am a family doctor, with no formal training in psychotherapy. But the parents had confidence in me, and they frankly did not want what they considered the stigma of having their daughter go to a psychologist. And so, a little, reluctantly, I agreed to meet with the girl. "Let's see how things go."

I met with the young woman weekly for a half hour. We talked. Actually, mostly she talked. She told me about her life, her insecurities, her worries, her dreams for the future. I listened a lot, didn't say too much. After about 2 months of weekly visits, the girl and her mother told me that they didn't think they needed to come any more. And then they thanked me, "Doctor, I don't think you even realize how much help you have been to all of us." And actually, I didn't, although today I better understand some issues in this story that I didn't appreciate as a younger physician.

WHEN DISCUSSING EVENTS IN THE PATIENT'S LIFE, HOW YOU FRAME THE QUESTION DETERMINES THE QUALITY OF THE RESPONSE

Here, I turn to a favorite topic – headache. For decades, my special area of clinical expertise has been headache. Many generalists have specific areas of interest – pain management, adolescent health care, maternity care, geriatrics, and so forth. My area is headache. Over the years, I accumulated a large number of headache patients, and for the past 15 years, I have taught a headache seminar to third year medical students every 5 weeks.

Events in a patient's life can affect the frequency and intensity of headaches, including migraine. Ask any migraineur. In fact, I believe – intuitively, and based on four decades of clinical experience – that when a patient comes to the doctor with a chief complaint of headache, not an incidental mention of the symptom, in that instance something significant is going on in the patient's life. The life event has exacerbated the headache, and, until the clinician identifies the life stressor, he or she is not really dealing with the root causes of the headache. Examples of such stressors have been job loss, financial reversals, impending divorce, pregnant teenage daughters, sons in trouble with the law, spouse abuse and more.

And so, we ask the patient to tell about their life outside our office, and here is where one's interviewing skills are crucial. I ask each group of students to tell me how they would ask a patient about noteworthy recent happenings. A question framed as, "Is there anything significant going on in your life?" gets a frown from the instructor – me. A patient is highly likely to answer "no," even if overwhelmed with life stresses, just to get off an uncomfortable topic and to be sure the physician doesn't think the problem is all "in the head."

More-open-ended queries are better. In the setting described, I like to add a little "permission-giving." My ideal question to the patient would be, "We all have problems in our lives. I do, and I am sure you do, too. And these problems can make physical illness worse. Tell me what is going on in your life that might be making your headaches worse."

ASSUME THAT THE PATIENT IS TELLING THE TRUTH

Start believing that the patient is telling the truth and wants your help. Beginning an encounter with the assumption that the described pain is imaginary or that the patient is malingering sets you up for a missed diagnosis or worse. With this said, I must admit that malingering occurs. Symptoms are sometimes exaggerated. Disabilities are overstated. And occasionally falsehoods occur.

Common clinical settings in which exaggeration or frank malingering might occur are personal injury and psychiatric illness, including posttraumatic stress disorder, in which there is considerable potential secondary gain. Military service, jails and prisons are classic venues for disease overstatement and fabrication. In fact, I have found one report of what the authors call "malingering by animal proxy." They report five cases in which pet owners bring animals to veterinarians, describing nonexistent ailments in an effort to obtain controlled substances for their own (human) use.[13]

Did you happen to see the same program I saw on television a few years ago? The tape showed a downtown city bus that had stopped following a minor traffic accident, an apparent low-impact fender-bender. The interesting item on the tape was the six people who quickly *boarded* the bus, a bus unlikely to move for quite a while, until after the accident investigation was concluded. Could it be that these persons hoped to file personal injury claims even though not on the bus at the time of the accident, and what do you think they told their examining physicians?

Nevertheless, instances of true malingering are rare, and an early assumption of untruthfulness will impede communication, introduce bias into your thinking, and may result in incorrect diagnoses and inappropriate therapy.

MEDICAL WORDS CAN HAVE DIFFERENT MEANINGS FOR PATIENTS AND PHYSICIANS

Wise physicians share their diagnostic impressions with patients, but are careful that everyone is using words the same way. For example, I treated a patient, a 60-year-old man, who had hypertension – high blood pressure. I treated him for a decade, and in all that time, I could never get him to understand that "hypertension" meant an elevation in blood pressure, and not anxiety.

Here are some clinical words and phrases that may be misunderstood or even cause unnecessary worry.

- Heart failure: We all know what *failure* means, and it's bad.
- Mass or tumor: To the clinician, these phrases mean a lump is present. Not every mass or tumor is cancer.
- Nerve: This refers to an anatomical structure, and has nothing to do with being "nervous."
- Shock: To the patient this word is likely to mean an acute emotional reaction. To the physician, shock is a syndrome characterized by plummeting blood pressure and racing pulse.
- Remission: Remission and cure are not the same.
- Internist: This physician is a specialist in internal medicine, not an intern.

■ Practice: We physicians practice medicine, but some persons interpret the term literally. That is, they think that we are practicing just as a basketball team might practice in preparation for a game. You might even hear, "I don't want any doctor practicing on me." In 2005, the specialty of Family Practice changed its name to Family Medicine; along with some other considerations, the potential for confusion about the word "practice" was a consideration in the decision.

TRY NEVER TO EXPRESS SURPRISE AT SOMETHING A PATIENT TELLS YOU

The gray-haired matron sitting across from you confides that she has been an intravenous drug user. A long-time patient tells of an instance of childhood sexual abuse. You learn that a respected community member has spent some time in jail. As a physician, you will hear all these tales and more. You have two responsibilities: The first is to maintain the patient's confidence, especially important in small communities, where everyone seems to know a great deal about everyone else. The other is to accept the revelation with the same impassiveness you would exhibit in a high-stakes poker game; that is, you show no telltale sign of a judgmental stance. Sometimes, the patient's story telling may be facilitated by an empathic expression such as, "That must have been difficult." But, generally, absent a medical reason to discover other details, that should be all. Any suggestion of disapproval or condemnation may block your chances of learning the patient's story.

SOMETIMES DOCTOR AND PATIENT ARE SEPARATED BY VALUES, LANGUAGE AND CULTURE

When I tell my British colleagues that I, a specialist in family medicine, am "certified," they snicker. To them my being "certified" means that I have a verifiable mental illness.

Some of my patients cannot read or write, in any language. Some new arrivals in the United States are encountering indoor plumbing for the first time. Can I, as an academic physician living in a large city, ever truly comprehend the experiences of, just as examples, a rural farmhand, an international captain of industry, or a recent immigrant from a developing country? All too often, as in much of the content of this chapter, we assume that we – patient and physician – both speak English as our native tongue, and that we share certain basic life experiences, such as attending grammar school at one time, having a passing knowledge of popular sports and their metaphors, possessing some ability with computers, having done some traveling, and so forth.

Consider what happens when clinical communication is confounded by differences in language and ethnicity. Following a review of the clinical literature on such differences, Ferguson and Candib concluded, "We found consistent evidence that race, ethnicity and language have substantial influence on the quality of the doctor-patient relationship. Minority patients, especially those not proficient in English, are less likely to engender empathic responses from physicians, establish rapport with physicians, receive sufficient information, and be encouraged to participate in medical decision making."[14] Of course, some of the markers of suboptimal doctor–patient relationships arise from cultural norms. For example, our patients who have recently immigrated to the US from southeast Asia tend to revere their physicians in ways seldom found in native-born Americans, and they tend to ask few questions, while seldom questioning recommendations. Nevertheless, most instances of poor rapport, insufficient information and lack of participation in decision making can be traced to the problem articulated by Paul Newman and the warden in the movie *Cool Hand Luke*: "What we have here is a failure of communication."

It is always a good idea for clinicians to check for comprehension from time to time. Asking the patient to restate what you have said is a good way to do so. "Just to be sure we understand each other, please tell me in your own words what you heard me just say." I suggest that verifying comprehension is especially important when there is a disparity in language and culture.

DON'T BE AFRAID TO SAY, "I DON'T KNOW"

A worthwhile phrase in the clinical interview can sometimes be, "I don't know." Often this is followed by, "I'll find out." Or even, "Let's look it up together."

I think that the "I don't know (at least, at this moment)" phrase sends the message that the physician is not omniscient, and is actually appropriately humble. It says, "Please don't hold me to a standard of knowing everything, because I don't and, what's more, nor does any other physician in the world." The value of this message occasionally becomes crucial when things go wrong. In a medical error setting, the patient may be more forgiving of the doctor who has expressed humility than of the more know-it-all, seemingly arrogant, physician.

Just don't say "I don't know" too often. I once knew a young doctor whose mentors had encouraged him to tell the patient openly when he did not know this fact or that. He took the advice to heart. It seemed that he said, "I don't know" very often, day after day. Before long, in the small town where he practiced, the general opinion was, "I won't go to Doctor Jones. He doesn't know anything."

AVOID THE USE OF MEDICAL SLANG

Aside from the fact that some of the terms doctors use to vent frustration are actually disrespectful of patients, there are other reasons to purge most medical slang from our daily vocabulary. First of all, patients often overhear what doctors say to one another, even when we think we can't be heard or that our medical argot is incomprehensible. Even worse is the inclusion of medical slang in the clinical record, which just might be read by the patient – or the patient's attorney – some day. Phrases such as bounce-back (a patient readmitted to a hospital shortly after discharge) and acronyms such as FLK (funny looking kid) may seem amusing, even if a little cynical, but they are not used in clinical practice by wise physicians.

BE SURE THE PATIENT HAS HAD A CHANCE TO SAY WHAT NEEDED TO BE SAID

The office visit really isn't over until the clinician has asked, "Is there something else we should talk about today?" In an interesting study, Heritage et al looked at the phrasing of the "what else?" question. They found that using the phrase "something else" rather than "anything else" was a subtle, but statistically significant difference. The "something else" query helped avoid unmet patient concerns, without increasing the length of the visit.[15]

However you phrase the query, checking for omissions offers the patient one last chance to add a few paragraphs to the clinical story being told. Here are some answers to this final question that I have received over the years:

- Can my family members catch this disease?
- Does this mean that I don't have cancer?
- Is this going to affect my ability to work?
- What is this test going to cost?
- Are you really sure of the diagnosis?
- Should I have a second opinion?
- Might this just get well if we do nothing?
- What has happened to others with this problem?
- Do you have to report this disease to anyone?

LEARN HOW TO PRESENT A PATIENT TO A COLLEAGUE

Not all clinical dialogue is with patients. Speaking with colleagues is a communication skill that should be learned in medical school. I spend a lot of time with medical students and residents, and I cringe when a senior student or resident presents a patient, beginning: "I have a sweet little lady who is here today with her daughter who has a cough and a lot of problems with her blood sugar." Is the lady 30-years-old and here with her 9-year-old daughter? Or is she 75-years old here with her adult daughter, who is actually her care-giver? How long has she had the cough, and is it severe or productive of sputum? Do we know her blood sugar levels, either on home monitoring or per office testing?

As for the word *little*, is she actually a "little person?" In fact, we are not really sure who has the cough and the presumed diabetes – mother or daughter.

At this point, I generally call "time out." Before going on with the patient's history, I suggest that the first sentence of the presentation would be more informative if phrased, "The patient is a 68-year-old female retired teacher with long-standing type 2 diabetes, diet controlled, who presents with a one-week history of moderately severe cough occasionally productive of some yellow sputum, accompanied by intermittent low-grade fever and blood glucose levels around 220 mg/dl on home monitoring." Now I have a clear picture of the patient, her presenting problem, and the clinical context.

WISE WORDS ABOUT CLINICAL DIALOGUE AND COMMUNICATION

- *Silence is a powerful weapon.* Sir William Osler (1849–1919) (Silverman et al, Page 29)

  A highly useful technique in the medical interview, the act of sitting quietly creates a conversational vacuum, often filled by the patient who may reveal the key fact in a diagnostic puzzle.

- *Good listeners are not only universally popular, after a while they know something.* (Meador, rule no. 33)

- *A doctor who cannot take a good history and a patient who cannot give one are in danger of giving and receiving bad treatment.* American physician Paul Dudley White (1886–1973)[16]

  Put two such individuals together in a clinical encounter, and mischief is likely to occur. Such a setting occurs, for example, in emergency rooms when the patient is flustered and the physician is rushed. If you sense this happening to you in a patient care situation, take some time to catch your breath, start over and elicit an adequate clinical history.

■ *Nowadays the clinical history too often weighs more than the man.* Martin H. Fischer (1879–1962) (Strauss, page 216)
Fischer, of course, referred to paper charts, sometimes delivered to the clinic or hospital floor in several volumes wheeled in on a shopping cart. Today paper charts are becoming anachronisms, but the electronic medical record is often still voluminous and daunting.

■ *History taking, the most clinically sophisticated procedure of medicine, is an extraordinary investigative technique: in few other forms of scientific research does the observed object talk.* American professor of medicine Alvan R. Feinstein (1926–2001).[17]
But is the elicitation of the medical history an investigative technique, or an opportunity for patients to tell their stories?

■ *The difference between patients describing their illnesses to their barbers or hairdressers and their physicians is the difference between a newspaper story and a chapter in a history book.* American family physician Gayle G. Stephens[18]
Except in the editorial pages, newspapers are vehicles for "just the facts." The clinical history should be a much richer narrative.

■ *Because of its richness, the history is one of the central moments in clinical medicine.* American physician Eric J. Cassell (1928) (Cassell, page 148)

■ *It is intellectual communication skills which will become the most crucial competency in health care.* British professor of public health and epidemiology R. J. Lilford.[19]

REFERENCES

1. Berger J. *A Fortunate Man: The Story of a Country Doctor*. New York: Random House; 1967:77.
2. Launer J. Narrative-based medicine: a passing fad or a giant leap for general practice? *Br J Gen Pract*. 2003;53(487):91–92.
3. Saito S. Narrative-based medicine and clinical knowledge. *Seishin Shinkeigaku Zasshi*. 2006;108(2):176–181.

4. Charon R. The patient–physician relationship. Narrative medicine: a model for empathy, reflection, profession, and trust. *JAMA*. 2001;286:1897–1902.
5. Tamblyn R, Abrahamowicz M, Dauphinee D. Physician scores on a national clinical skills examination as predictors of complaints to medical regulatory authorities. *JAMA*. 2007;298:993–1001.
6. Makoul G, Curry RH. The value of assessing and addressing communication skills. *JAMA*. 2007;298(9):1057–1059.
7. Groopman J. *How Doctors Think*. New York: Houghton-Mifflin; 2007.
8. Kahn MW. Etiquette-based medicine. *N Engl J Med*. 2008;359(19):1988–1989.
9. Seuss D. *You're Only Old Once*. New York: Random House; 1986.
10. Haidet P. Jazz and the art of medicine: improvisation in the medical encounter. *Ann Fam Med*. 2007;5:164–169.
11. Reik T. *Listening with the Third Ear: The Inner Experience of a Psychoanalyst*. New York: Farrar, Straus and Giroux; 1983.
12. Low CH. Reflection for young doctors and doctors of tomorrow. *Singapore Med J*. 1998;39(12):535–536.
13. LeBourgeois HS, Foreman TA, Thompson JW Jr. Novel cases: malingering by animal proxy. *J Am Acad Psychiatry Law*. 2003;31:394–395.
14. Ferguson WJ, Candib LM. Culture, language and the doctor-patient relationship. *Fam Med*. 2002;34(5):353–361.
15. Heritage J, Robinson JD, Elliott MN, Beckett M, Wilkes M. Reducing patients' unmet concerns in primary care; the difference one word can make. *J Gen Intern Med*. 2007;22:1429–1433.
16. White PD. *Introduction. Clues in the Diagnosis and Treatment of Heart Disease*. 2nd ed. Springfield, IL: Charles C. Thomas; 1956.
17. Feinstein AR. *Clinical Judgment*. Baltimore: Williams and Wilkins; 1967.
18. Stephens GG. A family doctor's rules for clinical conversations. *J Am Board of Fam Pract*. 1994;7(2):179–181.
19. Lilford RJ. Medical practice-what next? *J R Soc Med*. 2001;94:560–565.

4

The Art of Clinical Diagnosis

The precise and intelligent recognition and appreciation of minor differences is the real essential factor in all successful medical diagnosis. Eyes and ears which can see and hear, memory to record at once and to recall at pleasure the impressions of the senses, and an imagination capable of weaving a theory or piecing together a broken chain or unraveling a tangled clue, such are the implements of his trade to a successful diagnostician.
British physician and educator Joseph Bell (1837–1911)
Quoted in Strauss, page 96.

Recently I had lunch with some colleagues in the hospital cafeteria, and the discussion turned to teaching medical students. One of the physicians at the table, an internist, reported that rarely does he see a rectal examination described on a record of a hospital admission history and physical examination – and ours is a university teaching hospital! The surgeon then declared that the physical examination really isn't important anymore, and that now diagnoses are made in the laboratory and by imaging. I heartily disagree, and I still hold that the best physicians maintain keen physical diagnosis skills, even in the face of slights by the Philistines.

This chapter presents advice and methods regarding diagnosis. It is about the medical history, physical examination, laboratory investigation, and diagnostic imaging, and the conclusions that emerge following careful consideration of all that is found. As we begin, I call your attention to the quotation above. What is the story behind the quote and who was Dr. Bell? The source is a lecture to medical students by Dr. Joseph Bell, who was on the faculty of the University

R.B. Taylor, *Medical Wisdom and Doctoring: The Art of 21st Century Practice*, DOI 10.1007/978-1-4419-5521-0_4,
© Springer Science+Business Media, LLC 2010

of Edinburgh Medical School at the end of the nineteenth century. Dr. Bell's life might be a long-forgotten footnote in medical history except for one thing: He was fond of observing a person and then attempting – often successfully – to describe the subject's work and other activities. He is also reported to have been fond of using the word "elementary." In 1877, young physician Arthur Conan Doyle was working at the Edinburgh Royal Infirmary, where he met Dr. Bell, who became the inspiration for his fictional character Sherlock Holmes.

Bell, Doyle, you, and I are all diagnosticians – medical detectives. Our task begins with first contact with the patient which may be by telephone, via e-mail, or upon opening an exam room door, and from that moment the patient and we embark on what often becomes the search for a continually tentative and evolving diagnosis. This chapter is intended to help doctors in that task. To do so, I present a variety of precepts and methods: practical tips, diagnostic pearls, pathognomonic findings, "red flags," and clinical aphorisms – all with some attempt at documentation of their origins. In each group, I have not been inclusive, but instead have tried to offer just enough examples to inspire you to seek your own examples.

With that introduction, let us look at the art of clinical diagnosis:

THE PROCESS OF DIAGNOSIS BEGINS WITH THE PATIENT'S DECISION TO SEEK MEDICAL HELP

Knowing what has gone into that decision is generally an index of the patient's level of concern and may sometimes help make the diagnosis. Looking at early decisions to seek health care and the choices made by patients, Green et al examined "ecology of medical care" of people in the community.[1] The authors found that of 1,000 persons observed over one month, 800 reported some sort of symptoms, 327 of these persons considered seeking medical care, and 217 visited a physician's office, with half of these visits (113) being to a primary care physician. Significantly, there were 65 visits to complementary/alternative medicine providers.

Of those persons actually receiving medical care, what factors tip the scale toward professional versus home/self care? Or between allopathic and alternative care? Or toward visiting a physician's office rather than a hospital emergency department? One person with cough and recurring fever may be seen by a physician; a neighbor with the same symptoms may treat recent-onset cold symptoms with cough syrup and aspirin. In the end, the outcomes may not be very different. These "ecology" decisions, largely made before the medical team is aware of anything, are made on the basis of personal and family factors, including the extent of lay medical knowledge, past experience with the symptoms and with the health care system, the perceived severity of the problem, and advice from family and friends.

THE CIRCUMSTANCES OF THE PATIENT'S PRESENCE IN YOUR OFFICE CAN OFFER DIAGNOSTIC CLUES

Could there be a back-story to today's visit? Sometimes it helps to ponder on the circumstantial clues. Here are some questions wise physicians consider: Why is this patient here today, not last week, or not next week after giving the symptoms a chance to improve on their own? Why me as the physician and not some other specialist? If the patient is alone, with no spouse or children along, is that significant? Or, if the patient has asked a spouse to come into the exam room, does that person's presence have meaning? For example, an abuser is often reluctant to let the abused person out of his sight. Is the patient especially concerned about the meaning of today's problem, and might that indicate some as-yet-unexpressed concern? Does a change in the pattern of office visits – more frequent than usual, a different time of day or day of the week, even a different mode of transportation – have any diagnostic significance?

For example, I had a patient, a man who came to the office about every three months for his blood pressure check, usually in the late afternoon and accompanied by his wife. One day he arrived alone for an early morning appointment. His chief complaint, as recorded by the nurse, was to "check BP meds." But when asked, twice, about why he was in the office, it turned out that he had been having dizzy spells that were occurring with increasing frequency. He was employed as a delivery truck driver. He was worried that his blood pressure was high, which it was. But he specifically wanted treatment – "Give me something to stop this dizziness"—and he also wanted confidentiality. He feared, with good reason, that his wife would call his supervisor and that he might lose his job, or at least be prohibited from driving until the problem was solved.

THE ASTUTE DIAGNOSTICIAN MAKES CASUAL OBSERVATION PART OF THE PHYSICAL EXAMINATION

How often does the physician watch the patient walk down the hall? It certainly matters if he or she can walk briskly, or seem to be short of breath after a few steps. Is there a shuffling, antalgic, or unsteady gait? In a younger athletic person, gait may be the clue to an Achilles tendinitis or iliotibial band friction syndrome.

Once the patient has entered a small examination room, it is difficult to appreciate gait abnormalities, but there can be other indications of disease. Body language can provide important clues. Note if the patient attends brightly when you enter the room, or perhaps sits dejectedly, back bent and head bowed, perhaps suggesting the presence of depression. See how he or she gets up on the exam table, if there seems to be weakness, pain, or movements favoring some part of the body.

GREET YOUR PATIENT WITH A HANDSHAKE

Most patients prefer their physicians to greet them with a handshake. According to a study of 415 patients by Makoul, 78.1% reported that they wanted the physician to shake their hand.[2] In a similar study, Davis et al found, "Patients desire a degree of formality from their physicians in the form of a handshake ($61\% \pm 7\%$), greeting of family members ($69\% \pm 7\%$), and in addressing oneself as doctor."[3] Yes, there will be patients who feel otherwise, and the physician should be alert for interactive cues. But in general, our default beginning of a clinical encounter should include a handshake as part of the greeting.

Shaking hands is not only a social gesture welcoming the patient to the encounter. It might help with diagnosis. The following are some diseases that may be suggested by a handshake. Can you think of some others?

- Dupuytren contracture of tendons passing through the palm of the hand, affecting predominately persons of Celtic or Viking descent, and affecting men a decade earlier than women[4]
- Anxiety, manifested as a sweaty palm
- Hyperthyroidism, or perhaps fever, with a very warm palm
- Parkinsonism, with evidence of an intention tremor as the patient extends his hand toward yours
- Rheumatoid arthritis, exhibiting the characteristic deformities of a hand you should not squeeze tightly
- Chorea – of which there are a number of types
- Radial nerve paralysis with a wrist drop, perhaps due to "Saturday night palsy" or even lead poisoning.[5]

THINK ABOUT WHAT MIGHT BE THE TRUE PURPOSE OF THE MEDICAL ENCOUNTER

As a newly minted academic physician in 1978, fresh from 14 years in rural practice and keen to begin some scholarly endeavors, I recruited a research team of equally inexperienced faculty members. We naïvely embarked upon an unsophisticated and underfunded study to see if patients and physicians had consistent views of the "primary purpose" of the medical encounter.

After separate interviews of patients and physicians following 200 medical encounters, we found a number of visits in which "concern" as the patient's stated primary purpose was misperceived by the physician; that is, in these instances, the physician believed that the patient's agenda for the visit was relief of symptoms, while the patient's greatest wish was to understand the significance of the symptoms. That is, the physician failed to recognize that the patient was more interested in learning the cause of the headache or dizziness than in making the symptom go away.[6]

Here are some instances when learning the true purpose of the medical encounter was clinically relevant:

■ A 48-year-old woman with postural low back pain related to her work as a postal employee confided, a little sheepishly, that she had a lingering concern that the pain might be an early indication of multiple myeloma, the disease that caused her mother great suffering in the months before her death.

■ A 42-year-old man came as a new patient for treatment of his elevated blood pressure. But his "true purpose" in coming was to control his hypertension with a medication that would permit him to continue playing competitive full-court basketball. Knowing this helped guide the choice of antihypertensive medication.

■ A 16-year-old high school girl reported months of joint pains and fatigue following exercise. An extensive and expensive workup was unrevealing. The true purpose of the visit? She hoped to be excused from gym class, an activity she had come to hate because of her self-perception of her body image.

THE WISE PHYSICIAN DOES NOT READILY ACCEPT THE DIAGNOSIS OF ANOTHER

William Jenner (1815–1898), the English physician who first differentiated between typhoid fever and typhus, is quoted as saying: "Never believe what a patient tells you his doctor has said." (Brallier, page 213) As a good diagnostician, you should assemble your own fund of clinical narrative and physical examination data, perform any needed studies, and arrive at your own conclusions. There is a long list of why the offered diagnosis may be off base: First of all, you are seeing the patient at a later time; things change. Tumors grow and blood chemistries fluctuate. The physician who saw the patient earlier certainly elicited a different story; no two narratives are exactly the same, especially when elicited by two different historians. And the previous clinician may have used different diagnostic maneuvers than you employ, or not have used them at all.

The following is a personal lesson in why we should seek our own diagnoses: My colleague arrived back from an extended vacation to find that her patient, a 42-year-old married mother of three, had seen the resident three times for recurrent abdominal pain and some diarrhea. The resident's diagnosis was irritable bowel syndrome, and the patient was taking medication, although without much relief. During the first visit with her for this illness, my colleague asked if there was anything going on in the patient's life that might have to do with her symptoms. She began to cry and told of her husband losing his job, and how they were being forced to sell their home. Had the patient told this to the resident physician? No, she had not. She felt embarrassed by the family's financial reverses – she felt that she didn't know the young physician well enough to discuss this very personal issue – and she also didn't want the new doctor to think that the pain was imaginary. Had the doctor accepted the resident's diagnosis, she would have continued down an errant path. We physicians must think of each new problem as a "blank slate," and follow our own routes to diagnosis, which may not agree with what is on the clinical record.

PAY ATTENTION TO VITAL SIGNS

We call them "vital signs" because they represent the readily measurable function of body systems vital to survival. Always note the patient's blood pressure, pulse and weight and, when indicated by the nature of the chief complaint, the body temperature and respiratory rate.

Consider the following case: The patient was an overweight 60-year-old man who presented several times to his physician, complaining of waking up at night gasping for breath. His wife confirmed the episodes, and related that he was also often tired during the day. The provisional diagnosis was sleep apnea, empiric therapy was begun, and a sleep study scheduled.

What the physician failed to notice was that over three visits over about 8 weeks, the patient had a persistently rapid pulse rate recorded in the office, and he had progressively gained 13 pounds in weight. Had the physician attended to the vital signs, she might have considered the diagnosis of heart failure (HF), wondered if the episodes of shortness of breath at night might have been paroxysmal nocturnal dyspnea (PND), have asked about orthopnea and taken a close look for pedal edema, and perhaps have even obtained an echocardiogram. She might have been able to treat the HF successfully, and have avoided the subsequent episode of pulmonary edema that resulted in a 911 call to the home, an ambulance ride to the hospital, and several days in the intensive care unit.

ALWAYS EXAMINE THE AREA THAT HURTS

This may sound profoundly elementary, but I consider it a necessary admonition. In my epi-specialty of headaches, I find that most physicians treating patients for migraine or other headaches do not actually examine the head! They check the ears, eyes, nose, and throat. They look at the fundus of the eye. They listen for carotid bruits, and perform a general neurologic examination. But they don't examine the *head* itself. Some patients actually notice this deficiency, but seldom speak out. In 1928, American neurosurgeon Harvey Cushing remarked, "By a strange human frailty, auscultation of the skull seem to be the one thing most likely to be neglected in a routine neurological examination." And Cushing goes on to discuss possible causes of cranial bruits and vocal resonance. (Birnholz, page 33)

USE THE PRACTICAL METHODS THAT CAN ENHANCE YOUR PHYSICAL DIAGNOSIS

There are some techniques used by wise physicians, who are often the older clinicians who have not become dependent on the laboratory or diagnostic imaging to make their diagnoses. If you were fortunate to have one of these "dinosaur" educators teach you physical examination skills, you may have learned some of the following:

- If you suspect the presence of hyperthyroidism, you might dramatize the tremor by asking the patient to extend the arms and hands, and then place a single sheet of paper on the dorsum of each hand. With a tremor, the paper may seem to "flap" as though blown by a wind.
- Watch the patient's eyes when performing an abdominal examination. Persons with minor, nonspecific pain tend to close their eyes during the exam, but those with more serious abdominal disease keep the eyes open, fearful that the palpation will aggravate the pain.[7]
- Avoid attempting to elicit the patellar tendon reflex by striking on the bones of the knee joint; do so by using the index and middle finger of the left hand (assuming you are right-handed) to isolate the patellar tendon.
- If you cannot elicit deep tendon reflexed in the patellar or Achilles tendons, ask the patient to lock the curved fingers of both hands together, and then pull outward vigorously. This action lessens inhibition of the reflexes, and may allow neuronal recruitment sufficient to demonstrate deep tendon reflexes.
- The tuning fork has also been called the "back country bone scan." I learned this from a combat physician returning from Iraq, following which I searched the literature. Sure enough, I found a study by Lesho, done at Fort Richardson, Arkansas, who studied 52 patients with findings suggestive of a tibial stress fracture. He applied a 128-Hz tuning fork to the anterior surface of the tibia, and a report of marked exacerbation or reproduction of shin pain was considered positive. All patients then received bone scans. The tuning fork test was found to have 75% sensitivity and 67% specificity, with positive and negative predictive values of 77 and 63%, respectively. The author concludes that the tuning fork test is not sensitive enough to rule out a stress fracture on the basis of a negative test, but in appropriate settings, a positive test may be sufficient to institute treatment for tibial stress fracture.[8]
- If the tuning fork can be an improvised bone scan, the cell phone can – in a pinch – substitute for a tuning fork. Set the cellphone to vibration, and apply to bony sites just as you would a tuning fork.

▓ The dorsalis pedis pulse, important in the diagnosis of peripheral vascular disease, can be difficult to locate and, in fact, is absent in 2–3% of healthy young persons.[9] You can locate the artery on the dorsum of the foot by considering that, more or less, it forms an equilateral triangle with the medial and lateral malleoli. Of course, if you cannot find the dorsalis pedis artery, you can go to the posterior tibial artery, found just where its name suggests.

EXPERIENCED PHYSICIANS HAVE A "STRING" OF DIAGNOSTIC PEARLS THAT HELP THEM FROM TIME TO TIME

Clinical pearls represent the true folklore of medicine, often passed from the gray-haired elders to neophyte physicians, imparted in hushed tones in hospital corridors and coffee lounges. Hippocrates provided us with some timeless pearls, such as, "Sleep and watchfulness, both of them, when immoderate, constitute disease." (Strauss, page 551) Later, in the Middle Ages, Persian physician Avicenna described, "The rash of measles usually appears at once, but the rash of smallpox spot after spot." (Strauss, page 560)

Mangrulkar et al provide us with a perceptive analysis of medical pearls and how they relate to evidence based medicine.[10] The article begins with a vignette of a senior clinician attending an apparent stroke patient, who tells his residents and students, "A stroke is never a stroke unless it's had 50 of D50." This means, of course, that the astute clinician does not accept a stroke diagnosis without considering the possibility of metabolic causes, including severe hypoglycemia that would respond dramatically to the intravenous administration of hypertonic dextrose solution, a maneuver very unlikely to cause harm if the cause is other than stroke. The authors then go on to examine the characteristics of a good clinical pearl: (1) The teaching point is generalizable to other patients; (2) The source is a respected teacher, "lending validity to the information;" (3) The information is not common knowledge – in which case it would be a "glass bead;" and (4) The phrasing is sometimes catchy and easily recalled.

Early in your career is a good time to begin your own collection of clinical pearls. Here are a few examples. When available, I have cited evidence from the current literature:

▪ If you think you have detected multiple sclerosis in a patient over 50 years, seriously consider some other diagnosis.

This pearl, also from the paper by Mangrulkar et al emphasizes that the onset of multiple sclerosis in patients over age 50 is rare, "maybe nonexistent."[10]

▪ Nasal polyps in a child age 12 or under may be the tip-off to a diagnosis of cystic fibrosis.

In such instances, a thorough family history and a sweat chloride test should be considered.[11]

▪ Childhood carsickness can be the harbinger of adult migraine.

I have astonished a number of adult migraineurs by asking, "Did you happen to have carsickness as a child?" The reply is often, "Doctor, how in the world did you know that?" In fact, motion sickness occurs in approximately 50% of all migraine sufferers, and the childhood tendency may not abate, even when the headaches begin in adult life.[12]

▪ Think first of angina pectoris when a patient describes pain by pressing a closed fist to the sternum.

The "closed fist sign" is a treasured clinical pearl that has earned eponymous status as the Levine sign (Birnholz, page 39). Seeking to supply evidence to the clinical lore, Marcus et al looked at the Levine sign's utility in the diagnosis of angina pectoris.[13] They found a prevalence of 11% and a specificity of 78–86%, but the positive predictive value did not exceed 55%.

▪ Patients with acute pericarditis find their pain is better when leaning forward.

This long-respected pearl was reiterated in a review article by Goyle and Walling, noting that, "Patients with uncomplicated pericarditis have pleuritic-type chest pain that radiates to the left shoulder and may be relieved by leaning forward."[14]

■ Paroxysmal fibrillation should stimulate a search for underlying thyrotoxicosis.

This pearl from Reveno (page 34) highlights a treatable cause of atrial fibrillation.

■ Patients with gastric cancer lose their specific taste for meat.

I heard this pearl described when I was in medical school, and later found it again, without attribution, in Birnholz's book on *Clinical Diagnostic Pearls*. (Page 54). I have sought to confirm it, without success, on a PubMed search, and so here it is, a pearl seeking evidence to confirm or refute the assertion. A corollary pearl is that finding a Virchow sentinal node (an enlarged left supra-clavicular lymph node) should suggest the possibility of stomach cancer. (Ellerin and Diaz, page 99)

■ If the patient is hungry, a diagnosis of acute appendicitis should be questioned.

Patients with appendicitis have usually lost their appe-tites. This is a documented pearl. In a study of 267 patients operated upon for acute appendicitis, Gonclaves et al found that 86% had anorexia.[15]

■ Parkinsonism that begins with tremor runs a more gradual course than disease that starts with rigidity or hypokinesia.

In an evidence-based meta-analysis, Suchowersky et al concluded that, "Patients whose initial symptom is tremor may experience slower disease progression and may have a longer duration of response to levodopa therapy."[16]

■ The vast majority of varicoceles occur on the left, owing to the anatomy of the left spermatic vein, one of the body's longest.

In about a third of patients with varicocele, the abnor-mality will be bilateral. A unilateral right varicocele, however, should raise the suspicion of a mass lesion obstructing the inferior vena cava.[17]

▨ A young person with acute arthritis may have sarcoidosis.

This pearl from Nadeem highlights a possible cause of an arthritis – an uncommon problem in young persons.[18]

▨ Patients with Addison's disease are often suspected of being psychoneurotics.

Reveno's book on Medical Maxims (page 94) is the source of this pearl. An interesting historical note is that President John F. Kennedy had Addison's disease treated with corticosteroids during his tenure in the White House.

▨ Because forward flexion of the spine helps relieve the pain of lumbar spinal stenosis, these patients are unlikely to experience increased discomfort and may even report some relief when flexing the trunk while climbing stairs.

This phenomenon is in contradistinction to the person with vascular claudication who will probably experience pain while ascending a staircase.[19]

▨ It is easier for a patient with Parkinson's disease to bicycle than to walk.

Bloomfield and Chandler (Page 129) are the source of this bit of neurologic trivia. I have not had the opportunity to test the assertion in practice and have not found it in print elsewhere, but, given the characteristic gait abnormalities of Parkinsonism, it may well be true.

▨ Auditory hallucinations are likely to be psychotic in origin, while drugs and other chemicals tend to cause visual hallucinations. (Meador, number 157)

▨ If a pregnant woman near term has an umbilicus that seems to "go in," rather than being flat or protruding, think of the possibility that the baby is occiput posterior.

I heard this pearl at a clinical conference. I cannot find a literature citation, but it sounds very reasonable to me.

▓ A febrile person who has recently been traveling outside the US just might have malaria. Ask about a visit, however brief, to a malarious area. Then look for an enlarged spleen, thrombocytopenia and hyperbilirubinemia.[20]

With the world getting smaller every day, tropical diseases are no longer limited to foreign lands.

BEWARE OF "PLASTIC PEARLS" THAT LINGER AS PERSISTENT CLINICAL YARNS

Remember that there are also "plastic pearls," seemingly clever gems of wisdom that have not turned out to be exactly true, especially when examined in the light of current evidence based medicine. Here are a few plastic pearls:

▓ Night pain indicates severe disease.

Harding et al looked at the 1994 US Agency for Health Care Policy and Research suggestion that nighttime pain indicates a "red flag" in many diseases. They studied back pain in 482 patients, finding that of the 213 patients with night pain, with 90 having pain every night, none had serious pathology. They conclude, "Although it is a significant and disruptive symptom for patients, these results challenge the specificity of the presence of night pain per se as a useful diagnostic indicator for serious spinal pathology in a back pain triage clinic."[21]

▓ Pernicious anemia requires ongoing injections of vitamin B12.

We now know that oral treatment of pernicious anemia is as effective as injection therapy.[22]

▓ Administering narcotics to a patient with acute abdominal pain may make it difficult to determine the diagnosis.

Studies involving use of opiates in patients with abdominal pain indicate that pain relief not only may not interfere with diagnosis, but that the reduction in severity of physical signs may facilitate diagnosis.[23]

▦ Chest pain that decreases following use of sublingual nitroglycerine is of cardiac origin.

In fact, patients with pain that is or is not of cardiac origin may experience some pain relief with sublingual nitroglycerine, which cannot be relied upon to indicate ischemic chest pain.[24]

▦ Chest pain relieved by a "GI cocktail" (a mixture of viscous lidocaine, antacid and an anticholinergic) is due to gastrointestinal disease, and not myocardial ischemia.

I'm sorry to report that some patients with coronary artery disease may report relief after drinking the venerated GI cocktail.[25]

▦ Visual assessment by experienced physicians and nurses is a good way to assess the level of neonatal hyperbilirubinemia.

Contrary to popular opinion, a study by Riskin et al found that in evaluations of 1,129 jaundiced newborns by neonatologist and nurses, the level of serum bilirubin was misestimated two-thirds of the time, and there was considerable interobserver variability.[26]

KNOW THE PATHOGNOMONIC CLINICAL MANIFESTATIONS YOU MAY ENCOUNTER

A pathognomonic clinical finding is a symptom, physical sign, laboratory or imaging finding that is unique to a specific disease; its presence confirms a diagnosis. In a sense, the presence or absence of a pathognomonic manifestation is like the state of being pregnant – you are or you aren't. There is no gray zone. Yes, in a few cases, we state that such-and-such "is considered to be pathognomonic for" a certain disease, indicating that no serious challenge has yet arisen. An example of such waffle language is the bulls-eye rash seen with Lyme disease, described below. To quote Osler, "Although one swallow does not make a summer, one tophus makes gout and one crescent, malaria." (Bean and Bean, page 26) Our few recognized pathognomonic findings are well embedded in medical literature and have withstood the challenges of time and skeptical investigators.

Unless one chooses to wander in the wonderland of arcana – the distinctive magnetic resonance (MR) imaging findings in Balo concentric sclerosis[27] or the corduroy-like thickened trabeculae found radiographically in a vertebral body hemangioma[28] – there are actually not many pathognomonic clinical findings in everyday clinical practice. But there are a few:

■ Koplik spots. These tell-tale manifestations of measles were well described by Williamson in his 1961 book. He writes that, following nonspecific upper respiratory symptoms, fever and some conjunctival injection, "Within 12 h, Koplik spots usually appear on the buccal mucous membrane at the first molar teeth. About the size of a dot you make when dotting an 'I,' they are pearly or grayish white and are usually surrounded by a red or purplish halo. Koplik spots are evanescent and seldom last over 12–24 h in diagnosable form. For this reason it does not rule out measles if you do not see them." (Williamson, page 93) Because of the widespread and successful use of measles vaccine today, most physicians who entered medicine after the late 1960s have never seen measles or Koplik spots.

■ Bullseye rash of Lyme disease: Properly termed erythema migrans, the distinctive skin lesion is considered sufficient evidence to begin antibiotic therapy of Lyme disease. Malane et al write, "Approximately 75% of patients with lyme disease present with the pathognomonic skin lesion erythema migrans, an expanding erythematous lesion."[29] In several places where I read about this pathognomonic sign, however, I noted the qualifying phrase "is considered to be." Perhaps the ever-so-slight hedging comes from papers such as the one by Stanek and Strie, who write, "However, even erythema migrans might not be pathognomonic for Lyme borreliosis, especially in the southern part of the USA where there is no microbiological evidence for infection with the agent."[30] I note that this analysis of disease in the southern USA comes from the University of Vienna in Austria.

- Periungual fibroma of tuberous sclerosis. Sometimes called Koenen tumors, these pathognomonic smooth, firm lesions, found at the nail folds, were first described in 1903 by Richad (SIC) Kothe in Munich, Germany.[31]
- Negri bodies in rabies. Although not present in all cases, these inclusion bodies found on microscopic examination of nerve cells containing the virus are characteristic of rabies.[32]
- Gottron papules in dermatomyositis. Montemarano describes these pathognomonic lesions as "violaceous erythematous papules overlying the dorsal interphalangeal or metacarpophalangeal, elbow or knee joints."[33]

RECOGNIZE THE CLINICAL RED FLAGS THAT SUGGEST SEVERE DISEASE

In medicine, there are a number of clinical "red flags," danger signs indicating the possible presence of "must-never-miss" diagnoses. When encountered, a clinical red flag manifestation usually calls for prompt action.

- A patient with Herpes zoster infection of the trigeminal nerve and blisters on the tip of the nose (Hutchinson sign), suggesting a high risk for vision-threatening infection of the eye. The eye and the tip of the nose are both served by the fibers of the nasociliary branch of the trigeminal nerve.
- Acute unilateral testicular pain of sudden onset, very suggestive of testicular torsion, compromising blood flow and requiring emergency surgery.
- A child who has a fever, just doesn't seem well, and develops a petechial or purpuric rash, a combination of findings that should be considered meningococcemia until proven otherwise.
- An older person with unexplained weight loss that may be an early manifestation of cancer.
- Painless gross hematuria, which may be the first sign of a bladder or renal tumor.
- A child with an abdominal mass, which might be a Wilms tumor, aka nephroblastoma, the most common malignant renal tumor of childhood.

■ Unilateral visual loss described as "like pulling down a window shade," which is characteristically how retinal detachment is described.

■ Headache accompanied by one of several danger signs: paralysis; papilledema; or "drowsiness, confusion, memory impairment and unconsciousness," found by Lamont et al to be significant clues to intracranial pathology.[34]

■ Back pain accompanied by difficulty urinating, fecal incontinence, saddle anesthesia, or bilateral leg pain or weakness, signaling the possibility of a cauda equina syndrome.[35]

■ Unilateral pelvic pain in a woman 6–8 weeks pregnant, suggesting possible ectopic pregnancy.

■ An electrical burn found to have both an entry and exit site, indicating that the patient has had electric current pass beneath the skin and has sustained significant injury that may not be visible on initial examination.[36]

■ Any child with a croupy cough, especially if symptoms do not respond to the home remedy of sitting in a hot, steamy bathroom, suggesting that this is a child who might possibly be the one to go on to respiratory arrest.

■ Hemoptysis in an adult smoker, which may be an early sign of lung cancer.

■ A painful, injected, perhaps tense eyeball with a cloudy cornea, characteristic of acute angle-closure glaucoma. (Taylor 2003, page 598)

■ A young athlete with a family history of premature sudden death (i.e., younger than 50 years), which might suggest the presence of hereditary cardiac disease such as hypertrophic cardiomyopathy, coronary artery anomalies, or even Marfan syndrome.[37]

BE WARY OF OVER-ANALYZING A PROBLEM

Here, I offer a classic case of over-zealous and meandering analysis of a patient's medical symptom. Gordon (pages 202–213) tells the story of a humble English governess, living in Vienna, who sought medical care with the venerable Doctor Sigmund Freud in 1892. Her name was Miss Lucy Robinson, she was employed caring for the children of Dr. Schmitt, and her complaint was recurrent, annoying episodes of smelling an odor that seemed like burnt pudding. Freud begins by exploring her dreams, and goes on to inquire about her sexuality. He considers penis envy and the Electra complex. Still not satisfied that he has the correct diagnosis, he continues to believe, "There is a reason hidden deep in the mind for your smell of burnt pudding, Miss Robinson." (Page 209) Then he seems to have a moment of clarity. Freud states: "You have transferred an emotional dependence from your father to myself. You are in love with me." (Page 212)

In the end, the patient tells her theory: "I was going to tell you that Frau Schmitt's cook has secretly been attempting to perfect a *sachetorte* [a type of cake] for the doctor's own birthday, so far without success, and has been burning the evidence in the back yard under my window after the family was in bed." (Page 213)

The Miss Robinson and Dr. Freud story is a timeless example of the importance of letting the patient tell his or her full narrative before attempting to illuminate the clinical history with your own "burning" questions.

TRUST YOUR OWN CLINICAL JUDGMENT

Do not let clinical judgment be clouded by comments by emergency medical technicians (EMTs), nurses, and others who have seen the patient before you. Facts, yes, are important. Opinions are sometimes helpful, but the wise clinician tries very hard to resist bias and to make an independent and objective evaluation of each patient, disease, and clinical setting.

Here is an all-too-common example. The ambulance crew brings a somnolent and somewhat grimy individual found sleeping on the sidewalk. Just another drunk, the EMTs have concluded. The clerk at the admitting desk concurs. The patient is not quite coherent and needs assistance walking. If you, as the emergency physician, accept the proffered opinion, you may miss the diagnosis of subarachnoid hemorrhage – and the patient may fail to receive therapy that might literally be life saving.

SYMPTOMS OR SIGNS INCOMPATIBLE
WITH YOUR DIAGNOSIS MUST BE EXPLAINED

If a patient with apparent low back strain has a fever, the pyrexia deserves attention. Yes, the patient may have a second diagnosis – a concurrent respiratory infection – but diagnosticians who bet on the presence of two diseases are often wrong. A single diagnosis of viral influenza with a muscular backache may explain both symptoms, but the wise physician will consider the possibility that the "back strain" may, in fact, be a spinal epidural abscess, one of the "must-never-miss" diagnoses mentioned below.

AVOID CARELESSNESS, YOUR OWN
OR THAT OF YOUR STAFF

A few years ago, I consulted on a case involving a 76-year-old woman with nonspecific and puzzling symptoms including fever, fatigue, jaw claudication, headache, weight loss, muscle and joint aches, and a few brief episodes described as loss of vision in one eye. Her physician saw her several times, and ordered all the appropriate tests. The doctor's review of the laboratory and imaging reports did not suggest the cause of her symptoms, which were then treated expectantly for several weeks – until she experienced sudden blindness in her left eye.

Here is what happened. The doctor was smart. He had considered the correct diagnosis, along with a number of other possibilities, and had ordered the key test. But the doctor was not as careful as he should have been. When the test results came back, he somehow did not see the one report that would have offered the vital clue. He – or someone on his staff – overlooked the report of an erythrocyte sedimentation rate of 106 mm/h. The patient had giant cell (temporal) arteritis, with ischemia of the arteries serving the eye, which led to a disastrous result, permanent blindness in one eye – an outcome could have been possibly avoided had the patient received a timely diagnosis and treatment with corticosteroids.

TOMORROW'S DIAGNOSTICIANS WILL NEED TO MAINTAIN A HIGH LEVEL OF TECHNICAL COMPETENCE

The capable physician is able to read most types of X-rays, can recognize basic electrocardiographic changes, can comprehend ultrasound and other complex images, and knows how to locate and "manipulate" all of these on line. In the future, most of us will need to make sense of computed tomographic and magnetic resonance images, at least to the point where the clinician can discuss findings with a radiologist. The best physicians do not rely solely on X-ray reports; they look at the images, fortunately now much easier thanks to on-line availability.

Computers will increasingly become a mainstay of medicine, and the technology will become ever more portable. In the lifetime of many of today's practicing physicians, we have seen the shift from the huge mainframe monster housed in a frigidly air-conditioned room to bulky desktop computers with 25-pound monitors, to laptops, and most recently to wireless telephones with internet access. Technologic changes on the horizon will profoundly affect daily practice, and many of these changes will be in the realm of diagnosis: Internet-delivered images of electrocardiograms and roentgenograms, remote examinations of various body areas and orifices, the ability to view skin lesions and breathing patterns, and much more – some of which we cannot even imagine today.

The message for today's diagnostician is this: Keep your technological skills absolutely up to date, or you will quickly be left behind.

DO NOT OVERLOOK THE "MUST NEVER MISS" DIAGNOSIS – THE POTENTIALLY DISASTROUS BUT TREATABLE DISEASE

If a "must-never-miss" problem is in your differential diagnosis, be sure to take the steps necessary to exclude its presence. Sometimes the clues are subtle, and correct diagnosis depends on noting the clinical context. Of the many such diagnoses, here are a few examples:

▓ Slipped capital femoral epiphysis, which can lead to avascular necrosis of the femoral head.

This serious complication explains why Reveno (page 70) advises that, "Pain in the hip, knee or anterior thigh in a child between 9 and 15 years of age calls for X-ray study for slipped femoral epiphyses."

▓ Retrocecal appendicitis that presents with atypical pain.

In this setting, a positive psoas sign increases the possibility that the patient has appendicitis (Taylor, 2003, page 793).

▓ Spinal epidural abscess, generally presenting with back pain and fever, and typically found in an immunocompromised patient such as a person with cancer, alcoholism, diabetes, or acquired immunodeficiency disease.

Chao describes the disease in a 72-year-old woman with diabetes who had fallen three weeks earlier and who "presented with decreased appetite, severe low back pain, urinary incontinence and difficulty ambulating."[38]

▓ Meningococcal meningitis, treatable if detected early and potentially fatal if not.

Some four decades ago, long before the age of evidence-based-medicine and routine emergency room septic workups, I was on an evening house call. The patient was a 5-year-old boy, with a high fever, red throat and headache, but no stiff neck. He definitely lacked his usual energy, but was awake, well-hydrated, and paying attention to his surroundings. Almost in desperation, I rummaged in my black bag, gave him an injection of penicillin, offered advice about fever control, and instructed the parents to bring him to the office in the morning.

The next morning, the boy's fever was lower, but not absent, and he seemed a little less alert. The remarkable change was his neck, which was by then quite stiff. He was admitted to the hospital, treated for his meningococcal meningitis, and happily made a full recovery. In retrospect, I wish I had sent him to the hospital the evening before, and many physicians would do so today. And yet, looking back, and knowing how rapidly meningococcemia can progress, I have always wondered if my penicillin injection just might have saved his life.

▨ Abdominal aortic aneurysm (AAA) in the older individual with vague abdominal fullness, especially a man who has ever been a smoker.

The United States Preventive Services Task Force (USPSTF) currently recommends one-time AAA screening of men of age 65–75 who ever smoked, even if asymptomatic. The potentially catastrophic rupture of an AAA led Osler to comment, "No disease is more conducive to clinical humility than aneurysm of the aorta." (Bean and Bean, page 134.)

▨ Testicular tumor, which typically presents as a painless scrotal mass.

Because these cancers tend to occur in young men and because many are curable if detected early, prompt diagnosis is imperative. One day fairly early in my career, I received a call from a male patient I will call Ronald, age 29. "Dr. Taylor, it's probably nothing, but last night while we were having sex, my wife found that one of my testes seemed enlarged and "lumpy." Should I be worried about this?" Within 48 h, this man was in surgery. In Chap. 6, I'll return to Ronald and the rest of the story.

▨ Malignant melanoma.

Brittany Leitz, Miss Maryland, preparing for her appearance in the 2007 Miss America Pageant, spent hours in a tanning booth beginning at age 17. At age 20, she was diagnosed with melanoma, and she now counsels teens to avoid tanning salons.[39]

INCLUDE THE PATIENT AS A "CONSULTANT" WHEN DEVELOPING YOUR DIAGNOSTIC IMPRESSION

Ask the patient with chest discomfort, "What do you think might be the cause?" When a patient complains of tiredness, be sure to inquire, "A lot of things can cause fatigue, or make it worse. You have obviously thought about this. What is your opinion about the cause?" When I worked in North Carolina, a colleague once told me about an elderly woman with abdominal pain. When initial tests failed to reveal the cause, he asked the woman what she thought might be the cause. Her answer: "It's the Devil. I'm being punished for ..." She went on to describe her "sin" and how the Devil had been enlisted to punish her. Although the doctor never successfully refuted her "diagnosis," even when testing eventually revealed cancer of the gall bladder, knowing the patient's beliefs helped greatly in managing her disease.

REMEMBER THE WHIM – *WHAT HAVE I MISSED?* – EXERCISE

When leaving a hotel room after an overnight stay, I always pause at the door and ask, "What am I leaving behind?" (Yes, in the past, I had forgotten to repack items, prompting an emergency visit to a department store.) When reaching a diagnostic conclusion, I always ask myself if I am missing something. This exercise helps me avoid overlooking the answer to a clinical puzzle or even the "must never miss" diagnosis (see above). Some questions that may help you consider all diagnostic possibilities include:

■ Have I done an appropriate clinical investigation including the pertinent medical history, physical examination, laboratory and diagnostic imagining?

   Have I helped the patient tell me the story in his or her own words? Is there a diagnostic maneuver I should have performed? Have I considered that what may not be apparent today may be found later as the disease evolves, and thus kept the door open for the patient to return if things progress?

■ Could there be an important fact that the patient is hesitant to tell me?

   The key to the diagnosis may lie in what has not yet been told. This may be something the patient is embarrassed to tell me or to have on his or her medical record. One key area for conveniently omitted, but often pertinent, facts is the sexual indiscretion. Some years ago, I read the narrative of a businessman who had a series of problems, which began with a rash and low-grade fever, and then over many months evolved to nausea, headache, impaired vision, and eventually some hints of early dementia. He went from physician to physician, and was evaluated for Lyme disease, multiple sclerosis, psychoneurosis, and other possibilities, all without a firm diagnosis. At this point, I will pause to see if you, valued reader and astute diagnostician, have thought of what might be the key to the case. One hint is to note a provocative clue I provided above. "The rest of the story," as radio commentator the late Paul Harvey was fond of saying, is as follows: This happily married family man was on a business trip to a large city in Nevada – the city where what happens there stays there, as the slogan goes. While there, and after consuming a few alcoholic beverages, he had his first and only homosexual encounter with a total stranger. He would, perhaps literally, die before disclosing his misadventure. Fortunately, the patient had not acquired the human immunodeficiency virus, but he had a contracted syphilis, which was progressing through its classically predictable stages. Eventually, one insightful physician – later in the sequence of clinicians seeing the patient – ordered a serologic test for syphilis, and the diagnosis was made.

■ Could the problem be due to a medication or herbal remedy the patient is taking that was prescribed by another practitioner?

Herbal remedies can cause panoply of adverse effects. For example, the National Center for Complementary and Alternative Medicine of the National Institutes of Health lists side effects for the widely-used St. John's wort: "The most common side effects include dry mouth, dizziness, diarrhea, nausea, increased sensitivity to sunlight, and fatigue."[40] And these are only the "common" side effects. Consider also that the patient may, purposely, not tell you about taking herbal remedies, thinking that you, as an allopathic physician, might be critical.

■ Might some real or presumed environmental factor be playing a role?

Possibilities include sensitivity to various allergens such as airborne pollens, reactions to chemicals at work or in the home, or possibly even the sometimes-controversial multiple chemical sensitivity (MCS) syndrome. Magill and Suruda describe MCS as "characterized by the patient's belief that his or her symptoms are caused by very low-level exposure to environmental chemicals." Cited causes include allergy, toxic effects, and neurobiological sensitization. The authors state, however, that, "There is insufficient evidence to confirm a relationship between any of these possible causes and symptoms."[41]

■ Is it possible that the illness is providing some secondary gain that the patient, consciously or unconsciously, is reluctant to give up?

This often occurs in settings involving medicolegal, psychiatric, and pregnancy issues. For example, a study in the Netherlands found that 42% of outpatients attending a psychiatric hospital appear to harbor expectations of secondary gain and that they hide this from their psychiatrists.[42] Harris and Campbell interviewed 128 women in North London, and found that women with unplanned pregnancies were likely to have potential secondary gain, more so than women whose pregnancies were planned or who were not pregnant.[43]

■ Has it been a while since I did a physical exam on the patient, and should I do so again now?

Diseases evolve over time. For this reason patients with chronic and eventually progressive diseases should be examined regularly. These diseases include heart failure, diabetes mellitus, and chronic lung disease, just to name a few. It is all too easy to have a series of repeat visits in which you interview the patient, check a blood pressure or laboratory test, and renew medications without performing an actual physical examination. By doing so, you may miss the bibasilar rales, the incipient bedsore, or the early peripheral neuropathy.

THE DOCTOR WHO MAKES THE CORRECT DIAGNOSIS IS THE ONE WHO SEES THE PATIENT LAST

If you are tempted to criticize another physician who previously examined a patient with an "obvious" breast mass, recall that at some time not too long ago, the breast mass was too small to detect.

The patient who helps me remember this axiom was a young woman who had seen two different physicians over the previous several years, telling them at various times about diverse symptoms including changing mood, fatigue, sporadic dysequilibrium, and occasional urinary urgency, but displaying no physical abnormalities on repeated examinations. Her vague and variable symptoms, coupled with a labile affect, led these physicians to make the reasonable diagnosis of an anxiety disorder manifested as physical symptoms. The consensus seemed to be that the patient was a somatosizer.

Eventually she found her way to my practice, and by that time she had nystagmus and a clearly unsteady gait. These findings prompted me to get magnetic resonance imaging of her brain, which confirmed the diagnosis of multiple sclerosis. Was I a more brilliant diagnostician than her prior physicians? No, not at all, I happened to be the one to see her when the symptoms and signs had evolved to the point that the diagnostic picture was clearer than in the past.

Criticizing the community physician who has "missed the diagnosis" is a popular sport among medical students and residents in teaching hospitals, who sometimes record disparaging chart notes about the failings of the "LMD" (local medical doctor).Young physicians, remember that you are not seeing the hundreds of patients in whom the LMD has made timely, astute, and occasionally life-saving diagnoses. You are looking at a "series of one," in which you are fortunate to have drawn a lucky position in the line of physicians examining the patient over time. The next patient you see may be the one who later turns out to have suffered a "missed diagnosis" of an evolving myocardial infarction or an early cancer of the colon. That's right: you missed detecting the disease at a very early stage. I hope that the doctors who follow you in treating the patient will speak charitably of your efforts.

THINK FIRST OF HORSES, NOT ZEBRAS

By now we have all heard the zebra aphorism. My best on-line Google-powered research leads me to the following putative origin: The saying is attributed to Theodore E. Woodward, MD (1914–2005), who taught at the University Of Maryland School of Medicine.[44] It seems that the original advice to students in the 1940s was, "Don't look for zebras on Green Street." Where is Green Street? Green Street in Baltimore is the address of the University of Maryland Hospital.

There is no shortage of zebra examples. When you encounter a patient with the recent onset of lower abdominal pain, you will think of constipation, irritable bowel syndrome, appendicitis, diverticulitis, and some other causes; Meckel's diverticulitis may not be high on your differential diagnosis list. In the patient complaining of generalized weakness, a number of other items will appear on your differential diagnosis list before you come to a zebra such as myasthenia gravis. A patient found to have an enlarged spleen may, indeed, have histiocytosis X, but don't bet on it.

DON'T FORGET TO THINK ABOUT ZEBRAS

Considering the rare diagnosis is a stimulating academic exercise, keeping your diagnostic skills sharp. In fact, occasionally one will appear. Knight and Senior estimate that 6–10% of persons in the population have a rare disease.[45] To dramatize the ubiquity of the supposedly rare, I will tell you a story about my family. My grandmother lived on a farm in Ohio until she died at age 84. One day, in the 1950s my uncle, a formidable man who was then a successful football and basketball coach, was visiting grandma on the farm. As it happened, the farmer "down the road" had butchered a pig, and brought some sausages to grandma. She cooked the sausages, although apparently not thoroughly. Grandma and my uncle ate the sausages, and gave the scraps to the cat. My uncle later developed a severe febrile disease with muscle pain and eventual delirium that baffled everyone. Eventually, the clue of eosinophilia on a differential blood count prompted a muscle biopsy that confirmed the zebra diagnosis – trichinosis.

Following a long convalescence, my uncle recovered and returned to coaching. Grandma felt under the weather for a few days after the meal. The cat died.

And so, don't miss the occasional zebra diagnosis. Pay attention to clues – such as eosinophilia in the febrile patient. The patient with a papular rash just might have lichen planus. A person who calls complaining of weakness in the legs could be describing the first stages of Guillain–Barré syndrome. And once or twice in your practice lifetime, you may encounter a patient with Münchhausen syndrome, maple syrup urine disease, Waardenburg syndrome, pseudo-hypoparathyroidism, or hemochromatosis.

WISE WORDS ABOUT THE ART OF CLINICAL DIAGNOSIS

▪ *Diagnosis is founded upon observance of trifles.* (Meador, rule #53)

> Small things – an unexplained increase in weight, a faint but newly heard murmur, color changes in finger nails – can be important clues.

▪ *For every mistake in medicine made by not knowing, there are ten mistakes made by not looking.* (Lindsay, page 7)

> As an attending physician in a resident teaching clinic, I find that I am often asked to consult on patients with skin rashes. After all, it is much easier to look at a rash than listen to a wordy, and generally unclear, description. When entering the exam room with the resident, all too often I find the patient fully clothed, and the resident has been taking a peekaboo look at the skin. My bold diagnostic maneuver – and teaching point – is to invite the patient to disrobe sufficiently that the rash can be fully viewed.

▪ *All that wheezes is not asthma.* Attributed to Chevalier Jackson (1865–1958), Temple University School of Medicine. (Strauss, page 13)

> For me, one such instance involved a child who had inhaled a peanut after tossing it in the air and catching it in his mouth. He was afraid that his mother would be angry, and so he kept silent about the cause of his

recent-onset breathing problem. The generalization of this aphorism is that we should not be too quick to accept the seemingly obvious diagnosis.

■ *In malignancy, the easier the diagnosis, the worse the prognosis.* (Reveno, page 118)

■ *A smart mother makes often a better diagnosis than a poor doctor.* German anesthesiologist August Bier (1861–1949) (Brallier, page 146)

Bier also once said: "Medical scientists are nice people, but you should not let them treat you!" (Strauss, page 530)

■ *The fact that your patient gets well does not prove that your diagnosis was correct.* Attributed to Samuel J. Meltzer (1851–1921) (Strauss, page 97)

Over the years, I have treated thousands of patients with antibiotics for diagnoses of acute bacterial sinusitis. Virtually all my sinusitis patients recovered sooner or later. Were the therapeutic successes the result of my shrewd diagnosis of bacterial cause and my aggressive treatment? Did they have sinusitis at all?

■ *Interesting how we always think in negatives in medical history taking and physical examination. No this, no that; never good this or good that. No wonder the World Health Organization defines health as the absence of disease.* American physician and educator Richard C. Reynolds. (Reynolds and Stone, page 269)

■ *Uncommon manifestations of common diseases are more common than common manifestations of uncommon diseases.* (Anon)

Or to put it another way, the most common diseases occur most commonly.

REFERENCES

1. Green LA, Fryer GE Jr, Yawn BP, Lanier D, Dovey SM. The ecology of medical care revisited. *N Engl J Med*. 2001;344: 2021-2025.

2. Most patients refer their physicians to greet them with a hand-shake and introduction. http://www.Medscape.com/viewarticle/ 558511/; 2007 Accessed 19.08.07.

3. Davis RL, Wiggins MN, Mercado CC, O'Sullivan PS. Defining the core competency of professionalism based on a patient's perception. *Clin Experiment Ophthalmol.* 2007;35(1):51-54.

4. Brenner P, Krause-Bergmann A, Van VH. Dupuytren contracture in North Germany: epidemiological study of 500 cases. *Unfallchirug.* 2001;104(4):303-311.

5. Spinner RJ, Poliakoff MB, Tiel RL. The origin of "Saturday night palsy. *Neurosurgery.* 2002;51(3):737-774.

6. Taylor RB, Burdette JA, Camp L, Edwards J. Purpose of the medical encounter: identification and influence on process and outcome in 200 encounters in a model family practice center. *J Fam Pract.* 1980;10(3):495-500.

7. Gray DW, Dixon JM, Collin J. The closed eyes sign: an aid to diagnosing nonspecific abdominal pain. *BMJ.* 1988;297:837-838.

8. Lesho EP. Can tuning forks replace bone scans for identification of tibial stress fractures? *Mil Med.* 1997;162(12):802-803.

9. Robertson GS, Ristic CD, Bullen BR. The incidence of congenitally absent foot pulses. *Ann R Coll Surg.* 1990;72(2):99-100.

10. Mangrulkar RS, Saint S, Chu S, Tierney LM Jr. What is the role of the medical pearl? *Am J Med.* 2002;113(7):1-14.

11. Behrman RE, Kliegman RM, Jenson HB, eds. *Nelson Textbook of Pediatrics.* 17th ed. Philadelphia: Saunders; 2003:1388-1389.

12. Marcus DA, Furman JM, Balaban CD. Motion sickness in migraine sufferers. *Expert Opin Pharmacother.* 2005;6(15): 2691-2697.

13. Marcus GM, Cohen J, Varosy PD, et al. The utility of gestures in patients with chest discomfort. *Am J Med.* 2007;120(1):83-89.

14. Goyle KK, Walling AD. Diagnosing pericarditis. *Am Fam Physician.* 2002;66(9):1695-1702.

15. Gonclaves M, Martins AP, Leal MJ. Acute appendicitis in children. *Acta Med Port.* 1993;6:377-382.

16. Suchowersky O, Reich S, Perlmutter J, Zesiewicz T, Gronseth G, Weiner WJ. Practice parameter: diagnosis and prognosis of new onset Parkinson disease, an evidence-based review. *Neurology.* 2006;66:968-975.

17. Evaluation of nonacute pathology in adult men. http://www. uptodateonline.com/online/content/topic.do?topicKey=primne ph/7784&linkTitle=VARICOCELE&source=preview&selected Title=3~11&anchor=4#4/; Accessed 31.03.09.

18. Nadeem A. *Alarm Bells in Medicine: Danger Symptoms in Medicine, Surgery and Clinical Specialties.* London: BMJ Books; 2005.

19. Chad DA. Lumbar spinal stenosis. *Neurol Clin* 2007;25:407-418.

20. Bottieu E, Clerinx J, Van den Ender E, et al. Fever after a stay in the tropics: diagnostic predictors of leading tropical conditions. *Medicine (Baltimore).* 2007;86(1):18-25.

21. Harding IJ, Davies E, Buchanan E, Fairbank JT. The symptom of night pain in a back pain triage clinic. *Spine.* 2005;30(17): 1985-1988.

22. Berlin R, Berlin H, Brante G, Pilbrant A. Vitamin B12 body stores during oral and parenteral treatment of pernicious anemia. *Acta Med Scand.* 1978;204(1-2):81-84.

23. Attard AR, Corlett MJ, Kidner NJ, Leslie AP, Fraser IA. Safety of early relief for acute abdominal pain. *BMJ.* 1992;305:554-556.

24. Diercks DB, Boghos E, Guzman H, et al. Changes in the numeric descriptive scale for pain after sublingual nitroglycerine do not predict cardiac etiology of chest pain. *Ann Emerg Med.* 2005;45:581-585.

25. Wrenn K, Slovis CM, Gongaware J. Using the "GI cocktail:" a descriptive study. *Ann Emerg Med.* 1995;26:687-690.

26. Riskin A, Tamir A, Klugelman A, Hemo M, Bader D. Is visual assessment of jaundice reliable as a screening tool to detect significant neonatal hyperbilirubinemia? *J Pediatr.* 2008;152:782-787.

27. Caracciolo JT, Murtagh RD, Rojiani AM, Murtagh FR. Pathognomonic MR image findings in Balo concentric sclerosis. *AJNR Am J Neuroradiol.* 2001;22:292-293.

28. Bennett DL, El-Khoury GY. General approach to lytic bone lesions. *Appl Radiol.* 2004;33(5):8-17.

29. Malane MS, Grant-Kels JM, Feder HM Jr, Luger SW. Diagnosis of Lyme disease based dermatologic manifestations. *Ann Intern Med.* 1991;114(6):490-498.

30. Stanek G, Strie F. Lyme borreliosis. *Lancet.* 2004;362(9396): 1639-1647.

31. Borelli S. Koenen, Kothe and the periungual fibroma in tuberous sclerosis. *Hautarzt.* 1999;50(5):368-369.

32. Jogai S, Radotra BD, Banerjee AK. Immunohistochemical study of human rabies. *Neuropathology.* 2000;20(3):197-203.

33. Montemarano A. Dermatomyositis. *Am Fam Physician.* 2001; 64:1565-1572.

34. Lamont MS, Alias NA, Win MN. Red flags in patients presenting with headache: clinical indications for neuroimaging. *Br J Radiol.* 2003;76(908):532-535.

35. Kinkade S. Evaluation and treatment of acute low back pain. *Am Fam Physician.* 2007;75(1181-1188):1190-1192.

36. Electrical burns. http://www.burnsurgery.org/Betaweb/Modules/initial/bsinitialsec9.htm/; Accessed 19.08.07.

37. Giese EA, O'Connor FG, Brennan FH Jr, Depenbrock PJ, Oriscello RG. The athletic preparticipation evaluation: cardiovascular assessment. *Am Fam Physician.* 2007;75:1008-1014.

38. Chao D. Spinal epidural abscess: a diagnostic challenge. *Am Fam Physician.* 2002;65:1341-1346.

39. Miss Maryland: Brittany Lietz skin cancer survivor wins. http://www.thecancerblog.com/2006/07/02/miss-maryland-brittany-lietz-skin-cancer-survivor-wins/; Accessed 19.08.07.

40. St. John's Wort [hypericum perforatum] and the treatment of depression. http://nccam.nih.gov/health/stjohnswort/sjwataglance.htm/; Accessed 18.08.07.

41. Magill MK, Suruda A. Multiple chemical sensitivity syndrome. *Am Fam Physician.* 1998;58:721-730.

42. Van Egmond J, Kummeling I, Balkom TA. Secondary gain as hidden motive for getting psychiatric treatment. *Eur Psychiatry.* 2005;20(5-6):416-421.

43. Harris K, Campbell E. The plans in unplanned pregnancy: secondary gain and the partnership. *Br J Med Psychol.* 1999; 72:105-120.

44. Who coined the aphorism? http://www.zebracards.com/a-intro_inventor.html/; Accessed 19.08.07.

45. Knight AW, Senior TP. The common problem of rare disease in general practice. *Med J Aust.* 2006;185:82-83.

5

Disease Management and Prevention

The Laws of Medicine
A. If what you are doing is working, keep doing it.
B. If what you are doing is not working, stop doing it.
C. If you don't know what to do, do nothing.

Modified from Ref.[1] (Matz)

RESPECT THE RULES OF SENSIBLE CLINICAL PRACTICE

I begin this chapter on disease management and prevention by reminding readers – venerated senior physicians and neophyte clinicians alike – that we all should strive to employ wise practice methods in the examination room and hospital. A seminal study in sensible clinical practice was conducted by Viennese obstetrician Ignaz Semmelweis (1818–1865), who observed that obstetrical patients attended by medical students had a higher incidence of "childbed fever" than patients of midwifery students. The difference seemed to be that medical students came directly from the autopsy room to the delivery room without washing their hands, while the midwifery students had no such autopsy exposure. Semmelweis first had the medical students and midwifery students exchange wards; the higher infection rate followed the medical students. Then, in 1847, he had both groups wash their hands with chlorinated water prior to deliveries, and the rates of infection plummeted in both wards. Semmelweis' elegant experiment set the stage for today's sensible practice rules.

Today, medical students participating in Objective Structured Clinical Examinations (OSCEs) are careful to begin by washing their hands. During their medical school and residency training years they are taught the other rules

R.B. Taylor, *Medical Wisdom and Doctoring: The Art of 21st Century Practice*, DOI 10.1007/978-1-4419-5521-0_5, © Springer Science+Business Media, LLC 2010

of safe clinical practice, including universal precautions and proper isolation technique. Wise clinicians respect these rules and would never, for example, resheath a needle or enter an isolation room without gown and mask. A physician's seniority does not invalidate the work of Semmelweis nor confer exemption from the traditions of good clinical practice.

BE A BEDSIDE DOCTOR, NOT A "FOOT OF THE BED" DOCTOR

This maxim arose when most clinical teaching was in hospital wards, the locus of what we used to call "bedside teaching," but it really applies in all clinical settings. I think I can tell something about a physician making hospital rounds, based on where he or she chooses to stand in relationship to a patient's bed. When offering therapeutic advice, try to avoid physical obstacles (such as the foot board of a bed or a consultation room desk) or even excessive space between patient and physician.

INVOLVE THE PATIENT IN TREATMENT DECISIONS: WHEN REASONABLE AND APPROPRIATE

Ask a young clinician today, and you are likely to hear, "Of course patients should be involved in medical decision-making." Yet, there must necessarily be degrees of involvement. For example, Say et al performed a meta-analysis of patient preferences for participation in medical decision making. The authors found that patients most keen on having a role in health care decisions tended to be younger, female, and better educated. They also found that preferences regarding their role in decision making were influenced by patients' diagnosis, health status, experience of illness, amount of information they had about their disease, and their relationships with their physicians.[2]

In another study of patients' desire for participation in medical decision making, Strull et al interviewed 210 hypertensive patients and their 50 clinicians. They found that doctors in the study tended to underestimate patients' desire for information about diagnosis and therapy, and to overestimate their desire to be therapeutic decision makers.[3]

Young physicians are especially likely to present patients with a laundry list of clinical options, seemingly hoping for relief from the obligation to provide what the patient actually seeks – a therapeutic recommendation. "Yes, sir, for your prostate cancer the possible treatments include surgery, external radiation, the implantation of radioactive seeds, hormone pills, castration and, I almost forgot, watchful waiting." As clinical practice advice: Be open to involving patients in decisions about their health care, but be aware that there is a wide spectrum of patient desire to be active in the process. The wise physician, after telling the therapeutic possibilities, is prepared for the wise patient's key question, "Doctor, if you were I, what would you do?"

CONSIDER BOTH PATIENT AND PHYSICIAN EXPECTATIONS OF THERAPY

For the physician treating a young patient with an ankle fracture, a favorable outcome will be solid healing in good anatomic alignment with no residual posttraumatic arthritis. For the teen-aged patient, on the other hand, therapeutic success might mean a return to playing basketball in three months. Of all specialists, plastic surgeons are probably the most attuned to the risk of dissonance between patient and physician expectations, especially when cosmetic procedures are involved, and most tend to spend abundant time seeking agreement with their patients as to what will constitute successful outcomes.

BECOME AN EVIDENCE-BASED HEALER: WITH CARE

There are many sources of evidence-based-medicine (EBM) reports and clinical guidelines: Cochrane Reviews, the United States Preventive Services Task Force, Bandolier, the National Guideline Clearinghouse and others. Many guidelines are based on carefully constructed clinical studies and meta-analyses; others are the product of less rigorous methods. Some clinical guidelines are promulgated by special groups with narrow interests, and upon reviewing their published recommendations, a skeptic might wonder if some are actually self-serving. One type of recommendation is derisively called a GOBSAT guideline – an acronym standing for "Good Old Boys Sat Around a Table." Woolf writes, "Practice guidelines, although important in promoting quality, can be harmful if they do not advocate the best options for patients. The latter can occur because of uncertainties in scientific evidence, biases in guideline development, and patient heterogeneity."[4]

As clinical guidelines proliferate, there seems to be growing concern about their utility and objectivity. A 2009 *Journal of the American Medical Association* (JAMA) editorial by Shaneyfelt and Centor offered the opinion: "Current use of the term *guideline* has strayed far from the original intent of the Institute of Medicine. Most current articles called "guidelines" are actually expert consensus reports."[5]

Also, keep in mind that almost all research trials and clinical guidelines focus on a single disease entity.

DO NOT ASSUME THAT THE PATIENT HAS JUST ONE DISEASE

Our clinical guidelines, medical history templates, our continuing education lectures by experts, and even our medical specialty system seem to be based on a single-disease premise. A surgeon is likely to call another specialist for help when a post-operative patient develops hypertension or chest pain. Disease management protocols should really be termed "single-disease" protocols.

When a patient has several diseases, we are dealing not only with the interrelationships of concurrent disorders such as diabetes, hyperlipidemia, depression, and heart failure, but with the side effects and interactions of medicines used to treat the various ailments. For example, might a migraineur for whom clinical guidelines recommend triptan therapy also possibly have coronary artery disease? If so, following guideline therapy of migraine might result in a heart attack.

Is there a person over the age of 60 who doesn't have at least five entries on his or her problem list? If you are tempted to answer "yes," to this question, I will counter that you have not thoroughly examined the patient or are simply ignoring disease outside your area of specialization. Some patients can have so many diseases that their problem lists resemble a page from the index to a medical textbook. In these persons, clinical guidelines discussing just one disease can be almost laughable.

THINK ABOUT CLINICAL OUTCOMES AND RESOURCE USE IN TERMS OF SYSTEMS

At this point, I am going to take you, the reader, on a short journey into the ethereal world of systems theory – an approach to understanding how one small change in a body tissue or a single therapeutic decision can, in fact, have wide-ranging effects.[6] According to this model, there is a hierarchy of natural systems that originates with subatomic particles as the smallest known entities, and progresses to the biosphere, the most expansive system of all. Here is a version of the hierarchy of natural systems:

Biosphere
Homo sapiens
Society and nations
Community
Family
Person – your patient
Body systems, such as the cardiovascular system
Organs, such as the heart
Tissues, such as the myocardium
Cells, such as myocardial fibers
Molecules
Atoms
Subatomic particles

Now that I have briefly described the concept of the hierarchy of natural systems, consider what happens when a blood clot blocks the artery serving the anterior wall of the heart of a 55-year-old man. There is death of some myocardial tissue, including all its component cells, molecules and so forth. Then, as we ascend the hierarchy, the heart and cardiovascular system may malfunction – or may withstand the ischemic insult. On a "person" level, the patient experiences chest pain and rushes to the emergency room. His family's lives are suddenly disrupted. Community resources are used to minimize the effects of the heart attack. This resource use, including physician and nursing services, medication, oxygen and all the rest, has small, but significant impacts on all the systems above. In short, any care rendered our patient will employ natural, financial, and human resources that will not be available for use in some alternative setting.

I present this theoretical digression to highlight the truth that no illness occurs in just one organ and no therapy occurs in isolation. Every therapeutic decision has implications at each level in the hierarchy of natural systems, and wise physicians give thought to these effects from time to time. Understanding the effect of disease in the hierarchy is the theoretical foundation of systems-based medicine – health care that thinks of systems both "above" and "below" the affected organ.[7]

ACKNOWLEDGE THAT TODAY'S FAVORED METHOD MAY BE TOMORROW'S CONTRAINDICATION, BLACK BOX WARNING, OR AMUSING ABSURDITY

To begin, today's putatively scientific medicine, traced to its origins, was born in dark prehistoric caves. The first medical "miracles cures" followed well-intentioned incantations of shamans; our first medicines were forest gleanings and early physician-priests practicing their magic may well have harmed more than they helped.

We no longer attribute healing powers to snakes and we have given up treating wounds with boiling oil. A few centuries later, we come to Doctor Benjamin Rush (1745–1813), a member of the Continental Congress, signer of the Declaration of Independence, professor of medicine at the University of Pennsylvania, and sometimes called the "Founding Father of American Medicine." Dr. Rush was a champion of heroic bleeding and purging, techniques which he used to treat victims of the 1793 yellow fever epidemic in Philadelphia. Even in his day, Rush's methods were questioned. Rush's critics included no less than American president Thomas Jefferson (1743–1826). In a letter to Dr. Thomas Cooper dated October 7, 1814, Jefferson wrote: "In his theory of bleeding and mercury, I was ever opposed to my friend Rush, whom I greatly loved; but who had done much harm, in the sincerest persuasion that he was preserving life and happiness to all around him." (Strauss, page 425) One episode of bleeding as therapy resulted in Rush being sued, a harbinger of the professional liability morass we see today. (Taylor, 2008, page 215)

In the early 1960s, doctors treating Eleanor Roosevelt for tuberculosis gave her corticosteroids, a practice that would not be considered state of the art in the twenty-first century. (Taylor, 2008, page 218) Also in the 1960s, after chlorpromazine (Thorazine) came into widespread use, physicians and public health officials decreed that we had found the key to managing schizophrenia, and tens of thousands of medicated psychotic individuals were discharged from mental hospitals to unsuspecting and unprepared communities. (Taylor, 2008, page 219)

We have seen the consequences of giving diethylstilbestrol and thalidomide to pregnant women. We treated acne patients with irradiation, only to discover later that some developed thyroid cancer. We have advised the use of Vitamin E for cardiovascular disease, even though we now believe that tocopherols may be associated with *increased* mortality.[8] We have injected embryonic neurons directly into the brains of patients with Parkinson disease and we have used nerve cryoablation for pain control after hernia repair, procedures eventually proved to be no better than placebo or sham surgery.[9] Fortunately, most of our patients recover from their ailments, either because of or in spite of what we do, and when recovery occurs, patients tend to be convinced that the doctor cured them. Nevertheless, let us not, in our sincerest persuasion that we are helping our patients, continue disease management and prevention approaches that have failed the EBM test and that, like lumbar sympathectomy to treat severe hypertension, have been assigned to the dusty attics of medical history. Here are a few such clinical methods:

■ Routine prescribing of amphetamine-based appetite suppressants. Once upon a time, stimulant drugs were readily prescribed for overweight patients, but no longer. Yet today, there is an increasing use of such drugs to treat attention deficit disorder, especially in adults.

■ Routine use of hormone replacement therapy (HRT) at menopause. Menopause was once considered a deficiency state easily and safely corrected with a pill a day. A series of studies published in and shortly following the year 2000 highlighted the breast cancer and other risks of HRT, resulting in a rapid decline in the use of estrogen and progesterone products by menopausal women.[10]

■ The annual "executive physical examination." Writing in the *New England Journal of Medicine*, Rank has stated, "The executive physical is a perfect example of what American medicine should be working to expunge: the expensive, the ineffective, and the inequitable."[11]

■ Withholding beta blockers in patients with heart failure. We now know that, in selected heart failure patients, the addition of a beta blocker to the regimen can be very beneficial.

■ Bed rest for patients with acute back strain. Standard therapy for the "acute back" was once hospitalization with bed rest in Buck's extension traction – 5 pound weights attached to each leg of the supine patient. We now know that maintaining continued activity, as permitted by symptoms, is better than lying in bed.

■ Use of theophylline preparations as first-line asthma therapy. We now have better drugs with more favorable risk profiles.

KNOW THE QUIRKY RISKS OF MEDICINES YOU USE IN PRACTICE

Today's physicians, and patients, all know that almost any drug can cause the usual spectrum of side effects – nausea, abdominal distress, diarrhea, headache, somnolence, and so forth. In addition, there are some medications that cause idiosyncratic, but well-known side effects. One example is the tendency of the tetracyclines to cause dental staining during tooth development. All physicians who prescribe for children or for potentially pregnant women are – or should be – aware of this risk. Another peculiar side effect is the tendency of amoxicillin to cause a rash when given to a person with infectious mononucleosis. Niacin can cause wide-spread flushing, which limits doses that can be prescribed, and metformin can cause lactic acidosis, a familiar fact even if few of us have ever seen a case.

But there is a cluster of diverse medications that cause uncommon, even rare, side effects. For example, dopamine agonists are standard therapy in Parkinson disease. These drugs are known to sometimes cause "increased libido," sparking visions of sexually stimulated octogenarians earnestly seeking partners. Such manifestations are not every-day occurrences, but are noteworthy when they occur.

The following are some unusual medication side effects. Some, but not all of them, are dose-related and may actually be signs of toxicity. If you prescribe these drugs, you should know about these uncommon, but entirely possible, manifestations and risks:

- Acetazolamide (Diamox). This carbonic anhydrase inhibitor, often prescribed to prevent altitude sickness, can cause tingling of the fingertips and also lead to a bad taste when ingesting carbonated beverages.[12] I take this drug from time to time when traveling to high altitude destinations, and have experienced both side effects described.
- Alpha-1 blockers. Patients taking these drugs, typically for benign prostatic hypertrophy, may experience a unique complication – intraoperative floppy iris syndrome – when undergoing cataract surgery. Tamsulosin (Flomax), the most commonly prescribed drug in this class, is also the one most likely to lead to IFIS.
- Others in this class – terazosin (Hytrin), doxazosin (Cardura), and alfuzosin (Uroxatral) – can have the same result. Stopping the drug before surgery will not reliably prevent IFIS.[13]
- Aspirin. When taken in high doses, aspirin can cause agitation and confusion.[14] These drug effects can present a worrisome clinical picture in the setting of a youngster with fever and malaise. I encountered just such a picture one morning when called to the home of a 14-year-old girl who had had a fever for 2 days, and whose mother had diligently treated the fever with two adult aspirin every 4–6 h. At the end of 2 days, the girl's fever was low,

but she – a slight young woman considering the dose of aspirin she had received – was hyperactive and acting inappropriately. Observation and cessation of aspirin use were all the treatment needed.

■ While on the topic of salicylate poisoning, aspirin ingestion is not the only possible cause. Oil of wintergreen, which is 98% methyl salicylate, is a key component of over-the-counter products such as *Bengay Cream*, widely used for muscle aches. In 2007, a Staten Island high school track star died after using large amounts of salicylate-containing muscle-ache creams.[15]

■ Beta-blockers. Commonly prescribed for a variety of cardio-vascular disorders, beta blockers can cause or aggravate existing psoriasis or cause a psoriaform rash.[16]

■ Bisphosphates. Drugs in this family, such as alendronate (Fosamax), commonly prescribed for osteoporosis, can cause osteonecrosis of the jaw.[17]

■ Carbamazepine (Tegretol). This drug, used to treat epilepsy and bipolar disorder, has been reported to induce a shift in pitch perception – a zebra side effect that would be most distressing to musicians.[18]

■ Clomipramine (Anafranil). Patients taking this tricyclic antidepressant medication have been reported to experience unusual yawning-associated side effects – significant in that the symptom may affect compliance.[19]

■ Cyclophosphamide (Cytoxan). This cancer chemothera-peutic agent can lead to peculiar-appearing pigmentation of the nails.[20]

■ Cyproheptadine (Periactin). Generally used for its antihis-tamine and anti-serotonin properties, this drug can cause weight gain, and has occasionally been prescribed for this purpose. In fact, the drug has been suggested as being "useful in youths with attention deficit hyperactivity dis-order for stimulant-induced weight loss, pending future randomized controlled trials."[21]

■ Digitalis, digoxin (Lanoxin). A traditional remedy for heart failure, digitalis can cause yellow vision (xanthopsia). This side effect has been postulated to explain the vivid yellow hues used in some of the paintings by Vincent van Gogh, who took the drug as the contemporary therapy for his epilepsy. (Taylor, 2008, page 171)

■ Hydroxychloroquine (Plaquenil). Sometimes prescribed for rheumatic disease, antimalarials can cause corneal deposits that are reversible and, more rarely, retinopathy with visual loss.[22] On the plus side, the drug can cause hypoglycemia, and in fact, its use in patients with rheumatoid arthritis has the happy benefit of reducing their risk of diabetes.[23]

■ Hypnosedative drugs. Because of their favorable risk profile, nonbenzodiazepine receptor agonists – including zolpidem (Ambien) and zaleplon (Sonata) – have become widely prescribed. These drugs, however, can cause some peculiar side effects, such as sleep cooking, sleep eating, sleep driving, and sleep sex.[24]

■ Ibuprofen (Advil). Widely used as an over-the-counter analgesic, ibuprofen can cause a variety of skin reactions, including a fixed drug eruption, exanthematous pustulosis, and pemphigoid.[25]

■ Lithium. We are all aware that, when prescribing lithium for bipolar disorder, the patient may mention a fine hand tremor, mild thirst, and polyuria. But are you aware that a causal relationship has been suggested between the drug and idiopathic intracranial hypertension, aka pseudotumor cerebri? Recognition of early manifestations such as headache, papilledema, and constriction of the visual fields might prompt discontinuation of the drug and allow avoidance of possible blindness due to optic nerve atrophy.[26]

■ Mefloquine (Lariam). Many of us have both prescribed this drug and taken it ourselves as malarial prophylaxis. Are we all aware that the drug can cause a self-limited psychosis characterized by the acute onset of visual and auditory hallucinations, even in persons with no prior history of psychiatric illness?[27]

■ Minocycline (Minocin). Are you aware that minocycline, sometimes prescribed for long-term use to treat acne, can cause dark staining of the crowns of permanent teeth in adults, just as tetracycline can cause tooth-staining in children?[28]

▦ Phenytoin (Dilantin). Physicians are well aware that Dilantin often causes gum hyperplasia, a side effect that can be especially distressing to young persons with epilepsy. Less well known is the risk that when injected intravenously, the drug can cause purple glove syndrome, a rare complication manifested as pain, swelling, and discoloration of the hand distal to the injection site, a condition that may require surgery.[29]

▦ Phosphodiesterase type 5 inhibitors. This family of drugs, widely prescribed for erectile dysfunction, includes sildenafil (Viagra), tadalafil (Cialis), and vardenafil (Levitra). As a class, they have been reported to cause sensorineural hearing loss, prompting a 2007 warning by the US Food and Drug Administration (FDA).[30]

▦ Pramipexole (Mirapex). A dopaminergic agent used to treat Parkinson disease, this agent is currently being marketed as a remedy for restless leg syndrome. Pramipexole has an idiosyncratic side effect – pathologic gambling – and in July, 2007, a consumer-targeted television advertisement for the drug warned users about the risk of an urge to gamble.[31]

▦ Proton-pump inhibitors. These commonly prescribed drugs, when started within the past 30 days, may increase the risk of community acquired pneumonia.[32]

▦ Quinolones. The cartilage-damaging effect of quinolones on juvenile experimental animals has been known for almost two decades.[33] But are you aware that quinolone antibiotics such as levofloxacin (Levaquin) can cause tendinitis, sometimes leading to Achilles tendon rupture in adults? The complication is rare, but it happens, and was added as a "black box warning" in July, 2008. This is a risk you should know, and should consider sharing with your patients if you prescribe the drug, particularly elderly individuals or persons taking steroids.

▦ Rifampin (Rifadin). Used to treat tuberculosis and as prophylaxis for meningococcal meningitis, rifampin can cause a red-orange discoloration of the sweat, urine, and tears (and can stain contact lenses), which could alarm a patient who has not been alerted to the side effect.[34]

- Spironolactone (Aldactone). A diuretic useful in treating severe heart failure, spironolactone can cause gynecomastia, owing to alterations in the peripheral metabolism of testosterone.[35]
- Topiramate (Topamax). This antiepileptic drug, also a currently a popular migraine remedy, can cause hypohidrosis manifested as dry skin and even intermittent hyperthermia.[36]
- Trazodone (Desyrel). Occasionally male patients taking this drug for treatment of depression have experienced prolonged erections, even priapism.[37] Recently, I presented my collection of "uncommon side effects of commonly used drugs" at a continuing medical education meeting. Following the lecture, one of the attendees shared with me that she worked at a community psychiatric and drug abuse clinic, and that some of her male patients refer to the drug as "traz-erect."
- Varenicline (Chantrix). Widely use for smoking cessation, this drug can cause syncope and psychiatric side effects.[38] In the fourth quarter of 2007, the drug accounted for more reported serious injuries than any other prescription drug, prompting a February, 2008 FDA Public Health Alert about varenicline-induced psychiatric side effects.[39] Going further, in May 2008, the Institute for Safe Medication Practices published a Strong Safety Signal that read, "We have immediate safety concerns about the use of varenicline among persons operating aircraft, trains, buses, and other vehicles or in other settings where a lapse in alertness or motor control could lead to massive, serious injury. Other examples include persons operating nuclear power reactors, high-rise construction cranes or life-sustaining medical devices. Based on reports of sudden loss of consciousness, seizures, muscle spasms, vision disturbances, hallucinations, paranoia, and psychosis, we believe varenicline may not be safe to use in these settings. The extent to which varenicline has already contributed to accidental death and injury has not yet been investigated because these adverse effects had not been previously reported. The Federal Aviation Administration approved varenicline for use by airline pilots before most of these reports were available."[40]

KEEP UP TO DATE WITH POTENTIALLY DANGEROUS INTERACTIONS WHEN YOUR PATIENT IS TAKING BOTH YOUR PRESCRIBED MEDICATION AND HERBAL PREPARATIONS

Complementary and alternative medicine (CAM) is becoming part of mainstream medical practice, and many of our patients are taking dietary supplements, whether prescribed by you, recommended by a CAM practitioner, or bought over the counter by the patient, who may be following advice found in a magazine available at the grocery checkout counter. Nevertheless, herbal products have pharmacologic effects, side effects, and potential interactions with prescribed drugs.

The key to drug-herbal interactions is that patients often don't tell their physicians about their dietary supplement use. Perhaps the patient does not consider what he is taking to be "medication;" maybe he or she is embarrassed to tell the physician about taking something acquired outside the realm of allopathic medicine. Thus, you may wonder why your patient taking warfarin has an unexplained rise in the individualized normalized ratio (INR) level or why a patient taking a statin drug has begun to exhibit increased serum cholesterol levels. The answer to these and other clinical puzzles may lie in concomitant, but undisclosed, dietary supplement use. For example, problem bleeding in a patient taking warfarin may occur if the patient is also taking St. John's wort, fish oil, or cranberry juice. St. John's wort may lead to decreased levels of both digoxin and statin drugs, and the combination of ginseng and monoamine oxidase inhibitors can result in manic-like symptoms.[41] These few examples are provided to highlight the growing problem of herbal remedy related drug interactions, and the need for thoughtful questioning and constant vigilance.

CONSIDER THE PATIENT'S HEALTH LITERACY LEVEL

Health literacy refers to the patient's ability to comprehend printed handouts, instructions on prescription labels, and all the other written material presented to patients in the course of receiving health care. Some patients have dyslexia, some read English at a third grade level, some can read only some language other than English, and some cannot read at all.

Increasingly, health literacy has come to be regarded as a safety issue, especially when patients cannot decipher prescription warning labels, instructions on prescription bottles, or directions describing preparations for procedures. To assess health literacy levels, Davis et al interviewed 395 English-speaking patients, described as "mostly indigent populations," in waiting rooms in primary care clinics in three different states. Interviewees were asked their understanding of instructions printed on five container labels. Of those interviewed, 67.1–91.1% of patients had a correct understanding of the five labels. Patients with low health literacy were at the greatest safety risk. While 70.7% of these patients could correctly state the instructions "Take two tablets by mouth twice daily" only 34.7% were able to state how many pills were to be taken each day.[42]

THE UNFILLED PRESCRIPTION NEVER HAS A CHANCE TO HELP THE PATIENT

Are you shocked to learn that many of your prescriptions go unfilled? Unhappily, such is the case today. As I write this paragraph in 2009, America is in the throes of an economic crisis. Unemployment and underemployment are rampant. Today, the unimaginable is happening, with large national retail chains closing stores across the country, throwing thousands out of work. Computer giant Microsoft Corporation has announced plans to lay off thousands of employees. These newly unemployed persons have lost more than a paycheck; they have lost health care coverage for themselves and for family members. They have joined the army of Americans who have no health insurance or who have "discontinuous coverage" (covered only part of a year).

Lacking health insurance is a significant health risk factor, often involving a choice between buying food and needed medication. Olson et al reviewed a sample of 26,955 children age 17 and younger from the 2000 and 2001 National Health Interview Surveys. They found that of those children who had discontinuous health coverage, 9.9% of prescriptions were unfilled, and the number rose slightly to 10.0% for those who were uninsured for a full year. In the study, the authors also found that those insured only part of the year had 20.2% delayed care, and 13.4% reported unmet care, while those uninsured for a full year suffered 15.9% delayed care and 12.6% unmet care. (sic)[43]

THE FOUR CHARACTERISTICS OF THE IDEAL MEDICATION ARE: OLD, SAFE, CHEAP AND EFFECTIVE

Before investing the patient's hard-earned money in the latest wonder drug or expensive "gorillacillin," consider the following quote from the Rappaport and Wright 1952 book: *Great Adventures in Medicine* (page 23):

> The true physician uses everything ever found useful. And this leads me today to emphasize again the fact that a scientific physician today uses gladly any drug and any method of healing that he can hear of that was ever found really useful by anyone anywhere. Just let us go into a drug store and glance over the shelves. There we will find castor oil, senna, ox gall, aloe, and opium which were used in ancient Egypt; another purgative, magnesia, came originally from an ancient city of that name in Greece; jalap comes from Mexico, and cascara from California; the aspirin which is so popular today is first cousin to the smelly oil of wintergreen which our grandmothers used to put on flannel and tie around aching joints, and quinine and cocaine and ipecac come from South America."

One of the virtues of the older medications is that, by now, we are well acquainted with their risks. When prescribing a senna-based laxative or opiate derivative, we won't find later that there is some newly discovered side effect, such as the Achilles tendinitis and possible rupture we have found with the quinolones. (See above) Furthermore, most of the old, safe drugs are also long past patent protection, and thus tend to be inexpensive relative to the more recently developed pharmaceuticals. Of course, what matters most is efficacy, and the most expensive drug of all is the one that doesn't work.

Physicians and pharmacists can influence perceived effectiveness of medication. When you or I write a prescription, we must recognize the persuasive power of the act of prescribing. Handing the prescription to a patient represents the physician's unspoken message, "This is going to help you get well!" There is thus, in every prescription, a powerful placebo effect, which should never be underestimated. Take for instance, the problem of benign prostatic hyperplasia (BPH), a clearly anatomic abnormality, yet one which can cause annoying symptoms, including a decrease in the maximum urinary flow rate (Qmax). Nickel looked at 303 patients in the placebo arm of a placebo-controlled trial of the efficacy of finasteride therapy of BPH. The author concluded that placebo therapy produced a "significant improvement in Qmax and symptoms of BPH, but also causes clinically important adverse effects." The placebo group reported enhanced maximum urinary flow, a measurable entity. And, just to highlight the power of the placebo, 81.2% of patients receiving placebo therapy reported adverse events, including 6.3% who experienced impotence.[44]

One of my favorite aphorisms is: Nature, time, and patience are the best healers. (Anon) Given that most non-chronic illnesses improve eventually, that the cost of newer medications seems to have no ceiling, and that a great deal of our successful therapy (and some adverse effects, as well) can be ascribed to the power of the placebo, why not look first for a drug that is old, safe, cheap, and effective?

BEWARE THE MINEFIELD OF POLYPHARMACY

It is sad, but true, that the quickest way to end an encounter is to hand the patient a prescription. But this is often – perhaps usually – not the best thing to do. In Chap. 4, I discussed consideration of the "true purpose of the encounter." That is, often the patient seeks reassurance and the meaning of the symptom, and does not especially want or need "treatment." For example, the patient with a hip pain for a few months may fear that the cause is cancer, just as his uncle's bone cancer began with just that symptom a few years ago; this patient, once reassured by an examination and probably by appropriate imaging, is content to manage the pain with behavioral change, hot baths, and occasional use of ibuprofen.

Nevertheless, we physicians are trained from our first clinical encounter to take action, to identify the problem, and to have a plan to fix it. When faced with a patient with chest pain, fever, or abdominal distress, we are all too ready to do something. We develop *furor therapeuticus*, and begin searching for the ideal remedy for today's complaint. Yet too often, today's remedy becomes just one more entry on the patient's already-long medication list.

In a study of polypharmacy in older persons, Steinman et al looked at 196 patients age 65 and older taking five or more medications – not counting vitamins, minerals, herbal dietary supplements, and topical medications. These patients took an astounding average of 8.1 medications, with a range of 5–17 drugs. The authors found that 65% of these patients were using one or more inappropriate medications, and 57% were taking a medication that was not indicated, ineffective or duplicative. Interestingly, underuse was also common, and 42% of patients had both inappropriate use and underuse simultaneously.[45]

From the Steinman et al study, it appears that polypharmacy may have caused more mischief than benefit for many patients. Any patient who is taking five or more drugs lives in a pharmacologic Wild West, outside the boundaries of clinical science. When the time comes for a bold change in your approach to a patient's illness, the wisest course may actually be to discontinue a number of drugs on the medication list.

ACKNOWLEDGE THE LIMITATIONS OF MEDICATIONS

"He's the best physician that knows the worthlessness of most medicines," quipped American statesman Benjamin Franklin (1706–1790). (Quoted in Brallier, page 259) I tell headache patients that no analgesic will totally take away the pain of a migraine attack, and that all so-called painkillers carry some risk. In the case of headache, the risk is not only overdose or dependency, but also the risk of transforming episodic migraine to a chronic daily headache pattern.

Antispasmodic drugs don't stop all intestinal spasm; muscle relaxants really don't relax muscles very well; and vasodilators often fail to meet expectations. In truth, most of our medications work better when combined with the so-called lifestyle changes – diet, exercise, stress avoidance, and elimination of harmful habits such as alcohol overuse and tobacco in any form. In 1923, Lindsay wrote, "The treatment of high blood pressure is a regimen, not a drug." (Lindsay, page 86). The author wrote, of course, long before we had even a single drug effective against high blood pressure. Yet today, with the long list of allegedly potent, and potentially toxic, antihypertensive medications, we have no uniformly effective drug for high blood pressure. All the medications in our arsenal for hypertension and most other diseases have their limitations, and the best therapy today for many medical problems continues to be a regimen, not just a drug.

OFTEN THE DOCTOR IS THE "DRUG"

There is one "drug" that seems to have enduring effectiveness, and that is the person of the doctor. The concept of "the doctor as the drug" was first proposed in England by Doctor Michael Balint in his 1957 book, *The Doctor, His Patient, and the Illness* (New York: International Universities Press). Discussing what he calls the most frequently used drug in general practice – the doctor – Balint writes: "In spite of our almost pathetic lack of knowledge about the dynamics and possible consequences of 'reassurance' and 'advice,' these two are perhaps the most frequent forms of medical treatment. In other words, they are the most frequent form in which the drug 'doctor' is administered." (Balint, page 116)

The drug "doctor" is, of course, most likely to be effective in the context of a trusting relationship, and that generally involves an ongoing doctor–patient interaction. In a study of the personal doctor–patient relationship in general practice, Kearley et al concluded that the personal doctor–patient relationship was most valuable for more serious or for psychosocial problems.[46] In the realm of more serious problems, over the years, one patient after another has told me how the presence of the personal physician at the bedside of a patient undergoing surgery or suffering a heart attack can have a powerful therapeutic benefit. This is true even if the family doctor is not the attending surgeon or cardiologist. The value of the drug "doctor" and its connotation of a close bond between patient and physician, established over time, seems strong testimony to the importance of continuity in the doctor–patient relationship.

SOMETIMES CONSULTATION CAN AN IMPORTANT PART OF THERAPY

Whether you are a rural generalist physician or a big-city, academic medical center-based subspecialist, sometimes your best efforts and mine just don't seem to succeed. Diagnostic signs are confusing; the patient fails to respond to therapy; things go from bad to worse. When these events occur, it's time to consider the merits of consultation with a colleague.

Let me tell you a story about seeking consultation. When I was a medical student, on a clinical rotation at Philadelphia General Hospital, our team came across a patient where one thing after another had gone wrong. Today, house officers would call the case a "train wreck." In addition to multiple organ system failure, the patient's physical findings and laboratory results seemed only to obfuscate the diagnostic picture. In the midst of the confusion, some desperate resident had requested a consultation. In the blank where one should record "reason for consultation," there was a single word: "Help!" The best part of the story is that someone answered that consultation request.

Over the past decades, our most valuable medical instrument has been the telephone. Today, with email consultation and on-line reference sources, some would argue that the computer is now even more indispensible than the telephone. The Blackberry, iPhone and similar instruments seem to bring together the best of both instruments.

Physician willingness to seek consultation can be conceptualized as a bell-shaped curve. On one extreme is the physician whose extreme self-confidence can be just a little worrisome, and who views any consultation as an affront to his personal medical knowledge and skill. At the other end of the curve is the "traffic cop" physician, intellectually lazy and all too ready to seek specialty care for all but the most mundane illnesses. In between is the wise, but humble physician who recognizes when things aren't just going right, and seeks timely consultation, sometimes even when the referring physician suspects he or she knows the answer. (Manning and DeBakey, page 218)

Balint writes extensively about consultation and the relationships between the patient, the personal physician, and the consultant. One important point he makes is that the act of consultation should never blur the issue of who is responsible for the patient's care. A consultation is a request for recommendation; it is not a transfer of care, the latter properly called a referral. Yet sometimes, the personal physician and involved consultants become party to what Balint calls the "collusion of anonymity," a state in which, with many physicians and other providers making decisions and offering advice to patient and family, no one is really in charge. Balint holds that the *collusion of anonymity*, which he describes as a dilution of responsibility, dominates the field in medicine today. (Balint, page 93) Such a confusing diffusion of responsibility must be frustrating indeed for the heart attack, stroke or trauma patient and the patient's family.

Here is another thought regarding consultation. The personal physician must avoid excessive reliance on the consultant's advice. As a wise physician, you should thoughtfully consider the consultant's recommendations, and then use your own best judgment in planning the patient's care. One reason to view consultant recommendations with slight caution is summed up in the old saw: If your only tool is a hammer, then everything you see looks like a nail. When consulting with specialist colleagues, accept that what is recommended will be influenced by which specialist is consulted. If you send a back pain patient to a surgeon for a consultation, don't be surprised if the recommendation is for surgery.

All cautions considered, sometimes consultation is just what is needed. In the Kenny Rogers song, the gambler needs to know when to hold 'em, know when to fold 'em, know when to walk away, and know when to run.

To paraphrase for physicians: Know when to talk, know when to listen, know when to act, and know when to consult.

THINK PREVENTION AS WELL AS CURE

In his address to the Fraternal Association of Former Students of the *École Centrale des Arts et Manufactures* in Paris, May 15, 1884, French scientist Louis Pasteur (1822–1895) observed: "When meditating over a disease, I never think of finding a remedy for it, but, instead, a means of preventing it." (Strauss, page 451) In the long run, prevention is cheaper than cure, and Pasteur, an industrial chemist who discovered that partial heat-sterilization could prevent spoilage of beer and wine, was a strong advocate of cost-effective anticipatory interventions.

Today as the cost of disease treatment escalates each year, owing in part to increasingly expensive advances in therapy, many of our disease prevention strategies remain quite reasonably priced. Immunizations, whose prices are inflated by the absorbed costs of a tort liability system out of control, are still a bargain when compared to the expense of treating tetanus, diphtheria, hepatitis A and B, and herpes zoster.

Much less expensive are lifestyle changes – proper diet, tobacco avoidance, regular exercise, weight control, and moderation in alcohol use. In 1973, Belloc published a report of a 5½-year study of the health habits of 6,928 adults living in Alameda County, California.[47] Seven health habits showed a remarkable influence on longevity. A 45-year-old man who practiced three or less of the health habits had an expected life expectancy of 22 years; if he practiced five of the health habits, his anticipated longevity increased to 28 years; and if he engaged in six or seven of the health habits, he could expect to live another 33 years. Here are the seven health habits that can profoundly affect longevity:

1. Sleeping 7–8 h per night
2. Eating breakfast daily
3. Not eating between meals

4. Maintaining weight at a reasonable level
5. Exercising regularly
6. Using alcohol moderately or not at all
7. Never smoking cigarettes

As far as health habits are concerned, not too much has changed since 1973. Sensible health habits are still, by far, the most cost effective way to avoid morbidity and mortality. Whatever the presenting clinical problem, no wise physician discharges a patient without some consideration of lifestyle intervention, immunizations, and other aspects of disease prevention.

INFORM EVERY PATIENT OF WHAT TO DO IF THINGS GO WRONG

Murphy's laws often prevail, and things can go wrong. The infecting organism may resist the prescribed antibiotic, a surgical wound may pop some sutures, or a drug reaction can occur. We should especially warn the patient if the disease or the drug prescribed can have an unusual, but serious manifestation, for example if the patient with a cardiac arrhythmia begins to notice chest pain, or child with fever develops a stiff neck, or if the drug prescribed has one of the quirky side effects described above. A word of advice, carefully documented, is all it takes.

NEVER END A CLINICAL ENCOUNTER WITHOUT ADVISING THE PATIENT WHEN TO RETURN

The return appointment may be in a week, a month, even a year. You may contract to send a reminder card when it is time for the next visit. Or the patient may be counseled to call or return if not well in 10 days, if things get worse, or if something unexplained happens. Then, document in the record both the "what to do if things go wrong" and the "next appointment" advice. Careful anticipatory guidance, well documented, keeps the patient informed and, just occasionally, may head off a costly liability claim.

WISE WORDS ABOUT DISEASE MANAGEMENT AND PREVENTION

▨ *In prognosis, the patient being considered is not the average patient from whom statistics have been compiled.* (Reveno, page 105)

Every patient is different from the last in so many ways, including their respective genetic inheritances, life experiences, problem lists, medications in the drawer at home, and ability to tolerate discomfort and inconvenience.

▨ *Nickel-in-the-slot, press the button therapeutics are no good. You cannot have a drug for every malady.* Sir William Osler (1849–1919). (Bean and Bean, page 102)

Sir William had a gift for expressing axioms as metaphors.

▨ *The regular physician cures many a hysterical patient with a combination of pills, impressive apparatus, suggestion, and personal magnetism.* (Rapport and White, page 23)

By regular physician, I assume that the authors refer to the generalist, and that would be me. Yes, we generalists have a secret weapon in our clinical arsenal – the power of our personal therapeutic relationship with the patient – whether actualized as medication, a procedure or encouraging reassurance.

▨ *To write prescriptions is easy, but to come to an understanding with people is hard.* From the short story *A Country Doctor*, by Franz Kafka (1883–1924) (Quoted in Reynolds and Stone, page 95)

Unfortunately for busy clinicians, the coming to an understanding option takes more time than prescribing a pill. But doing so, however, is almost always better doctoring.

▨ *Every drug we prescribe is an experiment in applied pharmacology. (Anon.)*

Any medication prescribed can yield a desired therapeutic effect, an adverse reaction, both or neither. For example, if I take pseudoephedrine for a common cold, the drug's action clears my nose, but the side effect is a dry mouth making it difficult to swallow or even talk. This is an instance of "both" – a desired action, but a side effect limiting the usefulness of the drug.

■ *It is the patient rather than the case which requires treatment.* American surgeon and author Robert Tuttle Morris (1857–1938). (Quoted in Strauss, page 635)

■ *It usually requires a considerable time to determine with certainty the virtues of a new method of treatment and usually still longer to ascertain the harmful effects.* American surgeon Alfred Blalock (1899–1964). (Quoted in Strauss, page 637)

Best known for his innovations in pediatric cardiac surgery (Think of the Blalock-Taussig shunt for cyanotic heart defects), Blalock has provided us with a wise comment that is relevant to both novel surgical procedures and newly introduced medical therapy.

■ *Training programs can teach physicians to be their own instrument if they understand the task and its importance.* American physician and author Eric Cassell (Cassell, page 110)

Back in the days of pioneering American dancer and choreographer Martha Graham (1894–1991), I had a friend who was a modern dancer. My friend was fond of asserting, "My body is my instrument." She, of course, was using a dancer's performance metaphor, but the analogy is apt for physicians, whose clinical knowledge, skills and doctorly presence together is their most effective instrument – and not their scalpel, endoscope, or imaging device.

■ *In the ideal clinical encounter, the placebo effect begins when the patient enters the room.* Modified from American physician and ethicist Howard Brody.[48]

■ *It is best to use superior judgment – to avoid having to use superior skill.* (Anon.)

Carpenters live by the adage: "Measure twice, and cut once." This sort of carefully planned action minimizes the need for damage control, never a happy outcome in carpentry or in medicine.

REFERENCES

1. Matz R. Get ahead in medicine? Follow these simple rules. *Medical Econ*. 1978;16(9):119–123.
2. Say R, Murtagh M, Thomson R. Patients' preference for involvement in medical decision making: a narrative review. *Pat Educ Couns*. 2006;60(2):1020–1024.
3. Strull WM, Lo B, Charles G. Do patients want to participate in medical decision making? *JAMA*. 1984;252(21):2990–2994.
4. Wolff SH. Do clinical practice guidelines define good medical care? *Chest*. 1998;113:166S–171S.
5. Shaneyflet TM, Centor RM. Reassessment of clinical practice guidelines: go gently into that good night. *JAMA*. 2009;301(8):868–869.
6. Laszlo E. *The systems view of the world*. New York: Braziller; 1972.
7. Taylor RB. Family: a systems approach. *Am Fam Phys*. 1979;20(5):101–104.
8. Tatsioni A, Bonitsis NG, Ioannidis JP. Persistence of contradicted claims in the literature. *JAMA*. 2007;298(21):2517–2526.
9. Flum DR. Interpreting surgical trials with subjective outcomes: avoiding UnSPORTsmanlike conduct. *JAMA*. 2006;296:2483–2485.
10. Writing group for the Women's Health Initiative Investigators. Risks and benefits of estrogen plus progestin in healthy postmenopausal women. Principal results from the women's health initiative randomized control trial. *JAMA*. 2002;228:321–333.
11. Rank B. Executive physicals – bad medicine on three counts. *N Engl J Med*. 2008;359(14):1424–1425.
12. Burki NK, Khan SA, Hameed MA. The effects of acetazolamide on the ventilatory response to high altitude hypoxia. *Chest*. 1992;101(3):736–741.
13. Chang DF, Osher RH, Wang L, Koch DD. Prospective multicenter evaluation of cataract surgery in patients taking tamsulosin (Flomax). *Ophthalmology*. 2007;114(5):957–964.
14. Aspirin: Drug Information. http://www.uptodateonline.com. Accessed 4.12.2008.
15. Teen killed by muscle cream. New York Post. http://www.nypost.com/seven/06092007/news/regionalnews/killed_by_muscle_cream_regionalnews_austin_fenner.htm/ Accessed 2.9.2009.
16. Yilmaz MB, Turhan H, Akin Y, Kisacik HL, Korkmaz S. Beta-blocker-induced psoriasis: a rare side-effect. *Angiology*. 2002;53(6):737–739.
17. Gutta R, Louis PJ. Bisphosphonates and osteonecrosis of the jaws: science and rationale. *Oral Surg Oral Med Oral Pathol Oral Radiol Endod*. 2007;104(2):186–193.

18. Kobayashi T, Nisijima K, Ehara Y, Otsuka K, Kato S. Pitch perception shift: a rare side effect of carbamazepine. *Psych Clin Neurosci.* 2001;55(4):415–417.

19. McLean JD, Forsythe RG, Kapkin IA. Unusual side effects of clomipramine associated with yawning. *Can J Psychiatry.* 1983;28(7):569–570.

20. Dave S, Thappa DM. Peculiar pattern of nail pigmentation following cyclophosphamide therapy. *Dermatol Online J.* 2003;9(3):14.

21. Daviss WB, Scott J. A chart review of cyproheptadine for stimulant-induced weight loss. *J Child Adolesc Psychopharmacol.* 2004;14(1):65–73.

22. Rynes RI, Bernstein HN. Ophthalmologic safety profile of antimalarial drugs. *Lupus.* 1993;2(Suppl 1):S17–19.

23. Wasko MC, Hubert HB, Lingala VB, et al. Hydroxychloroquine and risk of diabetes in patients with rheumatoid arthritis. *JAMA.* 2007;298(2):187–193.

24. Dolder CR, Nelson MH. Hypnosedative-induced complex behaviors: incidence, mechanisms and management. *CNS Drugs.* 2008;22(12):1021–36.

25. Sanchez-Borges M, Capriles-Hulett A, Caballero-Fonseca R. Risk of skin reactions when using ibuprofen-based medicines. *Expert Opin Drug Saf.* 2005;4(5):837–848.

26. Levine SH, Puchalski C. Pseudotumor cerebri associated with lithium therapy in two patients. *J Clin Psych.* 1991;52(5):239–242.

27. Sowunmi A, Adio RA, Oduola AM, Ogundahunsi OA, Salako LA. Acute psychosis after mefloquine. Report of six cases. *Trop Geogr Med.* 1995;47(4):179–80.

28. McKenna BE, Lamey PJ, Kennedy JG, Bateson J. Minocycline-induced staining of the adult permanent dentition: a review of the literature and report of a case. *Dent Update.* 1999;26(4):160–162.

29. Chokshi R, Openshaw J, Mehta NN, Mohler E. Purple glove syndrome following intravenous phenytoin administration. *Vasc Med.* 2007;12(1):29–31.

30. Mukherjee B, Shivakumar T. A case of sensorineural deafness following ingestion of sildenafil. *J Laryngol Otol.* 2007;121(4):395–397.

31. Spengos K, Grips E, Karachalios G, Tsivgoulis G, Papadimitrous G. Reversible pathologic gambling under treatment with pramipexole. (Article in German). *Nervenarzt.* 2006;77(8):958–960.

32. Sarkar M, Hennessy S, Yang Y-X. Proton-pump inhibitor use and the risk for community-acquired pneumonia. *Ann Int Med.* 2008;149(6):391–398.

33. Stahlmann R. Cartilage-damaging effect of quinolones. *Infection.* 1991;19(Suppl 1):S38–46.

34. Rifampin. In: Lexi-Comp. http://www.uptodateonline.com/utd/content/topic.do?topicKey=drug/ Accessed 14.03.2009.

35. Rose LI, Underwood RH, Newmark SR, Kisch ES, Williams GH. Pathophysiology of spironolactone-induced gynecomastia. *Ann Intern Med.* 1977;87(4):398–403.

36. Cerminara C, Seri S, Bombardieri R, Pinci M, Curatolo P. Hypohidrosis during topiramate. *Pediatr Neurol.* 2006;34(5): 392–394.

37. Carson CC III, Mino RD. Priapism associated with trazodone therapy. *J Urol.* 1989;142(3):831–833.

38. Pumariega AJ, Nelson R, Rotenberg L. Varenicline-induced mixed mood and psychotic episode in a patient with a past history of depression. *CNS Spectr.* 2008;13(6):511–514.

39. Pharmacology Watch. December, 2008, page 2.

40. Moore TJ, Cohen MR, Furberg CD. Strong safety signal seen for new varenicline risks. The Institute for Safe Medication Practices. http://www.ismp.org/docs/vareniclineStudy.asp/; Published 21.03.2008

41. Gardiner P, Phillips R, Shaughnessy AF. Herbal and dietary supplement-drug interactions in patients with chronic illness. *Am Fam Phys.* 2008;77(1):73–78.

42. Davis TC, Wolf MS, Bass PF III, et al. Literacy and misunderstanding prescription drug labels. *Ann Int Med.* 2006;145(12): 887–194.

43. Olson LM, Tang SF, Newacheck PW. Children in the United States with discontinuous health insurance coverage. *N Engl J Med.* 2005;353(4):418–419.

44. Nickel JC. Placebo therapy of benign prostatic hyperplasia: a 25-month study. Canadian PROSPECT Study Group. *Br J Urol.* 1998;81(3):383–387.

45. Steinman MA, Landefeld CS, Rosenthal GE, Berthenthal D, Sen S, Kaboli PJ. Polypharmacy and prescribing quality in older people. *J Am Geriatr Soc.* 2006;54(10):1516–1523.

46. Kearley KE, Freeman GK, Heath A. An exploration of the value of the personal doctor-patient relationship in general practice. *Br J Gen Pract.* 2001;51(470):712–718.

47. Belloc NB. Relationship of health practices and mortality. *Prev Med.* 1973;2(1):67–81.

48. Brody H. Placebo. In: Post SG, ed. *Encyclopedia of bioethics.* New York: Macmillan Reference USA; 2004:2030–2031.

6

Caring for Dying Patients and Their Families

Cowards die many times before their deaths;
The valiant never taste of death but once.
Of all the wonders that I yet have heard,
It seems to me most strange the men should fear,
Seeing that death, a necessary end,
Will come when it will come.

From Julius Caesar, by William Shakespeare[1]

Whenever it comes, death is not optional. We all die, our patients, their families, our families and ourselves, the physicians. Freud once said, "The goal of all life is death."[2] On a more spiritual note, Coelho described death as a "beautiful woman," always sitting at his side (Coelho, p. 183).

I definitely prefer Coelho's image, and I am not sure I would use the word "goal." I think of my goal as the quest for my Personal Legend. But I do believe that dying is our last role on earth and the event of death surely brings down the curtain.

DEATH IS REALLY A PART OF LIFE

Dying and death are but the final chapter of a story that began with conception. The significance of this truism is that physicians should not necessarily equate death with failure. Marcus Aurelius wrote, "The act of dying too is one of the acts of life" (Meditations, VI.2. Quoted in Strauss, p. 268.)

That death is the natural culmination of life was eloquently stated by Alex Carrell: "Death resulting from old age, or natural death, is determined by the same factors

R.B. Taylor, *Medical Wisdom and Doctoring: The Art of 21st Century Practice*, DOI 10.1007/978-1-4419-5521-0_6,
© Springer Science+Business Media, LLC 2010

that cause the growth of the child and the maturation of the adult. The mechanisms responsible for the end of the old individual are already at work in the body of the embryo." (Rapport, page 851) In 1980, Fries calculated that the ideal average life span is approximately 85 years and that because many of the causes of nontraumatic, premature death (such as plague and smallpox) have been controlled or eliminated, "most premature deaths are now due to the chronic diseases of the later years." Stated another way, we are, and have always been, biologically programmed to live until about age 85, and the gradually sloping mortality curve that has been the historical norm has reflected the great plagues and often the outcomes of major wars. Over the past century, the composite morbidity curve of Americans has become rectangular; that is, unless we fall victim to some illness or injury causing premature death, most of us can expect to enjoy more-or-less good health until our mid-80s, when we begin a final and fairly steep downhill slide.[3]

Our job is to help patients postpone the date of demise as long as reasonably possible, and then assist the patient and family by helping see that the death is, to the greatest extent possible, appropriate, perhaps even noble, and attended by those closest to the patient.

THERE IS A SKILL TO MANAGING A DEATH

I have experienced the deaths of my wife's and my own parents at the end of long and full lives. In three of the four instances, the deaths were in hospital. In two instances, the physician bid us goodbye at about 5 pm and was not seen again. In the third instance, we did not set eyes on the attending physician at all. In each of these instances, my wife and I were left with our dying parent and a new shift of nurses every 8 h, busily fussing with lines and bags and ventilators. In one of the three instances, a neurologist was called to determine if the patient had any chance of return to a sapient state; he made his exam, wrote a short chart note, and exited through a back door without speaking with us, while we waited expectantly in the adjacent intensive care family room. Emboldened by my status as a fellow physician who had actually referred a few patients to the neurologist, I called him at home to get a first-hand report.

Later, at the time of death, someone we had never met before came from the emergency room to make the "pronouncement." And this was what happened to the family of a full professor in a medical school, who thought himself very savvy about how to get things accomplished in hospitals. I hate to think of what happens to "non-medical" persons in similar situations. What is described above is *not* how physicians should treat their dying patients and their families.

One of our roles as physicians is to help dying patients and their families deal with the practical elements of care – the seemingly inevitable tubes and machines. In the sense that the act of dying is finishing one's life story, another of the clinician's roles is to help the patient script the final hours and last moments. In a wisely managed death, the survivors tell a tale of dignity, respect, and perhaps even personal growth.

"PEOPLE DIE FROM VERY REAL THINGS"

The above is a direct quote from Doctor William J. Mayo (Mayo and Mayo, page 56). Another version that I have heard is: Even your most hypochondriacal patient will eventually die of a physical disease (Anon). Herein lie the land mines faced by the physician treating a person with a long list of nagging health problems or a patient with whom there are insurmountable communication difficulties.

A patient at special risk is the one with multiple illnesses managed by a phalanx of specialists. A few years ago, I reviewed medical records of one such case. A lady in her 60s whose past medical history included a hysterectomy suffered from diabetes, heart failure, osteoarthritis, depression, atherosclerosis, and psoriasis. She received ongoing treatment by five specialists in a large multispecialty practice, but this number did not include a gynecologist or family physician. None of these highly regarded specialists elicited the relevant history or did that physical exam that would have revealed that the remote hysterectomy was a supra-cervical hysterectomy, leaving the patient at risk for cervical cancer.

By the time she developed frank bleeding per vagina, her cancer had already spread throughout the pelvis, necessitating extensive surgery and eventually culminating in her death.

THERE IS ACTUALLY A "GOOD DEATH"

Since we all die, our goal should be a good death – one that occurs at the right time of life, in the right place, without undue pain and with the right cast of characters present. Physicians can help their patients in this regard by understanding what Goldsteen et al call the "normative expectations around death and dying."[4] The following are the authors' descriptors of five normative expectations concerning dying and death; the examples are mine:

Expectation	Example
Awareness and acceptance	Having appropriate prognostic information, including reasonable expectations regarding pain and pain control, as well as the possibility of future debility and the need for help
Open communication	When the dying process is attended by healthy family dialogue
Living one's life until the end	Maintaining robust and healthy relationships with family and friends
Taking care of final responsibilities	Getting one's estate plan up to date
Dealing adequately with emotions	Coping with anger, frustration, and depression, especially when the terminal illness is premature and "unfair"

Of course, each patient is different, and the doggedly rational person – like many physicians I know – will give a high priority to fulfilling final responsibilities. Some persons may not want prognostic speculation on what to expect next. On the other hand, other persons may want to know what the future is likely to hold, finding that knowing is the best way to deal with their feelings of impending loss. It is the physician's task to intuit how best to meet the patient's needs.

NO DEATH IS TRULY INSIGNIFICANT

Death is not only part of life, it is omnipresent in the media. We read of war deaths, flood and hurricane fatalities, and the demise of famous persons. We don't hear much about the deaths of ordinary people, nor of the faceless poor we see living on the street, nor of the tens of thousands of persons languishing in nursing homes today. Most of these persons see physicians, and we must keep in mind that each dying person – whether well-known or anonymous – has or had a family, friends, aspirations, dreams, and contributions to the lives of others.

Clinicians can honor the patient' life and death in several ways. One is to never allow the patient with a terminal illness to become depersonalized in the language of the staff or the physicians. The patient is never "the lung cancer in room 420;" he/she is a person with an identity and feelings. Because the opinion of the physician is truly important to the patient and family, you should take the opportunity to validate the patient's life and achievements. For example, family members may quote a comment by the physicians such as, "John will be remembered by all as a kind and generous man, especially for his years of work as a high school teacher, and for all he did for his family."

One of the ways physicians can honor their patients in death is attending their funerals. This is something small town doctors do, and that even "big city" physicians should consider. Physicians sometimes forget how much families value their presence, and showing up at an evening viewing or a funeral ceremony is silent testimony that the death was not insignificant. I learned in my early days in private practice that going to the funeral can make the physician aware of feelings that would not be learned any other way. I will next describe one such instance.

PATIENTS RECALL FOREVER EVENTS
THAT OCCUR AT A TIME OF A DEATH

During my very early days in private practice, I was a member of a 4-doctor practice, serving patients living in a 10–15 mile radius. House calls were common in those days, and our group assigned one physician to make all house calls each afternoon. In this setting, I had a patient I'll call Harold Brown. Harold had severe diabetes with peripheral neuropathy, hypertension in the days when we lacked truly effective antihypertensive therapy, and congestive heart failure that seemed to become a little worse each month. Harold and his wife lived in a trailer at the end of a wooded lane located about 15 miles of winding country roads away from our office. Because Harold shouldn't drive and his wife couldn't drive, I made monthly home visits.

One day Harold died. As was the custom at that time, a physician needed to go to the home to pronounce death before the local undertaker could remove the body. The day of Harold's death was not my day to make home visits. My physician partner, who had house call duty that afternoon, made the trip, pronounced death and comforted the widow.

I next encountered Harold's widow a few days later at the viewing in the funeral home. When she saw me, she began to weep, "Doctor Taylor, you should have come to our home the day Harold died. Not some other doctor Harold didn't know. Where were you?" I am sure, if she is still alive, that she still recalls how I failed her. And I clearly remember the events today, more than four decades later.

Families can also attach special meaning to words at the time of death. A colleague tells this story: (Some details have been changed to protect privacy.) The patient, Rosita, was a 29-year-old Latina woman, a grade school teacher and the first in her very large family to have finished college. Rosita was her mother's proof of the American dream, and thus it was devastating when this shining star of the family developed leukemia.

The doctors administered chemotherapy, but the disease persisted. Eventually, the patient received a bone marrow transplant from a sibling, and she enjoyed a period of remission. But her good fortune was not to last. She developed a fulminating infection, and antibiotics failed her. Surrounded by her family at the bedside, Rosita died quietly at home.

My friend tells that when the mother saw the death certificate, she objected to the presence of the word *leukemia*, and asked if it could be removed. At this point, I will quote my colleague: "And it was clear in my conversation with her mother over the death certificate that there was overwhelming pride in all the ways this daughter had overcome – getting through college, being an inspiration to nephews and nieces (unmarried, childless) and in the final analysis, she even *beat leukemia*."

THE AGED OFTEN HAVE A DIFFERENT VIEW OF DEATH THAT OF THEIR DOCTORS

Writing two and a half millennia ago, Herodotus (484–424 BCE) observed, "Death is a delightful hiding place for weary men."[5] Young physicians are sometimes surprised – and often appalled – to hear the aged state that they are ready to die. More mature physicians are seldom so astonished. When you think of it, perhaps the ready-to-die patient is being more rational than the physician. Metaphorically, there is always the right time to leave the party – not too early and certainly not too late. Patients who professes readiness to die are not necessarily just weary; they may also have done all they want to do in life, have made peace with family relationships, have very likely outlived most of their lifelong friends, and have, in the words of the estate planners, "their affairs in order."

The "different view of death" is part of what has prompted voters in my home state of Oregon to support the Oregon Death with Dignity Act (DWDA) enacted October 27, 1997. This legislation allows terminally ill Oregonians to end their lives through the voluntary self-administration of lethal medications, expressly prescribed by a physician for that purpose. The bill called for stringent safeguards and administrative oversight. According to the latest report, from 1998 to 2007, 341 DWDA patients have died after ingesting a lethal dose of medication.[6]

The differing viewpoints about death held by patients and their doctors are often not discussed. The physician, seeing death as the enemy, makes an all-out assault in the final days of life. Patients, and perhaps the family, welcome the end of what has often been a long, weary process of dying. Sadly, an open conversation, perhaps beginning with the words of Herodotus, might bring consensus. In writing about our ability to prolong biologic life through the use of technology, Slomka states that ideally, "The patient's demise becomes a negotiated death, a bargaining over how far medical technology should go in prolonging life or prolonging death."[7]

WHEN CARING FOR A DYING PERSON, SEEK THE GOLDILOCKS APPROACH TO CARE: NOT TOO LITTLE, BUT NOT TOO MUCH

Slomka's comments on the negotiation of death and clinical decision making at the end of life brings us to practical aspects of patient care. On his deathbed, Alexander the Great (356–323 BCE) is reported to have said, "I die with the help of too many physicians" (Strauss, p. 257). American president George Washington (1732–1799) may have died of a throat infection, perhaps epiglottitis; on the other hand, his actual cause of death may have been related to the use of tartar emetic, vigorous purging, and the heroic blood-letting of five pints of presidential blood (Taylor 2008, p. 215). On the other hand, we all know of instances of inadequate care, especially instances of failure to control pain, as well as instances of "benign neglect." The best way to find the Goldilocks approach to managing dying and death is through open discussion with the patient, meetings with family members, and team conferences involving all key persons involved in the patient's care.

CONSIDER THE POSSIBLE CLINICAL MEANING WHEN A PATIENT TELLS OF A DEATH, EVEN ONE THAT OCCURRED SOME TIME AGO

If the patient has suffered a loss, such as a death of a family member, allow him/her to tell you about it, even if it takes a little time. Telling you, the caring physician, about events can be an important part of healing. Be sure to express your sincere sympathy. If the patient seems to want to talk about the death, listen attentively. The introduction of the topic of death may be a plea to discuss a concern, perhaps about a symptom that matches one described by the person who died. Or it may be the patient's way of telling you another anecdote in his/her life story.

IF AN ELDERLY PATIENT BEGINS TO PREDICT HIS OWN DEATH, TAKE THE PROGNOSTICATION VERY SERIOUSLY

The patient foretelling his own death may be correct. In my early years of practice, I cared for a 79-year-old man I will call Herbert, who lived with his wife in a small home not too far from my office. He came to me several times, telling me he was going to die and that he was ready to do so. In thinking about what happened, I am sure he was clinically depressed, at least to some degree. But most depressed people don't just die. As the good clinician I thought I was, I examined Herbert thoroughly, performed blood tests and X-rays, and eventually informed him that he was in surprisingly good physical health for his age. He thanked me for the effort, and reiterated his belief that he would die soon.

Of course, Herbert went home and died quietly in the night about a week later. Perhaps he suffered a heart attack or fatal arrhythmia. No specific physical cause of death was ever discovered. His demise was a message to me that I wasn't as smart as I thought I was. Today, I clearly recall the lesson learned, and now I take seriously any hint that the patient believes that death will come soon.

NEVER PREDICT DEATH – OR RECOVERY – TOO PRECISELY

Only a foolish physician would tell a patient that he/she has 6 months to live. Osler once remarked, "Gentlemen, if you want a profession in which everything is certain you had better give up medicine" (Silverman et al, p. 75). In no sphere of medicine is certainty more elusive than in attempting to foresee the course of an apparently terminal illness.

On one hand, we have statistical tools to predict risk of death from various diseases. And we know the life expectancy of persons with various cancers. But the person in the office in front of you is not the "average patient" in the studies you read. Yes, the accountants must love medicine's research-validated scores used to predict the risk of death from various ailments such as cardiovascular diseases.[8]

In the office and hospital, we physicians earnestly wish to provide needed guidance to patients and families, thereby inviting the occasional memorable error. If tempted to prognosticate life expectancy in the setting of terminal disease, consider that, at least in one prospective cohort study, we seem to overestimate life expectancy in 63% of instances.[9] Are we overestimating our abilities to sustain life in the face of grim realities?

Siegler describes a method of dealing with the urge to prognosticate death, remission, or recovery.[10] The technique, admittedly a little devious, involves describing the most dire and pessimistic prognosis. Thus if the patient dies, the physician has not only prepared the family, and not incidentally has proved to be an astute prognosticator. But if the patient survives, everyone is happy. The strategy harkens to the "Necessity of the Wager" essay, written by French philosopher Blaise Pascal (1623–1622). Pascal's Wager, sometimes called Pascal's Gambit, was described in *Pensées*, a collection of his notes published after his death. According to the Pascal's wager, we should "bet" that God exists, even though His existence cannot be proved concretely. If you so believe and God exists, you will gain eternity, while betting only one life on earth. In the end, if there is no God, you have wagered only your brief earthly existence. Yes, the analogy between clinical crepe hanging and Pascal's wager may be slightly flawed, but I think we can see the similarities.

RECOGNIZE THE ISOLATION OFTEN FELT BY A DYING PERSON

I learned from a friend and patient a valuable lesson about death. In Chap. 4, I introduced you to Ronald, whose testicular tumor was detected by his wife, confirmed by me, and promptly removed surgically. Postoperatively he received chemotherapy, but survival was in doubt.

Ronald and his family lived in a small community – one traffic light – where he was well known. Everyone in town knew that Ronald had cancer. One day in the office, Ronald told me of how people he had known all his life seemed to be avoiding him. "I watch in the grocery store as long-time friends change aisles just so they won't pass by me." Many persons with terminal illness have related how family and staff will converse in their hospital rooms just as if they were not present. This sort of isolation amounts to a *premature declaration of death* and it can make the process of death just that much more difficult.

Ronald, of course, fooled them all. At this writing 40 years later, he is living, cancer-free and happily retired in his home town.

TRY TO FIND SOME WAY TO BE HOPEFUL

Ambroise Paré (1517–1564), the military surgeon who revolutionized wound care by finding a better method than cauterizing flesh, has given us some memorable aphorisms. One of these is this: "Always hold out hope to the patient, even if the symptoms point to a fatal issue." When I was a very young family doctor, I once asked an oncologist how he could do what he did in his career, as I pointed out that so many his patients die of their cancers. His answer was, "No matter how bad things seem, there is always something we can do." Today I find the positive, can-do attitude to be a model we should all emulate.

WHEN DEATH IS NEAR, YOU SOMETIMES NEED TO DO WHAT NEEDS TO BE DONE

Anthony was a 68-year-old man, a veteran of World War II, and like so many veterans, a long-time heavy smoker. He and Hanna, his wife (or so I assumed), both retired, had assumed the responsibility of raising two young grandchildren after their single mother, a drug addict, departed 3 years earlier for who knew where.

All was fine, and I treated the blended-generation family members for the usual health problems, until one day, Anthony was diagnosed with lung cancer. Before long the cancer had metastasized to his brain, and he suffered some loss of both neurologic and cognitive function.

Despite his problems, Anthony liked to walk about town, until the day he stepped in front of a large truck, which struck him squarely. No one will ever know if the event was truly an accident or an attempted suicide. Whatever the circumstances, Anthony was admitted to the intensive care unit with severe injuries to many areas, including brain trauma, and death seemed imminent. Although in great pain, he seemed to have periods of mental clarity.

At this time, Hanna confided, "Doctor, you didn't know this, but Anthony and I were never married. We just never got around to it. The problem is that our only income is his veteran's pension, and when he dies, the pension will stop because we aren't married. The kids and I will have nothing to live on."

What would you do? As their physician, I suggested a remedy. We obtained a marriage license, arranged for a hospital chaplain to visit during one of Anthony's lucid times, and Hanna and Anthony were married in the intensive care unit; several nurses were witnesses and I gave the bride away. Anthony died a week later, and I am sure he was comforted knowing that his family would be cared for in his absence. As health care professionals and caring human beings, the intensive care staff and I did what needed to be done.

AVOID EXPRESSIONS THAT CAN BE MISUNDERSTOOD BY PATIENTS AND FAMILIES

Especially worrisome are comments that may be interpreted as conveying hopelessness or abandonment. Here are a few such seemingly objective remarks and how they may be misinterpreted by the patient and family:

Comment by the Clinician	What the Patient Might be Thinking
"We're doing what's appropriate and cost-effective."	I may be getting "bargain-basement" treatment to save the hospital money.
"The medicine just isn't working."	Things may be even worse than I thought."
"We've tried everything I know."	My doctor is losing interest in me.
"We need to move you to a chronic care bed."	The doctors are giving up.
"Are you familiar with hospice care?"	I don't like this at all. My pain is going to get worse and I am going to die.
"We should discuss circumstances under which we would stop treatment. That is, we need to review your Advance Directive, your living will."	That's it. I'll be dead before long.

RECOGNIZE THAT DEATH IS NOT THE WORST THING IN THE WORLD

"Death is better than disease," wrote American poet Henry Wadsworth Longfellow (1807–1882). Now when I came across this quotation and looked into the life of the poet, I anticipated finding that, like so many of his day, Longfellow suffered the progressive wasting of tuberculosis or perhaps some other chronic infection. In fact, he seems to have enjoyed good physical health until dying of peritonitis at age 75, far exceeding the usual life expectancy of his day. His chief affliction was persistent grief over the death of his wife Frances ("Fanny"), killed when her dress caught on fire in 1861, sadness that Longfellow sometimes assuaged with laudanum.

Death as a possibly preferred option brings us to pneumonia, the time-honored terminal event allowing an apparently easy exodus at life's end. Pneumonia, the final common pathway for many of our patients, is described by Dowell as "the leading infectious killer worldwide."[11]

Writing circa 1892 in his epic reference book, *The Principles and Practice of Medicine*, Osler observed, "Pneumonia may well be the friend of the aged. Taken off by it in an acute, short, not often painful illness, the old man escapes those 'cold gradations of decay' so often distressing to himself and to his friends" (Silverman, p. 137.). Considering that for the very aged and infirm pneumonia can allow the easy exodus, are we doing some aged patients a disservice when we administer the pneumococcal vaccine and even the annual influenza vaccine? Is it ethical to withhold these vaccines in the nursing home patient with, for example, advanced Alzheimer disease?

SOME OF YOUR PATIENTS WILL DIE UNEXPECTEDLY

Sudden death, such as that of Herbert, described above, is quite different from managed death. Writing about the dying role, Emanuel et al describe three key elements: the practical element, involving specific preparatory tasks; the rational element, the process of engaging with others; and the personal element, including tasks that foster personal growth and completing one's life story.[12] When a person dies unexpectedly, as in an auto accident or owing to an unanticipated heart attack, the three key elements are, for all practical purposes, denied.

When there is sudden death of your long-standing patient or mine, we must deal with both with the family's acute grief and also with our own feelings of professional angst. Could I have made a difference and might I have prevented this death? Was there undetected depression that played a role in the fatal crash? Did I overlook early signs of coronary artery disease? Did I, the physician, somehow fail my patient? Wise physicians know that feelings of professional inadequacy are sometimes most acute following an unexpected death.

SOME OF YOUR PATIENTS WILL COMMIT SUICIDE

"The thought of suicide is a great comfort. It's helped me through many a bad night," is a saying attributed to German philosopher Friedrich Nietzsche (1884–1900)[13] Suicide was the 11th leading cause of death in the United States in 2008, and I suspect that this figure is artificially low because of under-reporting. How many one-car accidents, drownings and "accidental" overdoses were really suicides? Was Anthony, described above, an accidental death or a suicide?

Today all clinicians know that when a patient reports suicidal ideation, there should be an inquiry about intent, means, and plan. Wise physicians also avoid saying things that could tempt suicide, such as stating that the doctor has no influence over a patient's actions or even exhibiting a lack of empathy for the emotions being expressed. Perhaps the most effective suicide prophylaxis in a clinical setting is the physician's strongly expressed wish that the patient will not suicide, will make a personal vow not to do so, and will promise to call the physician if there seems to be change of heart.

BE CAREFUL WHEN INFORMING A FAMILY OF A DEATH

In 1961, when I was a senior medical student, I was employed by a private hospital in Philadelphia to serve in an "intern" role, reporting to a senior resident. Today, such a role sounds improbable, but it happened in the early 1960s. Most of my time was spent taking calls overnight on a private medical service.

Because I worked only about one night a week, I was never fully aware of the full stories of the many patients I covered. In addition, my resident back-up support was variable, and my contact with the private attending physicians was, to be charitable, not very good. They must have had great faith in my abilities, because although I talked on the telephone with a few private physicians, I seldom saw them in the hospital during my shifts.

My job on the private medicine floor was to respond to the nurse's calls overnight, whether it was for a laxative order or because a patient had gone into pulmonary edema. In a few instances, patients died, and it fell to me to tell the family, who were sometimes at home in bed. Still today, I recall the advice of a senior resident: "If a patient dies and the family is not in the hospital, don't inform them of the death over the telephone. Say that your family member has 'taken a turn for the worse, and you need to come to the hospital right now.' If necessary, repeat this phrase over and over, but don't say that the patient died." His reasons were twofold. The first was that we would need a family member present to request a post-mortem examination – a trophy considered quite important at that time. The other reason was more practical: "If you tell the person by telephone that his family member has died and he or she is not ready for the news, the next sound you may hear on the line is the person you were talking to hitting the floor after passing out." Although now the resident's advice may seem a little as though from Shem's book, *The House of God*, it did not sound fully irrational or overly cynical at the time.[14]

I have since resigned myself to the fact that, owing to long distances and other factors, we sometimes must convey bad news – even the report of death – over the telephone. When this must be done, I am careful to inquire, "Is there someone at home with you?" If not, I try to insist that I will wait to tell the news until someone else is present.

CONSIDER THE MEANING OF A DEATH TO VARIOUS FAMILY MEMBERS

Every death has meaning to family and friends, but sometimes the significance is not quite what we physicians would anticipate. At the time of death we would, in most instances, predict profound loss and grief. But perhaps there are other feelings. Possibilities include relief, vindication, and even triumph.

The patient was Clyde, a man in his early 70s with severe hypertension and arteriosclerosis and who had survived several strokes. Sadly, he had lost much of his brain function and his ability to walk unassisted. He needed to be spooned every mouthful of food he consumed. Dutifully, his wife installed a hospital bed in the dining room of their small home, and nursed him day and night. The children helped out as much as they could, but they had jobs, children, and busy lives. As family gatherings on weekends, the children helped Clyde to a chair so he could be present, even though he was not fully aware of the events and he sometimes fell out of his chair.

From time to time, he had another stroke or episode of atrial fibrillation. His young physician would rush Clyde to the hospital, heroically save him from death once again, and then return him home to "family care."

One day Clyde finally died. The family gathered for the funeral and dutifully paid their respects. Nevertheless, the dominant mood was relief that the ordeal was ended. Clyde, as they knew him, had "died" years before, and the dependent soul that had remained represented a sad family burden, one which had now been lifted.

DYING AND DEATH CAN BRING OUT THE BEST OR THE WORST IN FAMILY MEMBERS

When an elderly person, especially one with some financial resources and without a functional family nearby, develops a terminal illness, it seems that a number of distant nieces, nephews, and cousins suddenly develop intense feelings for their distant relative, as well as a keen interest in how care is managed. Matters can become complicated if one or more of these concerned relatives show up at the hospital or nursing home. Somehow, they sense that criticizing how care is rendered by hard-working physicians and nurses can compensate for decades of avoidance and neglect. I sometimes think that there is an inverse relationship between the love of family for a patient and the amount of concern they express (and sometimes the disruptions they cause in the patient's care).

REMAIN ALERT TO THE POSSIBILITY
OF PATHOLOGIC GRIEF FOLLOWING A DEATH

Like everything else in life, sometimes things don't go as we would hope. Following a death, patients' families go through more-or-less predictable stages of grief, described by Kübler-Ross in her 1969 book *On Death and Dying*[15] But not all family members experience, sequentially, the stages of Denial, Anger, Bargaining, Depression, and Acceptance. Simply stated, following a death, some survivors follow a very long journey on their way to acceptance, and a few seem never to arrive at the destination. The result is that a survivor becomes bogged down in denial, anger, or agonizing depression, resulting in pathologic grief.

Sometimes pathologic grief can be traced to an event occurring around the time of death. A classic example would be suicide, especially of a young person. Another would be a family quarrel or a confrontation with a medical caregiver. One example I encountered was an older, powerful man, one who made the decisions for both his wife and himself. The couple had no children and were actually quite close, despite what some might consider a dysfunctional relationship. Then he died following a short illness. One of his final decisions was that there would be no viewing, no funeral, and no memorial service – nothing. The result was that the wife was denied the opportunity to grieve, and thus settled into a pathologic state of simmering anger that lingered until her death a few years later.

Pathologic grief can be subtle, and difficult to detect. Meador suggests, "When a grieving patient's spouse died more than 6 months ago, find out, gently, where the patient is living and sleeping, and what disposition, if any, was made of the spouse's clothes." (Meador, No. 97) This advice may afford us a handy indicator to open dialogue regarding progress through the stages of grief.

RECOGNIZE THE EMOTIONAL RESPONSES
OF PHYSICIANS TO THE DEATHS OF THEIR PATIENTS

In his humorous, yet intensely cynical book *The House of God*, the author, pseudonymous Samuel Shem, MD describes the adventures of young medical residents working at an inner-city hospital. On page 420, he lists the "Laws of the House of God." In this list, Law Number IX is: "The only good admission is a dead admission."[14] Perhaps the indifference to death described in Shem's book can be attributed – but not excused – by the herculean work schedules and sleep deprivation that characterized postgraduate medical training in the 1960s and 1970s.

Physicians, as well as surviving family members and friends, can have unhealthy responses to death. At one end of the spectrum is excessive grief, a special danger when the physician senses that more could have been done or even that some sort of error occurred. The other extreme is an absence of sadness when a patient dies, a state that probably occurs more often than physicians would care to admit. Berry has reflected on factors that may contribute to physician indifference to death: One is clinical distancing, separating oneself from the patient's pain. Others cited include "the atrophying effect of perceived hopelessness, insincerities in the establishment of the original relationship, and an inability to imbue the sedated or unconscious patient with human qualities." Berry holds that recognizing these adverse factors may help protect physicians against "what might be an otherwise insidious process of dehumanization."[16]

FROM TIME TO TIME, PHYSICIANS SHOULD REFLECT
ON THE BRAVERY OF THE DYING AND THEIR FAMILIES

Somehow, as we grow older, we become more like we really are. The optimistic, cheerful person becomes a joy to be around, and these qualities only seem to be enhanced with aging. On the other hand, the person who was never satisfied and always seemed to find fault can, in old age, become a truly crabby individual. In time, these evolving personal characteristics may become fully revealed during the act of dying.

Happily, as death approaches, we don't encounter too many angry, bitter faultfinders. I have found that most dying persons face death with laudable equanimity; asking for cheerfulness would be asking too much. The nobility with which many of my patients faced dying is reflected in the words of English author W. Somerset Maugham (1864–1965), who studied medicine for 5 years in London before launching his writing career: "Even now that forty years have passed I can remember certain people so exactly that I could draw a picture of them. Phrases that I heard then still linger on my ears. I saw how men died. I saw how they bore pain. I saw what hope looked like, fear and relief; I saw the dark lines that despair drew on a face; I saw courage and steadfastness. I saw faith shine in the eyes of those who trusted in what I could only think was an illusion and I saw the gallantry that made a man greet the prognosis of death with an ironic joke because he was too proud to let those about him see the terror of his soul."[17]

WISE WORDS ABOUT DYING AND DEATH

▧ *Death is a debt we all must pay.* Ancient Greek philosopher Euripides (484–406 BCE) (Strauss, page 91)

▧ *In acute disease it is not quite safe to prognosticate either death or recovery.* Hippocrates (ca 460–377 BCE)[18]

▧ *Pale Death with foot impartial knocks at the poor man's cottage and at the prince's palace.* Horace [65–8 BCE]. Odes, I.iv.13. (Quoted in Strauss, page 91)
   Yes, death has a perverse leveling effect.

▧ *As a well-spent day brings happy sleep, so life well used brings happy death.* Italian artist Leonardo Da Vinci (1452–1519)[19]

▧ *It is the duty of a doctor to prolong life; it not his duty to prolong the act of dying.* British physician Lord Thomas Horder (1871–1955) (Strauss, page 159)
   Explaining this distinction has often been what helps families to work with physicians in making wise end-of-life choices. And for physicians, this is an instructive axiom to ponder when one is tempted to initiate a "code" on a

patient who has lost any redeeming human quality and is already near death.

▓ *Dying is a very dull, dreary affair. And my advice to you is to have nothing whatever to do with it.* English physician and author W. Somerset Maugham (1874–1965).[20]
Unfortunately, Maugham was, in the end, unable to follow his own advice, although he did avoid death until his 91st year.

▓ *Dying is an art like everything else.* American writer Sylvia Plath (1932–1963), as reported to have said not long before she committed suicide.[21]

▓ *There is no cure for birth and death other than to enjoy the interval.* Spanish-American philosopher George Santayana (1853–1962)[22]

▓ *A single death is a tragedy. A million deaths is statistics.* Leader of the Soviet Union Joseph Stalin (1878–1953).[23]
Surely this statement, which Uncle Joe translated into action, must receive the Academy Award for cynicism regarding death.

▓ *The difference between sex and death is that with death you can do it alone and no one is going to make fun of you.* American actor Woody Allen (1935–).[24]

REFERENCES

1. Shakespeare W. Julius Caesar, II, ii, 32.
2. *New York Times Magazine,* May 6, 1956; source, Evans B. Dictionary of quotations. New York: Delacorte:148.
3. Fries JF. Aging, natural death, and the compression of morbidity. *N Engl J Med.* 1980;303:130-135.
4. Goldsteen M, Houtepen R, Proot IM, Abu-Saad HH, Spreeuwenberg C, Widdershoven G. What is a good death? Terminally ill patients dealing with normative expectations around dying and death. *Patient Educ Couns.* 2006;64(1-3):378-386.
5. Herodotus. Histories, VII.xlvi.
6. DWDA 2007 report. http://www.oregon.gov/DHS/ph/pas/docs/yr10-tbl-3.pdf. Accessed 8.06.2008.
7. Slomka J. The negotiation of death: clinical decision making at the end of life. *Soc Sci Med.* 1992;35(3):251-259.

8. Pocock SJ, McCormack V, Gueyffier F, Boutitie F, Fagand RH, Boissel JP. A score for predicting risk of death from cardio-vascular disease in adults with raised blood pressure, based on individual patient data from randomized controlled trials. *BMJ*. 2001;323:75-81.

9. Christakis NA, Lamont EB. Extent and determinants in terminally ill patients: prospective cohort study. *BMJ*. 2000;320:469-473.

10. Siegler M. Pascal's wager and the hanging of crepe. *N Engl J Med*. 1975;293(17):853-857.

11. Dowell SF. Surviving pneumonia-Just a short-term lease on life? *Am J Respir Crit Care*. 2004;169:895-896.

12. Emanuel L, Bennett K, Richardson VE. The dying role. *J Palliat Med*. 2007;10(1):159-168.

13. Aphorisms. http://littlecalamity.tripod.com/Quotes/D.html/ Accessed 12.11.2007.

14. Shem S. *The House of God*. New York: Dell; 1981.

15. Kübler-Ross E. *On Death and Dying*. New York: Macmillan; 1969.

16. Berry PA. The absence of sadness: darker reflections on the doctor-patient relationship. *J Med Ethics*. 2007;33(5):266-268.

17. Maugham WS. *The Summing Up*. Garden City, NY: Doubleday; 1946.

18. Bioethics discussion blog. http://bioethicsdiscussion.blogspot. com/2005/06/more-hippocratic-aphorisms.html/. Accessed 12.11.2007.

19. Da Vinci L. The Notebooks.

20. Quote DB. http://www.quotedb.com/quotes/3355/. Accessed 13.04.2009.

21. Medical quotes and anecdotes. http://easydiagnosis.com/secon-dopinions/newsletter12.html/. Accessed 27.09.2007.

22. Use Wisdom. http://www.usewisdom.com/sayings/death.html/. Accessed 12.11.2007.

23. Famous aphorisms. http://www.aphorisms-galore.info/category/life-and-death/. Accessed 12.11.2007.

24. Aphorisms Galore! http://www.ag.wastholm.net/aphorism/F66L57-IYZ/. Accessed 12.11.2007.

7

Making a Living as a Clinician

My office is only two blocks from the hospital. At five minutes to nine I walk in [after making hospital rounds]. My office staff has been there since 8:30. The first two patients are already there. The first one is in the examining room. I glance at the appointment book. The day is full. I see that Mrs. D is scheduled at 10:30 for fifteen minutes. There is no way that I can see that woman in fifteen minutes. It takes her longer than that to recite her neatly written list of complaints.

From "*A Day in the Life of an Internist,*"
by American physician and educator
Richard C. Reynolds (Reynolds and Stone, p. 268)

One of the weaknesses of contemporary medical education is that we seem to lead medical students to believe that they won't actually need to make a living as doctors. We teach them the basic sciences, share our clinical knowledge and skills, and even help them ponder medicine's ethical dilemmas. But we somehow fail to tell students how to earn the money needed to eliminate their education debts, how to pay on a mortgage and feed their families, and how to manage the funds they haven't spent by the end of the month. Instead we present medical students with diplomas asserting their proficiency to practice medicine and surgery, and cast them adrift like ships without rudders, left at the mercy of bankers, investment advisors, third-party payers, office equipment salespersons and, of course, the well-meaning but typically ill-informed family member with investment advice.

Part of being a wise physician is learning how to control your own financial destiny. There are at least two topics related to this advice. The first is learning the day-by-day

R.B. Taylor, *Medical Wisdom and Doctoring: The Art of 21st Century Practice*, DOI 10.1007/978-1-4419-5521-0_7, © Springer Science+Business Media, LLC 2010

economics of the practice of medicine. This advice may seem a little anachronistic, since today most young physicians join groups with existing office protocols, contracts and salaries. Not many newly minted physicians begin new practices from scratch – renting or buying an office, purchasing office equipment, setting up medical records, hiring staff, creating a billing system and all the other details needed to see patients and get paid for doing so. Today, the physician fresh from residency signs more or less the same contract as the last physician hired by the group, assumes that a business manager will take care of all financial matters for the practice and – other than an occasional discussion about billing codes and productivity – remains financially naïve about what happens between the time of seeing a patient and the paycheck at the end of the month.

The second topic related to controlling your financial destiny concerns saving and investing for your children's education, a secure retirement, or whatever else is important to you. In this chapter, I will focus chiefly on practice management. However, I urge you learn everything you can about both topics – running a practice and investing your money. I'll discuss investing in Chap. 13 in the context of planning for tomorrow.

DO YOUR BEST TO UNDERSTAND EVERYTHING THAT GOES ON IN YOUR OFFICE

If you don't understand something that is done in your office, then you – and your income – are at the mercy of the person who has the knowledge you lack. This admonition includes the telephone protocols, the appointment scheduling system, the process of "rooming" patients, the workings of any medical equipment in the office, the medical record system, the check-out process for patients, and the billing and collections procedures. Some enlightened residency training programs have residents spend a few days at the front desk and in the billing office, just to learn a little about how things work.

HIRE STAFF MEMBERS WHO HAVE BOTH PROFESSIONAL SKILLS AND A SERVICE ORIENTATION

Today, not all physicians are directly involved in hiring those who work with them – support staff, administrators, nurses, nurse practitioners, physician assistants, and even fellow physicians. To the greatest degree possible, however, I urge all physicians to seek a voice in the hiring process, because your colleagues in the office are not only who you will spend your working days with, but they are also the face of your practice that the public sees.

I recommend a timely book, *Applebee's America: How successful political, business, and religious leaders connect with the new American community* (Sosnik et al, p. 85.). In this book, the three authors, all with a political background, discuss the depersonalization that has come with the rise of technology and look at the current desire for human contact and the need for a sense of community. Their model for success is the Applebee's restaurant chain, which values customer satisfaction as well as profit. From their study of Applebee's comes a lesson that has relevance in today's political campaigns and in your medical office. The authors report: "Applebee's has brought a bit of science to the task of finding employees willing to give customers what they want: a friendly encounter." They go on to tell of a 150-question psychological test given to prospective employees. The goal is to uncover the personality traits likely to influence on-the-job performance. An Applebee's executive states: "We're looking to see if you love your mother. Think about it; if you don't love your mother, then you have some baggage we don't want to deal with."

In hiring staff – and associates – I have never administered a formal psychological test, but I certainly do consider the applicant's ability to connect with me and with others encountered during the interview day. Office culture is important – visitors can sense the "community spirit" of the workplace – and the patient's friendly encounter begins with hiring the right people. It isn't about identifying extroverts and seeking the sparkling personality, it is about finding the person who enjoys life and is committed to serving others. Such hiring is often intuitive, and when I encounter a job applicant with outstanding clinical skills, but with whom my current team and I just don't connect, then I keep looking.

TREAT YOUR PATIENTS WITH RESPECT

Every patient is a valued "customer" who is, in a sense, your employer who can "fire" you by simply not ever returning to see you. If for no other reason than this, the wise physician respects all patients in the practice. But there is more.

In researching the topic of respect in medical practice, I came across a paper by Beach et al from the Berman Institute of Bioethics at Johns Hopkins University in Baltimore. In this paper, the authors write of respect as a moral obligation of health professionals that involves "recognition of the unconditional value of patients as persons," including as persons whose autonomy must itself be respected. They advocate for respect with the cognitive dimension of believing in the value of patients and the behavioral dimension of acting in concert with this belief.[1]

I always admire the ability of scholars to consume three journal pages elucidating what should be part of the fiber of every seasoned and reasonable physician. Perhaps the fact that such apparent pedantry finds its way into print is testimony that many clinicians fall short of the ideal when it comes to respecting patients.

Of course, sometimes patients don't make it easy. There are patients who fail to keep scheduled (and often confirmed) appointments, who treat our staff rudely, who argue with our best advice, and who don't pay our bills. Nevertheless, they are humans with health problems who have somehow ended up in our offices, hoping that we can help. Showing respect in the most difficult situation is the mark of a professional, and by this I mean a professional in the true sense of the word: one who has *professed an oath* to serve humanity.

SEEK WAYS THAT PATIENTS CAN GET TO SEE YOU

You should look at your appointment scheduler as someone whose job is to facilitate patient access to you – their physician – and not as a gatekeeper that patients must overcome in order to get care. What's more, you need to do your best to see that your patients get to see you whenever possible, and not be shunted to someone else.

Today's current answer to the problem of patients getting to see their physician when needed is open access scheduling. Simply stated, "open access" means that a patient can call the office today and be seen that day or perhaps the next. It's the scheduling application of the axiom, "Do today's work today." In my solo practice years, I always subscribed to this philosophy, at least to the degree possible in a very busy small town office. Our office mantra was: If you are sick today and call us *early*, we will get you in today. Of course, the patient who had been mildly ill all week and called at 4 p.m. might not enjoy the benefits of open access scheduling that day. What is most important is having the person scheduling, or not scheduling, the end-of-day, work-in appointment be capable of making a wise decision.

Yes, open access scheduling can certainly lead to occasional feelings of "feast or famine," and can tend to make for slack early mornings and busy afternoons. Nevertheless, patient satisfaction with open access scheduling is generally high and studies of measurable outcomes seem to show benefits. One such study looked at the impact of open access in a pediatric clinic, showing a decrease in missed appointments and an increase in timely administration of childhood immunizations.[2]

INVEST IN THE SPACE AND EQUIPMENT YOU NEED FOR EFFICIENT PRACTICE

You should never struggle with cramped quarters or with outdated or poorly functioning equipment. Life is too short. Furthermore, proper space and equipment will usually pay off in increased productivity.

DEVELOP SYSTEMS TO MANAGE THE MOUNTAINS OF DATA

How many of us have struggled with old hospital charts almost too heavy to lift? These relics contained page after page of chart notes by physicians and nurses, lab and imaging reports, and endless documentation of vital signs and urinary output. In the clinic setting, our paper charts have been cluttered with prescription refill documentation and managed care authorizations, making it difficult to find clinically pertinent data.

The electronic medical record (EMR) has come to the rescue. We are trying to believe this, but not everyone is quite sure. Himmelstein and Woolhandler at Harvard Medical School write about today's lofty expectations with the EMR. Observing little benefit from large investments in EMRs, they report, "Indeed, computing at a typical hospital has not gotten much beyond what was available 25 years ago." In their opinion, the EMR has behind it a "disturbing array of unproven assumptions, wishful thinking, and special effects."[3] Yes, the study cited is from 2005, but was that really so long ago and have we made breakthrough innovations in the meantime?

Balancing the skepticism is a report by O'Neill and Klepack telling about what happened when a family practice in rural New York went to EMRs. They tell about more efficient prescription ordering, more efficient billing, and enhanced quality management. In the second year after introducing the EMR, practice revenue jumped 20%, ascribed to better documentation.[4]

As for me, as both clinician and patient in a university hospital setting, I have had mixed feelings. When we first learned that an EMR was on the way, the speaker at the initial meeting said, "In the beginning you will hate the electronic record. In the end you will come to love it." Although the EMR and I have not yet developed an amorous relationship, I have liked the easy access to up-to-date chart notes and lab data. There is no waiting for reports to be filed; the clinician types in the note and it is there if an emergency occurs that evening. And when I was recently a surgical patient, I liked that on my journey through the pre-admission process and on the hospital floor, every clinician had access to my problem list, medication list, and current laboratory data.

SEEK WAYS TO MAKE THE PATIENT'S VISIT JUST A LITTLE MORE PERSONAL AND INFORMATIVE

There are a number of ways to make the patient's visit to the doctor a less stressful and perhaps even a little enjoyable:

- Be sure that your waiting room is a pleasant place to be. Go and sit there for a while some day, just to get the feel of the space.
- See that patients are informed if there will be a delay in being seen. One clinic has a dry-erase board in the waiting room, telling expected wait times for clinicians in the office. Not a bad idea.
- Encourage your staff to speak to patients using their names.
- Consider employing bilingual employees if warranted by your practice population.
- Check for patient preferences and comfort with the examination gown, room temperature, and the presence of others (family or learners) in the room.
- Print copies of pertinent reports for patients. For example, the ECG tracing, X-ray and key laboratory reports.
- Wrap up by asking if everything has been covered and if the patient understands what has been said.

SUPPORT YOUR OFFICE STAFF MEMBERS IN THEIR DEALINGS WITH PATIENTS

Team members must be empowered to make certain operational decisions and even offer appropriate medical advice. No physician can field every appointment request or respond to every health care question received by telephone. Most such issues will be staff responsibilities, but such delegation to staff members, of course, must come after careful coaching and observation. In the jargon of leadership theory, what happens is building task-related maturity. The new office nurse may not be ready to field questions from Mrs. Jones about suspected reactions to the many medications she is taking, but in time, and after getting to know Mrs. Jones, the then-experienced office nurse may be Mrs. Jones' go-to advisor.

BE WILLING TO LEARN FROM THE CUSTOMER SERVICE EXPERTS

We clinician don't make or sell widgets, a word used since 1924, when playwrights George S. Kaufman and Marc Connelly presented a comic hero torn between his love of writing music that earned no income and the prospect of a mind-numbing, but salary-paying job in a factory where "widgets" were made.[5] The play was *Beggar on Horseback*, and widget was never explained, but I am quite happy that I need not make nor sell them for a living. Instead, you and I are physicians and what we offer to our patients – our customers – is service. A few years ago, I ruminated about how often our patients encounter poor customer service in our offices and hospitals and, as is my weakness, I wrote an article, summarized below, describing some of the service experts in my life.[6]

- My mechanic. After working on my car, Dimitri always gives me a document showing just what was done. Why aren't we better about giving patients documentation of what we did and what was found, such as lab and X-ray results?
- My dentist. When I get my twice-yearly dental checkup, the receptionist signs me up to receive a reminder for the next appointment. There is no way they will let me forget to come back on time. Why don't we physicians make the full use of reminders?
- The hotel staff on my vacation. Not long ago, my wife and I stayed at a small resort hotel in southern Oregon. As we checked in, the desk clerk was careful to learn our names and how we preferred to be addressed. From then on, everyone on the hotel staff seemed able to address us by name, a remarkable feat that can only be achieved with focused effort. For us, it should be much easier with a medical record in hand.

■ My mattress salesman. Last week we bought a new mattress, which was delivered yesterday. Today we received a telephone call from Jim, our salesman, hoping that we had had a good night's sleep. We had. Now why don't we call our patients more often to see how things are going the day after an office visit?

■ The salesperson at Nordstrom Department Store. When my wife shops at Nordstrom's the salesperson is only too happy to go with her from department to department, helping her find just what she is looking for. How often do we go the extra mile to guide our patients through the health care maze?

■ My accountant. I have quick access to my accountant by email, with prompt replies to questions. Why don't we physicians offer such service more often?

LEARN TO MANAGE TIME EFFECTIVELY

One key to having a satisfying practice each day is learning how to take control of your own time. Here, I am reminded of one of Murphy's Laws: Work will expand to exceed the time allotted (More on Murphy's Laws in Chap. 11). In fact, time is a precious commodity, which you should value highly. Your patients certainly value your time – and their own.

A good first step is a time analysis. Get a small notebook, and record what you do each waking hour for a week. Then review your findings by asking four questions:

1. What are the time wasters? These include handling papers more than once, pacing in the hall while the patient changes into an examination gown, and allowing interruptions that aren't urgent situations.
2. What am I doing that should be done by someone else? This may include photocopying, logging routine data on the computer, answering everyday telephone inquiries, and setting up for procedures such as suturing and casting.
3. What could I be doing differently to get control of my time? Are you fully booking your day, knowing that there will be emergencies that must be accommodated?

Are you scheduling patients so late in the afternoon that working overtime is a certainty for everyone?

4. What is recorded in the time log that should come "off my plate" entirely? Are you attending meetings that serve no useful purpose? Do you see your favorite pharmaceutical representatives monthly even though you are learning nothing new?

In a study of time management problems, König and Kleinmann used vignettes of typical time management decisions.[7] The authors found that "people discount future consequences of their time management decisions, meaning that they work on tasks with smaller but sooner outcomes rather than on tasks with larger but later outcomes." For example, a harried physician is more likely to save a few appointment slots for emergencies (small, but rapid results) than undertake a change to open access scheduling (a much larger change with later and greater results).

Fundamentally, time management begins with distinguishing *controllable* from *uncontrollable* time (most physicians need to travel each day from home to office, and perhaps from office to hospital). Callan estimated physician-controllable time to be 20–50% of the working day, and adds that it should be higher (Callan, p. 90). Your job and mine is taking charge of our controllable time while doing our best to steal a few hours from the so-called uncontrollable group.

BE AWARE WHEN YOU ARE LOSING TIME CONTROL OF AN ENCOUNTER AND THUS YOUR SCHEDULE

Some patients just take longer to see than others, as acknowledged by Dr. Reynolds contemplating a visit by Mrs. D in the introductory quote to this chapter. The difficulty is not necessarily that they have a long problem list, although that is often true. The problem arises in the patient's lack of time urgency; in fact, the patient has all the time in the world and is very happy to spend it with you. In addition to the patient with an extensive problem list, ready and willing to discuss each ache and pain in great detail, there is the person who cannot answer a question in less than six paragraphs.

As likeable as these individuals often are, we come to see them as "heartsink" patients – your heart sinks when you see the name on the appointment list.

Part of managing your day calls for orchestrating the visit by the patient who repeatedly consumes more than his/ her allotted time. One method is simply to schedule longer appointments for this person; then document and charge for the time. I have found that the best way to cope with a patient with a list is to take the list in your hand, and then decide which complaints will be addressed today. Setting limits may work: "Mrs. Waverly, we have 15 min scheduled. Let's make the best use of them, because at the end of 15 min, my nurse will knock on the door to remind me that the next patient is waiting." Whatever you do, time management success and your professional equanimity require that you – and not the time-consuming person – maintain control of the encounter.

AVOID CREATING TIME PROBLEMS FOR YOURSELF

Sometimes we create our own time management difficulties. For me, this has often happened when I decide to do more than was planned. The patient here to follow up on diabetes care has a mole on his arm. Why not remove it today? A youngster with a sore throat needs a school physical? Why not do it today – with all the hearing and vision checks and the review of immunizations? These extra services are kindly gestures, and the patients are genuinely grateful, but they are sure to take longer than the scheduled visit, meaning that you and your staff will be under time pressure for the rest of the session.

When I am serving as preceptor in our clinic and a resident suggests doing an unscheduled elective procedure, I suggest that he/she thinks like a dentist. Imagine that you have gone to your dentist for a regular checkup, and the dentist has just discovered that you have a cavity that needs to be filled. What will the dentist do? Will he fill the cavity today? Not a chance. You will be asked to return for a later appointment, when there is scheduled time for the procedure. When tempted to perform the time-consuming unscheduled service, think "dentist," and schedule the separate appointment, which will both keep you on schedule today and also clarify your billing for the two separate services.

COMPLETE TODAY'S CHARTING TODAY

Record your clinical notes in the office, ideally after each encounter while the facts are fresh in your mind. Next best is completing your notes at the end of a session. The wise physician does not write notes during family time in the evening, even though the EMR may allow access at your home. Ideally you should never let the sun set with unfinished chart notes, a threat to precise and complete documentation, an invitation to errors, and an admission that time management has eluded your control.

NOT ALL YOUR DAILY TIME WILL BE SPENT PRODUCTIVELY: AT LEAST AS WE TEND TO DEFINE PRODUCTIVELY

Sometimes the clinician actually needs a little break. This can be a coffee break, a walk in the fresh air outside, or even – horrors – a short nap in your comfortable desk chair. Look upon these diversions as recharging your batteries, and don't hesitate to include them in your schedule, if that works for you.

And while you are contemplating relative productivity of various times of the day, keep the Pareto principle in mind.

PARETO 80/20 PRINCIPLE WILL BE EVIDENT IN MANY FACETS OF YOUR PRACTICE

The story begins with Vilfredo Pareto, an Italian economist and gardener. As a gardener, he observed that 20% of his pea-pods yielded 80% of his harvest of peas. He also noted that 20% of the population owned 80% of the land. He went on, as an economist, to discover that 20% of the population of Italy controlled 80% of the wealth. From these observations comes the Pareto principle, an eponymic descriptor created by American industrial engineer Joseph M. Juran (1904–2008). Succinctly stated, the Pareto principle holds that 20% of a set is responsible for 80% of a related outcome.[8]

What, then, are some medical practice management implications of the Pareto 80/20 principle?

▓ Twenty percent of your patients will cause 80% of your staff complaints.
▓ Eighty percent of your missed appointments will be traced to 20% of your patients.
▓ Twenty percent of your patients will be make 80% of your night and weekend telephone calls.
▓ Eighty percent of your most important and satisfying work will be done in 20% of your time.

DO YOUR MOST IMPORTANT WORK AT YOUR PERSONAL BEST TIME

Implicit in this precept is considering if you are a morning or evening person. One often-overlooked step in effective time management is planning your day to be consistent with your biorhythm. You and I need to reconcile our practices with our personal biologic clocks. For each of us there is a time of day when we are most creative, intense, and alive. These best times of day allow us divide the world into two types of people: *Morning Persons* and *Evening Persons*. About two-thirds of generalist physicians are morning persons and about one-third are evening persons. What is my basis for asserting this? At least once a year for the past 15 years, I have presented a talk on leadership to groups of generalist physicians; usually, the audience is about 100–200 persons. At one point in the interactive session and in the context of learning to manage one's own life, I ask for a show of hands: How many of you are morning persons? Evening persons? How many of you are just good all day? For the most part there is no hesitation; almost everyone knows. As the hands go up, the breakdown is remarkably consistent: Morning persons: 60+ percent. Evening persons: 30+ percent. And in each group, there will be a few "undecideds," who have no strong morning vs. evening preference.

Now, as I mentioned, my sample in this somewhat unscientific survey is generalist physicians, mostly family physicians. Would the numbers be different in a large group of surgeons, whose specialties are relentlessly morning oriented? Might obstetricians be more evening oriented? Would emergency physicians have a higher number of "undecideds?"

Now, why do I take the space to present the topic of circadian biorhythms in some detail? Because it can have a lot to do with your professional productivity and, in fact, with your life. I will consider professional life and time management first.

You and I will achieve our best professional results by doing what is most challenging – that which calls for alertness, concentration, and sometimes innovation – during our best times. The "best time" concept may explain a recent study showing that colonoscopies performed early in the morning resulted in the detection of significantly more polyps and more histologically confirmed polyps than procedures performed later in the day.[9] I urge that you protect that "best time" from the mundane issues that can threaten it. As for me, I am a strong morning person, and my day as an academic physician has a wide variety of tasks and opportunities – teaching, patients, meetings, mentoring, writing, and more. I know that the one activity that involves the most creativity and requires the freshest mind is writing. For this reason, I guard my morning, especially the first few hours. No routine meetings or mind-numbing conference calls at that time. No unnecessary interruptions. No mundane paper-work. All of those can come later in the day. If I were a night owl, I suspect my priorities regarding "best time" would be different.

While on management and "best times," I suggest that you seek to work with key staff members who share the same biorhythm as you. In job interviews, there are a number of prohibited questions; these concern personal illness, sexual orientation, family issues, and so forth. But I don't see any reason why you and I cannot ask a prospective employee whether he/she is a morning or evening person. I don't know about you, but I would prefer working with someone whose biorhythms are in the same cycle as mine.

Then there is your personal life and mine. Most of us will marry, and although I have no survey data to cite, anecdotal evidence suggest that morning persons and evening persons will marry one another – and each will spend the rest of their married lives trying to change the other.

RESPECT YOUR PATIENT'S TIME AS VALUABLE

Here, we return to the patient's perception of time. Our patients, like us, perceive themselves as having very busy lives. They value their time, just as we do, and they resent any system that seems to waste treasured minutes of their days.

In a study based on an emergency department (ED) setting, Cassidy-Smith and colleagues looked at patient satisfaction and "throughput" times – the patient's time from first arrival to walking out the door at the end of the encounter.[10] Their study used the Disconfirmation Paradigm, psychological jargon for the profound thesis that people become unhappy with service expectations that are not met. Intuitive as this thesis may seem to us, it remained for the authors to supply some numbers, based on interviews of 1,118 patients. They concluded that throughput time that exceeded expectations led to general dissatisfaction with the ED visit.

In a medical encounter, patients have two time values – their own time and the time spent with the physician. I have been fortunate to visit a number of countries abroad and to look at their health care systems, many of which are government controlled. Without identifying the countries and offending my friends there, I will report that in several settings I have heard the lament: "Three hour wait; three minute visit." In case there is any confusion, this is not intended as praise for the system.

A study by Anderson et al offers an interesting insight. The authors surveyed 5,030 patients on their experiences with their primary care encounters. I will quote the conclusion, which I find instructive: "The time spent with the physician is a stronger predictor of patient satisfaction than is the time spent in the waiting room. These results suggest that shortening patient waiting times at the expense of time spent with the patient to improve patient satisfaction scores would be counter-productive."[11] One way to operationalize this finding might be to use waiting room time for teaching sessions with staff members or interactions with students instead of providing old issues *National Geographic* magazine for patients to read.

RESPECT THE PERSONAL TIME OF YOUR STAFF

The best physicians do not have office hours that run late every afternoon. If this occurs, there is something dysfunctional happening. Smoothly running medical teams stay more or less on time. They also end the day when promised, which I consider one index of a humane and smoothly functioning practice. Staff members are likely to have kids arriving home from school, meals to prepare, and family events scheduled. Come to think of it, perhaps you do, also. Thus, it is helpful to keep everything moving on schedule.

Show your team how to use time more effectively by anticipating your needs. Here are some useful methods by which your professional staff can help everyone be more efficient and get home in time for dinner:

- Logging the visit into the EMR
- Obtaining a preliminary history, at least learning the chief complaint and duration of the symptom
- Gowning patients, so that the doctor can complete the visit without having to leave the exam room while the patient changes attire
- Obtaining a urine specimen when the patient complains of urinary symptoms
- Preparing the operative site and setting out needed instruments in anticipation of a procedure
- Seeing that patient's name and address are preprinted on Rx blank (if you are still using paper prescriptions)
- Learning to give instructions to patients, such as in proper use of the diaphragm or care of a wound site

ACKNOWLEDGE STAFF ACHIEVEMENTS

Your staff members spend many of their waking hours working to help you be a successful clinician. For this dedicated hard work, a paycheck is not enough. The wise physician finds ways to say "Thank you," and does so in creative ways. In research for my leadership talk (mentioned above in connection with morning and evening persons), I came across the axiom that the creative use of rewards is one of the characteristics that distinguishes the best leaders.

One way to be sure our staff members are rewarded is to institutionalize the process. This can be done by the use of "applause cards." Your practice can have some cards available for patients or family members to note instances of exceptional service. Then the lead clinician can read the comments at the next staff meeting, and perhaps quote them in an annual performance review.

SEEK FEEDBACK FROM YOUR PATIENTS ABOUT HOW WELL YOU MEET THEIR NEEDS

One often underutilized practice management tool is the customer service feedback report. From time to time, the physician should survey a sample of patients in the practice, asking some open-ended questions intended to determine how well patient expectations are being met and how service could be better. Not being an advocate of long and wordy questionnaires, I suggest that you use some iteration of three general questions:

1. What are we doing right?
2. What could we do better?
3. What ideas or suggestions do you have to offer us?

Eliciting customer feedback can not only help the practice but also provide an occasional bright idea that changes the way things are done, such as the suggestion of sending a monthly practice newsletter. Patient feedback with attention to responses may help assure your continuing success in a competitive environment. After all, employers and managed care companies sometimes drop medical practices when they believe that customer care standards are not being met.[12] On the other hand, if things are going well, feedback from patients can give you the personal satisfaction that comes with leadership of a harmonious and efficient team.

WISE WORDS ABOUT MAKING A LIVING AS A CLINICIAN

Medicine is not a lucrative profession. It is a divine one.
John Coatley Lettsom (1744–1815) (McDonald, p. 60)

▧ *Beware of the men who call you "Doc." They rarely pay their bills.* Sir William Osler (1849–1919) (Silverman et al, p. 64)
One of my greatest surprises in private practice was when personal friends neglected to pay my bill.

▧ *It is because we have begun to act like merchants, and in many instances to observe the same hours, that the public expects us to be regulated by the same restraints.* John L. McClenahan (1915–) (Strauss, p. 385)
Merchants! It began with "practice announcements," and now we have giant billboards and commercials on television telling of successful cosmetic surgery.

▧ *Our patients hire and fire us at every visit.*[13]
Doctor William Jackson Epperson, practicing in Murrells Inset, South Carolina, obviously has a keen awareness that we are purveyors of a service – albeit a very essential service – and our patients are customers who can choose to deal with us, or not.

▧ *Never hire an employee or adopt an office strategy to save yourself from talking with patients.* (Meador, number 84)
Your employees are there to facilitate your contact with patients, not to shield you from them.

▧ *If you can't be smart, at least be organized.* (Anon)

▧ *Treat every patient the way you would want your own mother to be treated by her doctor.* (Anon)

REFERENCES

1. Beach MD, Duggan PS, Cassel CK, Geller G. What does "respect" mean? Exploring the moral obligation of health professionals to respect patients. *J Gen Intern Med.* 2007;22(5):692–695.
2. O'Connor ME, Matthews BS, Gao D. Effect of open access scheduling on missed appointments, immunizations, and continuity of care for infant well-child visits. *Arch Pediatr Adolescent Med.* 2006;160(9):889–893.
3. Himmelstein DU, Woolhandler S. Hope and hype: predicting the impact of electronic medical records. *Health Aff (Millbrook).* 2005;24(5):1121–1123.
4. O'Neill L, Klepack W. Electronic medical records for a rural practice. *J Med Syst.* 2007;31(1):25–33. Score one for the EMR.

5. New plays. Time; March 25, 1924. <http://www.time.com/time/ magazine/article/0,9171,736212-1,00.html/> Accessed April 13, 2009.
6. Taylor RB. Learning from the service experts. *Female Patient*. 2005;30(1):7–8.
7. König CJ, Kleinmann M. Time management problems and discounted utility. *J Psychol*. 2007;141(3):321–334.
8. Pareto principle – how to apply it, and what to avoid. <http://www.pinnicle.com/Articles/Pareto_Principle/pareto_principle.html/> Accessed April 13, 2009.
9. Finn R. First colonoscopy of the day yields more polyps. *Fam Pract News*. Aug. 15, 2008;38(16):26.
10. Cassidy-Smith TN, Baumann BM, Boudreaux ED. The disconfirmation paradigm: throughput times and emergency department satisfaction. *J Emerg Med*. 2007;32(1):7–13.
11. Anderson RT, Camacho FT, Balkrishnan R. Willing to wait? The influence of patient wait times on satisfaction with primary care. *BMC Health Serv Res*. 2007;7:31–34.
12. Zimmerman D, Zimmerman P, Lund C. Customer service: the new battlefield for market share. *Healthc Financ Manage*. 1997;51(10):51–53.
13. Epperson WJ. Radiating courtesy and professionalism. *Fam Pract Manag*. 2007;14(3):16.

8

Staying Up To Date

Certainly the doctor who thinks his student days are over when he gets his medical diploma, or even his certificate of hospital internship, is unfortunate – but his patients are more unfortunate than he. In no other profession in the world is it so necessary to keep up with the times.

American physician W. M. Johnson[1]

Is there a being more deserving of scorn and pity than the physician whose medical knowledge is outdated, and whose clinical skills have withered? The choice of a medical career connotes a commitment to lifetime learning. And what was true when Dr. W. M. Johnson wrote the introductory paragraph above in the 1930s is even truer now, owing to the accelerating pace of change in medical knowledge and techniques. Each year, we physicians and scientists encounter literally thousands of new scientific factoids, pharmaceutical agents, and drug interactions. I am fond of telling my medical students that, with the exception of a very few drugs such as salicylates and digitalis, the medications I use today were all introduced after I finished medical school and postgraduate training. Only diligent attention to continuing medical education (CME) keeps us from becoming professional dinosaurs.

One of my favorite perspectives on keeping up-to-date is by Doctor C.H. Low, presented as part of a medical school commencement address and subsequently published in the Singapore Medical Journal[2]:

Once upon a time, I was a young medical student like you; and to a great extent, I am still a medical student today – perhaps an old one. The moment you take up medicine, you are committed to be a student all your life. When I was in medical school, there

R.B. Taylor, *Medical Wisdom and Doctoring: The Art of 21st Century Practice*, DOI 10.1007/978-1-4419-5521-0_8, © Springer Science+Business Media, LLC 2010

was no such thing as flexible gastroscope, ultrasound, or CT scan. Laparoscopic and laser surgery were still in the realms of imagination. Yes, dear friends, unless you are committed to learning all your life, you'll be exiled into the wilderness of medical ignorance and antiquity. We do not need other people to tell us that continuing medical education is good for us. Indeed we know that CME is an absolute necessity – it is an essential part of our medical survival kit.

AVOID PROFESSIONAL ISOLATION

From time to time in my career, I have been involved in retraining senior physicians who have become out of touch with current medical practice. Most are not physicians who have had an illness or injury. They suffer no cognitive defect. They are not lazy; in fact, they have often been exceptionally hardworking. The common thread is that they have become isolated from their fellow physicians, and consequently they approach today's disease with yesterday's methods.

Solo practice is a prominent risk factor. So is rural practice, with few physicians nearby. None of the out-of-date physicians I have encountered cared for hospital patients or worked in urban group practices; instead, they examined and treated patients in a sort of professional time capsule, uninfluenced by the scrutiny of colleagues. In addition, the out-of-date physicians seldom attended CME conferences or review courses.

The lesson to be learned is to stay connected with other physicians. Ask their opinions about clinical entities you encounter. Discuss complex cases during chance encounters and at medical staff meetings. Talk about recent advances in the literature. In short, use your professional interactions as one of the ways you stay up-to-date in medicine.

MAINTAIN YOUR CLINICAL SKILLS

You worked hard to learn what you know and what you can do with your hands today. Do not casually abandon hard-earned skills. I especially worry about young physicians who are abandoning hospital care and doing only office practice. Medicine changes quickly, and a few years away from hospital practice is all you need to become dangerously out of date. We are now creating retraining programs for physicians who, for various reasons, have been away from hospital practice for a few years.

As medicine becomes progressively more fragmented, I also have grave misgivings about the clinical judgment of some physicians, especially self-proclaimed generalists who spend their days doing cosmetic procedures, prescribing herbal medications, or doing routine physical examinations. Some day soon a person will come to one of these physicians in the early stages of coronary artery disease, heart failure, cancer – during the golden time when early detection and intervention might avert the massive heart attack, the ventricular thrombus that results in an embolic stroke, or the lethal metastasis. Will the physician with atrophied clinical skills be able to make a timely diagnosis?

DO NOT COUNT TOO HEAVILY ON YOUR EXPERIENCE

I am fond of the old saying that experience is what we rely on when we haven't read anything for a while. When we are young clinicians, we are rich in textbook knowledge and we yearn for experience. As we near the end of our careers, our data base of knowledge may be a little dated, but we are rich in experience. The only trouble is, in the words of American surgeon J. Chalmers DaCosta (1863–1933): "What we call experience is often a dreadful list of ghastly mistakes." (Taylor 2008, p. 145) And learning from mistakes is a costly way to gain knowledge.

Unconvinced of the merits of experiential learning, medical students and residents are rightfully skeptical of anecdotal advice. I well know that when a resident asks me for help with a clinical problem and I begin my reply, "In my experience …," the young physician is rolling his or her eyes and hoping I will get around to an evidence-based response.

RECOGNIZE YOUR BEST LEARNING STYLE

If we can't count on experience as the best teacher, then we must seek other ways of learning. These alternatives to experience will involve reading, listening, or using our hands.

For generations, medical students have endured seemingly endless lectures on basic science and clinical topics, while practicing physicians have dutifully attended lectures and workshops at CME conferences. These activities supplement personal reading of medical journals and books, plus focused Internet searches. Through all these activities, we sometimes wonder, "Is this the best use of my time, and am I really learning anything?"

The wise physician asks: "What is my best learning style?" For some, the answer is solitary reading. For others, it is interactive learning, participating in workshops, or using on-line CME programs. Still others of us seek the presence of experts – derisively defined as people from out of town with slides (now PowerPoint, of course). Today it is fashionable to proclaim that the traditional medical CME model – referring to the lecture series with "talking heads" – is broken, an attitude reflected in declining attendance at medical specialty teaching conferences. Nevertheless, I urge you to consider a few facts about the lecture-based medical conference: First of all, some of us still learn the best while hearing a lecture, watching slides on a screen, and taking notes about pertinent facts. Then, at a conference, there is no competition from daily patient care demands; the doctor is generally out of town and having practice phone calls fielded by a colleague. Finally, there is the camaraderie of the conference – the opportunity to speak with fellow physicians, often from other areas of the country.

The message of these few paragraphs is as follows: Make your personal assessment of your best learning style. Devote your CME time to quiet reading, if that is what works best for you. Or perhaps search the web-based literature for new information about a few cases you see each day. But if you enjoy medical conferences, and feel that you learn from the presentations there, then by all means, go and enjoy them.

READ, READ, AND READ SOME MORE

Sir William Osler once stated, "It is astonishing with how little reading a doctor can practice medicine, but it is not astonishing how badly he may do it." (Osler, p. 75) Osler cited books, perhaps because there were few medical journals in his day. If he were writing today, Osler might advise reading current refereed medical journals and consulting the reliable sites on the World Wide Web.

Young physicians should cultivate the reading habit early in their careers. Furthermore, they should understand the various categories of educational resources available. There are texts such as the textbook of anatomy or physical diagnosis you used early in medical school; textbooks are generally read as part of a formal course of learning. There are books and, increasingly, web reference sites, such as *Harrison's Principles of Internal Medicine* that we consult to be sure we are using the latest medical evidence; we go to Harrison's and similar sources to find answers to specific questions. Has anyone but the editor of *Harrison's* ever read it cover to cover?

From here, we turn to journals. Below, I will name five journals. The ones listed are generally considered to be the top general-interest medical journals in the world. This designation is based not only on the sentiment of knowledgeable physicians, but on a slightly arcane device called the Impact Factor. Very simply stated, the impact factor measures how often a journal's articles are cited in other publications. Devised in 1955 by Eugene Garfield to "evaluate the significance of a particular work and its impact on the literature and thinking of the period," the impact factor has become a means to rank journals.[3] Among the broad based journals examined by Chew et al, those with the top impact factors, presented in ranked order, were:

New England Journal of Medicine
The Lancet
Journal of the American Medical Association (JAMA)
Annals of Internal Medicine
British Medical Journal (BMJ)

The five mentioned above are broad-based journals. There are hundreds of others, most of which are more narrowly focused, competing for your attention, and keeping up can be a challenge. Next, I will offer some tips on how to read these journals and avoid information overload.

LEARN TO APPROACH THE MEDICAL LITERATURE EFFICIENTLY

English essayist Joseph Addison (1672–1719) once observed, "Reading is to the mind what exercise is to the body." I think that we can expand the analogy by stating that both activities should be done efficiency. Neither you nor I would undertake an unstructured, excessively rigorous and otherwise inappropriate exercise program. Nor should we do so with our medical reading. But consider that there are more than 20,000 medical and scientific medical journals in the world, with more added each year. Manning and DeBakey suggest that physicians may receive some 5,000 pages of journal material each month. (Manning and DeBakey, p. 60) Clearly, planning a sensible approach to medical reading takes some thought.

Above, I briefly described the leading peer-reviewed, broad-based medical journals – *New England Journal of Medicine (NEJM)*, *The Lancet*, *Journal of the American Medical Association (JAMA)*, *Annals of Internal Medicine*, and the *British Medical Journal*. I recommend that you select and subscribe to the two that seem to be most consonant with your needs. My personal favorites have been the New England Journal of Medicine and JAMA – perhaps reflecting my ethnocentrism as an American, or maybe my resistance to change after many years of faithful reading. Then, add the two leading journals in your specialty. If you are a cardiologist, for instance, I suspect that one of your specialty-specific choices will be the *American Journal of Cardiology*.

Now that we have selected and subscribed to our four favorite journals – two broad-based and two specialty-focused – it's time to plan our reading, no small task since issues arrive on our desks relentlessly. NEJM comes weekly; JAMA is published 48 times a year, almost weekly; and the American Journal of Cardiology arrives 24 times a year. And I have not mentioned the advertiser-supported journals that show up uninvited in your mailbox and that actually sometimes contain provocative and well-documented articles. How do wise physicians keep up?

I looked at this issue a few years ago, beginning with a literature search from which I concluded that physicians tend to spend 3–5 h a week reading journals, and sometimes books and medical sites on the Internet.[4] In doing so, we shift between three reading styles – gorging, grazing, or hunting. *Gorging* refers to the attempt to read it all, thumbing through every page of every journal, analogous to beginning a fitness program by hoisting barbells exceeding your body weight. Such activity delights the paid advertisers, but soon proves to be exhausting and unproductive.

Experienced physicians soon learn the skill of *grazing*. They scan the table of contents for articles of interest. (As an aside to medical authors, this means that the article title may be all your reader ever sees of your report, and hence you need to make every word count.) From the titles, the physician will then turn to the first page of an article or two or even three in an issue. Here, he or she reads that abstract, and often stops there. Some articles are read in their entirety, when the reader wants to know details of methods and subtle result findings.

What about *hunting*, the targeted search for the answer to a question? Years ago, I kept files of papers ripped from journals, and even today I retain the last year or two of the print journals to which I subscribe, the latter an anachronistic habit that sometimes still proves useful. Hunting, however, has become an Internet sport, using *PubMed* or occasionally *Google*. My paper files were shredded long ago. I can't promise what will eventually happen to my big bookcase full of recent journal issues, but I am sure that your future and mine lies in acquiring information mastery skills that include very little paper.

HONE YOUR INFORMATION MASTERY SKILLS

A book about medical wisdom and doctoring would be incomplete without a discussion of evidence-based medicine (EBM), which is really a systematic approach to "hunting" for answers to clinical questions. The skill set needed to navigate the oceans of scientific data is called "information mastery." (Taylor 2003, p. 34.)

Sackett et al have provided us with a handy definition of EBM: "the conscientious, explicit, and judicious use of current best evidence in making clinical decisions about the care of an individual patient."[5] Note the key words and phrases in the definition – explicit, current best evidence, and individual patient. Thus, the physician employing an EBM approach will follow five steps: The first step is the development of a focused, answerable clinical question, such as: Is an eye patch appropriate therapy for a corneal abrasion? Next comes a search for the best evidence available regarding the topic, classically involving peer-reviewed reports of well-designed clinical trials. The third step, evaluation of the quality of the evidence found, calls for some skill and for an avoidance of bias. Once the evidence has been evaluated and interpreted, the conclusion – e.g., current clinical evidence does not support the once-favored use of an eye patch for the treatment of an otherwise uncomplicated corneal abrasion – and applying the conclusion in practice.[6] The fifth and final step is assessing the impact of any resulting change on one's clinical outcomes.

Not all clinicians are ardent fans of EBM, which DeSimone has dubbed "reductionist inference-based medicine."[7] Some hold that EBM favors biomedical data and ignores the psychosocial aspect of clinical care. Rogers asserts that the current processes of EBM are biased against women; she states, "The biomedical model of health that underpins most medical research used by EBM ignores the social and political context which contributes to the ill-health of women."[8] Older physicians, if asked, might reveal feelings that EBM seems to devalue their wealth of practice-based experience, and that it represents a threat to clinical freedom – the prerogative to make clinical decisions based on the totality of each clinical situation. In the end, of course, EBM is concerned with answers to focused questions about clinical entities, and how these answers may apply to a specific patient in your office. Thus EBM, used thoughtfully, is a tool that can enhance the doctor's clinical freedom; it is a reasonable consideration in the complex process of decision making, along with one's personal experience, patient preferences, and the psychosocial context of the clinical setting.

One of the current efforts of EBM and information mastery advocates is the cataloging of "validated" answers to pertinent clinical questions, thus sparing the busy practitioner the need to undertake the "five steps" each time a clinical dilemma is presented. Instead, at least in the primary care setting, clinician scholars are seeking answers to key questions in settings that might actually change practice, developing evidence based answers, and validating the information in practice. One such endeavor is identified as "Problem Oriented Evidence that Matters," or POEMs. (Taylor 2003, p. 34.) Recently studied questions have been:

- Can warfarin therapy be safely interrupted for an elective procedure? Answer: Yes, warfarin can be withheld for up to 1 week in patients at risk of bleeding because of an invasive procedure such as colonoscopy or dental surgery.[9]
- Should clinicians use duplex ultrasonography to screen for clinically significant carotid artery stenosis in asymptomatic patients? Answer: No, the procedure is unhelpful and likely to cause harm.[10]
- Are there any effective topical medications for childhood eczema that don't contain steroids or calcineurin inhibitors (e.g., tacrolimus), and that are available over the counter?
- Answer: Yes. There are three useful emollients: tar products, gamma-linoleic acid preparations such as borage oil and evening primrose oil, and MAS063DP (Atopiclair).[11]
- Is biphasic, prandial, or basal insulin best for poorly controlled type 2 diabetes mellitus? Answer: Basal insulin, focusing on patients with an initial glycosylated hemoglobin exceeding 8.5%.[12]

The emerging dilemma, as the numbers of valid POEMs increase, is finding a way to organize the information into a format that is easily accessible by clinicians – the next horizon in information mastery.

MAINTAIN YOUR PERSONAL REFERENCE LIBRARY, WHETHER PAPER OR WEB-BASED

Even with the best information mastery skills, we still need our favorite reference sources. If using actual "hold-in-your-hands" books, be sure that you are using current editions. Today, most reference sources can be found on the web. Here is my bare-bones list of recommendations:

- *Medical dictionary*: Every clinician needs access to a comprehensive medical dictionary. There are two clear leaders available: *Dorland's Illustrated Medical Dictionary*, published by Saunders, and *Stedman's Medical Dictionary*, published by Lippincott, Williams and Wilkins. Both include the etymologic derivation of medical terms and both are available on-line.
- *General medical reference source*: A classic is *Harrison's Principles of Internal Medicine*, published by McGraw Hill, also available as *Harrison's Online*. My current favorite is *UpToDate*, available only online, a searchable source covering a broad scope of clinical topics and drugs, and offering hyperlinks to reference sources cited.
- *Comprehensive drug reference source*: The classic reference source is the *Physicians' Desk Reference* (PDR), currently a hefty 3,500 pages in length. Fortunately for those who cannot manage the hefty 8½ pound tome, the PDR is available online. Today, most young physicians use *Epocrates*, a free on-line source of drug information. Another option is the *Quick-Look Drug Book*, revised annually, and available both in print format and as a CD-ROM.
- *Specialty-specific reference book*: Buy the best reference book in your specialty, whether in print or on-line, and become familiar with how to use it. (Yes, each reference book has some peculiarities that you must learn in order to use it efficiently.) Then buy each new edition as it is released.

BECOME AN INTERNET "POWER USER"

This chapter on staying up-to-date would be incomplete without emphasizing the need to prepare for the telemedicine revolution we will experience throughout the twenty-first century.

Sometime in the future, we will look back in amazement at the primitive status of today's electronic medical records and online search capabilities. To prepare for the future, each clinician must begin today to work toward "power user" status. We need to augment our computer skills, to learn more and more about what the machines in front of us can do, and keep current with current innovations. In short, we, as clinicians, need to become as skilled in our computer use as our 15-year-old children.

Especially relevant to this "keeping-up-to-date" chapter is the probability that much of tomorrow's continuing education will be virtual E-learning. For example, Harden describes the International Virtual Medical School (IVIMEDS) in Dundee, Scotland.[13] The author describes guided-learning resources, a virtual practice with virtual patients, peer-to-peer learning and "ask-the-experts" opportunities. The school's philosophy is based on learning activities customized to the needs of the individual physician and "just-in-time" learning – making learning available to physicians when needed. To at least some degree, this is the CME of the future. If interested, you can access the school's web site at www.ivimeds.org.

Pappas and Falagas hold that "the future may see entire educational courses being conducted on the World Wide Web, unifying the medical community, provided some forms of free access are implemented."[14]

I'll return to the topic of the e-medicine of tomorrow in Chap. 13 to discuss what future office and hospital practice might look like.

KEEP A NOTEBOOK (OR NOW A COMPUTER FILE) OF WHAT'S NEW IN MEDICINE

Record the new information and also the source, so you can find it again in the future. Here are a few entries I made in my notebook while working on the manuscript for this book:

- "Among patients with stage III colon cancer receiving adjuvant chemotherapy, a family history of colorectal cancer is associated with a significant reduction in cancer recurrence and death," according to a study by Chan et al.[15] This finding seems paradoxical, but will be some comfort to stage III colon cancer patients with positive family histories.

■ In a West Virginia study, fatally injured drivers were more likely to have prescription drugs – notably opioid analgesics and depressants – than illegal drugs.[16] Sobering as this report should be for we who prescribe opioid and depressant medications, the leading culprit in the West Virginia study was alcohol.

■ Metformin can be prescribed, along with lifestyle modifications, to promote weight loss in patients who gain more than 10% of their pretreatment body weight while taking antipsychotic medications.[17] I'm not sure I am ready for this sort of polypharmacy, but the innovative use of metformin is intriguing.

■ In patients with atrial fibrillation and congestive heart failure, controlling rhythm (to maintain sinus rhythm) does not yield better clinical outcomes than rate control, making the simpler rate control the treatment of choice in these patients.[18] This is a clinically relevant study, given that patients with heart failure are at increased risk for atrial fibrillation.

■ Men with lower levels of plasma 25-hydroxyvitamin D are at increased risk of having a heart attack.[19] With this finding, can a recommendation for supplementary vitamin D be far behind?

PERHAPS ADD SOME "GEE-WHIZ FACTS" TO YOUR "WHAT'S-NEW" NOTEBOOK OR FILE

Gee-whiz facts are tidbits of information, generally bits and pieces of epidemiologic data that are interesting, and often are found on the initial PowerPoint slides of lectures on clinical topics. Gee-whiz facts often don't seem to have much clinical relevance ... until they do. Here are some examples of gee-whiz facts:

■ Approximately one third of the world's population is latently infected with *Mycobacterium tuberculosis*.[20]

■ Community-acquired methicillin-resistant *Staphylococcus aureus* causes almost three quarters of skin and soft tissue infections in United States communities.[21]

- Nearly a third of American adults are obese, a figure that has doubled in the past two decades.[22]
- The landmark article in the US medical literature that statistically linked smoking and lung cancer, written by Ernst L. Wynder and Evarts A. Graham, was published as recently as 1950.[23] (Some insist that there were earlier reports in the European medical journals.)
- There are 300–500 new cases of malaria annually, causing an estimated 1.5–2.7 deaths worldwide each year. The most likely victim is a child living in sub-Saharan Africa.[24]

CONSIDER EACH CONSULTATION AS A LEARNING OPPORTUNITY

Consultation, the opportunity to share the clinical care of a patient, can be one of the joys of medicine. In addition to the patient probably getting better care – two heads being better than one, or so they say – you have the opportunity to *learn*. I think of each consultation as a personalized educational experience, and I try to prepare accordingly.

First of all, I carefully frame the questions I want to be answered, and I make sure that both the consultant and the patient know what these questions are. Then, I often follow the advice of Manning and DeBakey and look up the subject in a standard reference source, just to refresh my knowledge. (Manning and DeBakey, p. 219) Then comes the most stimulating exercise of all: I try to imagine that I am the consultant faced with the problem involved. What would be my recommendation to the patient and to the primary care clinician? It is fun to see how close my hypothetical recommendation agrees with what the consultant says.

For example, one of our family medicine residents presented a patient – a 44-year-old male patient seeking a referral to a urologist. He was in general good health, except for his chief complaint – premature ejaculation. The patient had heard of a topical cream that is available, or maybe there were some pills that would help. He was adamant in his insistence on obtaining a referral to a urologist. And so, our learning-exercise question was: What would be the best therapy for this man? An online search showed that the

American Urological Association recommends antidepressants, notably the serotonin specific reuptake inhibitors (SSRI), as first line treatment, while also recommending prilocaine–lidocaine cream (EMLA).[25] The resident and I put our bet on an SSRI, and sure enough, the urologist recommended sertraline (Zoloft), a drug which we, of course, would have prescribed had the patient not insisted on a consultation.

Over the years, by following these steps, and especially after framing my imagined responses, I think my patients and I need a few less consultations than in the past.

THINK ABOUT WHAT YOU DO EACH DAY AND PERHAPS WRITE ABOUT IT

Scholarly contributions should not be the exclusive domain of academicians. Each of us sees interesting cases, develops handy techniques, and creates office innovations that might help fellow physicians, if only we would share our experiences. By doing so, we also might just become wiser physicians. Writing in 1954, Buck offers the opinion, "A physician who writes, other things being equal, is a better doctor than one who does not. This does not refer to *belles-lettres* (an avocation that has attracted a good number of indifferent and a few excellent physician authors) but to medical writing in the course of professional activity."[26]

Happily, writing opportunities exist in many settings: books, refereed journals, medical magazines, web sites, and the lay press. For me, writing as an avocation began by writing about my solo country practice in *Medical Economics* magazine, followed a few years later by writing trade books: My first was a health care guide for the senior citizen, cleverly titled *Feeling Alive After 65*.

J. Willis Hurst, MD tells of his mentor Paul Dudley White, pioneer cardiologist and a renowned and wise physician I was once privileged to meet, if only briefly. Hurst describes how, in the early 1900s, White collected data about his patients, recorded on 4 × 6 in. note cards. His notes on his cardiac patients included etiology, abnormal anatomy and physiology, and functional heart status – a system subsequently adopted by the New York Heart Association.

White, "took this large collection of cards, along with his bride, Ina, to the Isle of Capri, and wrote his first book, published in 1931." (Hurst JW. In: Manning et al, p. 45) I found no record of Ina's thoughts about Paul taking his card collection along on their honeymoon on Capri.

Now, very few of us will undertake such a heroic, even romantic task. Yet, any physician can submit a case report, write a letter to a medical journal commenting on a recent article, or post a comment on line at scholarly web sites such www.bmj.com, on which the British Medical Journal (BMJ) encourages "rapid responses" to articles published in the journal. For example, Vreeman and Carroll published a very nice article in the BMJ titled "Medical Myths," debunking popular misconceptions such as the notion that reading in dim light can ruin your eyes, showing that there is a place in the clinical literature for common-sense wisdom.[27] JAMA has regular sections titled "Poetry in Medicine" and "A Piece of My Mind," with no academic credentials needed for submission. Or, closer to home, this morning my local newspaper – The Oregonian – published a letter signed by two physicians, commenting on pending legislation regarding businesses allowing nursing mothers time during the work day to breast feed or pump.

KEEP YOUR MIND ACTIVE BY THINKING ABOUT THE POSSIBLY UNRECOGNIZED CONNECTIONS IN WHAT IS SEEN EACH DAY

Don't miss what may be the once-in-a-career opportunity to make a clinical connection that no one had made before, and perhaps taking some meaningful action. Pasteur has told us, "Chance only favors the mind which is prepared...."[28] Certainly John Snow (1813–1858), actually an anesthesiologist, had both a prepared mind and a penchant for epidemiology when he encountered the London cholera epidemic in the 1850s. Going from door to door to determine where people obtained their drinking water, Snow found that the incidence of cholera was much less in persons whose drinking water came from the Thames river upstream from the site where the city sewage was dumped into the river, while the cholera incidence was enormous in those whose drinking water came from sources downstream from the sewage outpouring. Today we remember John Snow because he recognized that, in own neighborhood of Soho, there was a high incidence of cholera in persons who drew water from the Broad Street pump. In a bold stroke of interventional epidemiology, Snow removed the handle of the Broad Street pump. His action helped lower the neighborhood cholera incidence rate, bringing it more in line with the incidence in employees of the nearby Lion Brewery, whose apparent resistance to cholera is attributed to their daily consumption of malt beverages to the virtual exclusion of drinking water.[29]

American geneticist Francis S. Collins (1950–), best known for his work on the human genome, has written an intriguing book titled *The Language of God*. In this book, he tells, "One of the most cherished hopes of a scientist is to make an observation that shakes up a field of research. Scientists have a streak of closeted anarchism, hoping that someday they will turn up some unexpected fact that will force a disruption of the framework of the day. That's what Nobel Prizes are given for." (Collins, p. 58). In addition to scientists, there is some of this "closeted anarchism" in most practicing clinicians. For example, in 1941, Australian ophthalmologist Norman McAlister Gregg first recognized the link between maternal rubella in early pregnancy and the development of congenital cataracts in infants.

In 1993, Indian Health Service physician Dr. James Creek was serving in a frontier area called the "Four Corners" because it included pieces of four states: Arizona, Colorado, New Mexico, and Utah. His observation of two young persons who died after developing acute dyspnea led to the discovery of a new species of hanta virus and what we now call the Hantavirus cardiopulmonary syndrome.

Then in 2007, Doctors Mukherjee and Shivakumar, working at the Command Hospital Air Force in Bangalore, India, described what they believed to be "the first case report of sildenafil-induced sensorineural hearing loss in the world literature."[30] Today, the televised consumer-directed advertisements for phosphodiesterase type 5 inhibitors warn of this uncommon side effect.

Even if you never find the publishable connection, your mind and your clinical skills will benefit from the intellectual exercise of just looking.

TEACH

Sir William Osler once wrote, "I desire no other epitaph ... than the statement that I taught medical students in the wards, as I regard this as by far the most useful and important work I have been called upon to do." (Silverman et al, p. 222.) A good teacher needs a reasonable fund of knowledge, the ability to communicate clearly, a willingness to insist upon high standards, a high level of energy, and a ready sense of humor – also, incidentally, attributes that help make one a successful practicing physician.

As I approach the final years of my career, I find it a little difficult to recall the many patients whose health I have improved, and even whose lives I have saved by timely diagnosis and insightful management of disease – all the instances of hyperlipidemia my statin prescriptions have improved, all the pneumonias I have treated with antibiotics, and all the fractures I have casted. What does come to mind is some of my teaching. In my role as medical educator since 1978, I have taught some 30 classes of students the diseases a skilled clinician might suspect based on a handshake (page 76), the best way to elicit the patellar reflex (page 81), and the diagnostic pearl that the patient with acute appendicitis is unlikely to be hungry (page 84). I have taught these students the correct way to present a patient to a colleague – for example, "This is a 73-year-old male retired school teacher with a 2 day history of recurrent substernal chest pain unrelieved by sublingual nitroglycerin." (page 69) I have helped them learn to sort the horses from the zebras, and how to recognize a zebra when one appears.

Today, part of medical education takes place in the community setting. For example, at our medical school, during any given week, some 250 of our medical students have clinical experiences in the offices of local physicians. If you live within a tank-of-gas drive from a medical school, there is probably an opportunity for you to teach some of tomorrow's physicians. And, as I tell my medical students, I want to do a very good job as teacher and make them the best doctors possible, because I'm not getting any younger and some day, one of them might just be my physician.

WISE WORDS ABOUT STAYING UP TO DATE

▨ *To teach is to learn twice.* French moralist Joseph Joubert (1754–1824)[31]

Curiously, Joubert was a gifted teacher and aphorist who wrote letters and handwritten notes, but did not actually publish anything during his lifetime.

▨ *The education of the doctor which goes on after he has his degree is, after all the most important part of his education.* American humorist Josh Billings (the pen name of Henry Wheeler Shaw) (1818–1885).[32]

In the 40 years of practice after receiving our MD degrees, we will gain a lot of experience and even learn a few new facts.

▨ *The killing vice of the young doctor is intellectual laziness.* Sir William Osler (1849–1919) (Bean and Bean, p. 73)

What would Osler have to say about physicians whose chief concern is lifestyle?

▨ *Once you start studying medicine you never get through with it.* American surgeon Charles H. Mayo (1865–1939) (Mayo, p. 15)

If you are not committed to lifelong learning, then choose a less challenging career such as investment banking or national politics.

▨ *It is not hard to learn more. What is hard is to unlearn when you discover yourself wrong.* Martin H. Fischer (1879–1962) (Strauss, p. 261)

Of course, the first step is realizing when one is wrong. Then comes the unlearning, and the replacement of flawed "knowledge" with current information, a little like unlearning "hunt-and-peck" to master touch-typing on your keyboard.

■ *Never consult a textbook that is older than the youngest medical student in your service.* From Meador, number 204. Today the useful life of a medical reference book is about 3 years, and with the availability of online resources, even 3 years may be too long.

REFERENCES

1. Johnson WM. *The True Physician: The Modern Doctor of the Old School*. New York: Macmillan; 1936:58.
2. Low CH. Reflection for young doctors and doctors of tomorrow. *Singapore Med J*. 1998;39(12):535–536.
3. Chew M, Villanueva EV, Van der Weyden MB. Life and times of the impact factor: retrospective analysis of the trends for seven medical journals (1994–2005) and their editors' views. *J R Soc Med*. 2007;100:142–149.
4. Taylor RB. How do we read the medical literature? *Female Patient*. 2004;29(1):8–10.
5. Sackett DL, Rosenberg WMC, Gray JAM, Haynes RB, Richardson WS. Evidence-based medicine: what it is and what it isn't. *BMJ*. 1995;312:71–72.
6. Turner A, Rabiu M. Patching for corneal abrasion. *Cochrane Database Syst Rev*. 2006;19(2):CD004764.
7. DeSimone J. Reductionist inference-based medicine, i.e. EBM. *J Eval Clin Pract*. 2006;12(4):445–449.
8. Rogers W. Evidence-based medicine and women: do the principles and practice of EBM further women's health? *Bioethics*. 2004;18(1):50–71.
9. Garcia DA, Regan S, Henault L, et al. Risk of thromboembolism with short-term interruption of warfarin therapy. *Arch Intern Med*. 2008;168:63–69.
10. US Preventive Services Task Force. Screening for carotid artery stenosis. US Preventive Services Task Force recommendation statement. *Ann Intern Med*. 2007;147:854–859.
11. Yates JE, Phifer JB, Flake D. Do non-medicated topicals relieve childhood eczema? *J Fam Med*. 2009;58(5):280–281.
12. Holman RR, Thorne KI, Farmer AJ, 4-T Study Group, et al. Addition of biphasic, prandial or basal insulin to oral therapy in type 2 diabetes. *N Engl J Med*. 2007;357:1716–1730.
13. Harden RM. A new vision for distance learning and continuing medical education. *J Contin Educ Health Prof*. 2005;25(1):43–51.
14. Pappas G, Falagas ME. Free internal medicine case-based education through the World Wide Web: how, where, and with what? *Mayo Clin Proc*. 2007;82(2):203–207.

15. Chan JA, Meyerhardt JA, Niedzwieki D, et al. Association of family history with cancer recurrence and survival among patients with stage III colon cancer. *JAMA*. 2008;299:2515–2523.

16. Centers for Disease Control and Prevention. Alcohol and other drug use among victims of motor vehicle crashes – West Virginia, 2004–2005. *MMWR Morb Mortal Wkly Rep*. 2006;55:1293–1296.

17. Wu RR, Zhao JP, Jin H, et al. Lifestyle intervention and metformin for treatment of antipsychotic-induced weight gain: a randomized controlled trial. *JAMA*. 2008;299:185–193.

18. Roy D, Talajic M, Nattel S, et al. Rhythm control versus rate control for atrial fibrillation and heart failure. *N Engl J Med*. 2008;358:2667–2677.

19. Giovannucci E, Liu Y, Hollis BW, Rimm EB. 25-Hydroxyvitamin D and risk of myocardial infarction in men: a prospective study. *Arch Intern Med*. 2008;168(11):1174–1180.

20. Inge LD, Wilson JW. Update on the treatment of tuberculosis. *Am Fam Physician*. 2008;78(4):457–465.

21. Centers for Disease Control and Prevention. Health-care-associated methicillin resistant *Staphylococcus aureus* (MRSA). <http://www.cdc.gov/ncidod/dhqp/ar_mrsa.html/> Accessed April 4, 2009.

22. Silver L, Bassett MT. Food safety for the 21st century. *JAMA*. 2008;300(8):957–959.

23. Wynder EL, Graham EA. Tobacco smoking as a possible etiologic factor in bronchiogenic carcinoma; a study of 684 proved cases. *JAMA*. 1950;143(4):329–336.

24. Suh KN, Kain KC, Keystone JS. Malaria. *CMAJ*. 2004;25:693–702.

25. Montague DK, Jarow J, Broderick GA, AUA Erection Dysfunction Guideline Update Panel, et al. AUA guideline on the pharmacologic management of premature ejaculation. *J Urol*. 2004;172:290–294.

26. Buck RW. Reading and writing. In: Garland J, ed. *The Physician and His Practice*. Boston: Little, Brown; 1954.

27. Vreeland RC, Carroll AE. Medical myths. *BMJ*. 2007; 335(7633):1288–1289.

28. Pasteur L. Inaugural lecture, University of Lille, December 7, 1854. In: Vallery-Radot R, ed. *The Life of Pasteur. Devonshire RL, trans*. Garden City, NY: Garden City Publishing; 1923:76.

29. Hempel S. *The Strange Case of the Broad Street Pump: John Snow and the Mystery of Cholera*. Berkeley: University of California Press; 2007.

30. Mukherjee B, Shivakumar T. A case of sensorineural deafness following ingestion of sildenafil. *J Laryngol Otol.* 2007;121(4): 395–397.
31. Taylor RB. *Academic Medicine: A Guide for Clinicians.* New York: Springer Verlag; 2006:120.
32. Billings JS. Educating the physician. *Boston Med Surg J.* 1894;131:140.

9

Mentoring Tomorrow's Physicians

> *Medical training is transformative. I promise you that when you come out of training, you will in some sense divide the world into doctors and non-doctors, and you will identify as a doctor.*
>
> American physician and author Perri Klass[1]

What makes a caring, empathic, and wise physician is not medical school. These qualities have their origins in our early environment – one's upbringing, grade school teachers, scout leaders and coaches, and later educators who take a special interest in one's personal development, and, of course, mentors.

This chapter is about mentoring aspiring and neophyte physicians – medical students, residents, and recently-minted practitioners who still recall their earliest patient care experiences and who are learning how to actually function as a physician. It tells about donning the mantle of a healer, and the obligations that act entails.

As a start, let us set the stage. Being a physician is like no other profession. A century before the time of Klass, English writer Rudyard Kipling (1865–1936), author of *Gunga Din* and *The Man Who Would Be King*, wrote about doctors and their self-identity. In *A Doctor's Work*, an address to medical students at London's Middlesex Hospital in 1908, He stated: "There are only two classes of mankind in the world – doctors and patients" (Strauss, p. 383). I tell medical students and residents that they and I have chosen the former, being a doctor, and will strive to put off patienthood as long as possible. And, since these young persons have elected to be physicians, I challenge them to be the very best they can.

R.B. Taylor, *Medical Wisdom and Doctoring: The Art of 21st Century Practice*, DOI 10.1007/978-1-4419-5521-0_9,
© Springer Science+Business Media, LLC 2010

In the words of Martí-Ibáñez (Martí-Ibáñez 1958, p. 195), "Ever since the first day you said those magic words, 'I want to be a doctor,' you have been wrapped in the colorful fabric of the history of medicine, a fabric woven from the ideals, wisdom, endeavors, and achievements of our glorious predecessors in medicine." The author throws down the gauntlet of a strong challenge to your aspirations and commitment to purpose. Will you measure up? Will you give every bit of professional energy needed to serve your patients and humanity? Martí-Ibáñez, still writing for medical students, goes on to state, "You are embarking on a noble career where there is no room for amateurs or dilettanti, a career in which we must all aspire to be masters of whatever we undertake, for the mistakes of medical carpenters and pre-scribers' apprentices can have tragic results" (Martí-Ibáñez 1958, p. 200).

In this chapter I tell some thoughts I think we might all share as mentors for those students and young physicians who look to us for advice and counsel.

ADVISE THOSE YOU MENTOR TO CONSIDER OUR PROFESSIONAL INHERITANCE AND THEIR OWN EVENTUAL LEGACY

Today's medical students, residents, and young physicians are the beneficiaries of the generations of physicians that have gone before them, their accomplishments and their character. These predecessors include the pantheon of Great Doctors: Hippocrates, Galen, Sydenham, Hunter, Jenner, Semmelweis, Snow, Osler, and more. What you inherit as a young physician also comes from the generations of unsung physician heroes, which, if you were fortunate, may include the personal physician you recall from your childhood. These doctors treated their patients with dignity, respect, and the best care they could offer at the time. This is their legacy to you – that people generally hold physicians in high regard, and respect their efforts. Because of this legacy that you have inherited without yet earning a bit of it, you can meet a person in an examination room and that stranger will tell you the secrets that he or she would not tell his or her mother, will let you look at the unclothed body, and will respect what you have to say, even if you had just begun a medical school last week.

And so, what about your newly-acquired mantle of power and privilege? Should society accord you esteem because you have completed college and perhaps hold an advanced degree, because you have even written a paper or two, or because some of your professors even hold that you have "promise?" But being "promising" does not, in itself, confer wisdom or merit respect. Here I quote the comic strip character Pogo, who once commented, "A promising future is a heavy burden."

In *Faust*, Johann Wolfgang Goethe (1739–1832) writes, "What you have inherited from your fathers, you must earn in order to possess." As a physician, this will be your burden. Accepting the legacy of the distinguished healers and scientists who have gone before you means that you accept the obligation to maintain their high standards, continue their tradition of service, and endeavor in some small way to advance the understanding of medicine for the benefit of those who will follow you.

At the end of your career, the legacy that you leave to the generation of young physicians to follow will be the skill and perseverance you have exhibited and your passion for work you bring to the office or hospital every day. You may make a discovery that advances medicine just a little, as did otolaryngologist John Epley who developed a maneuver to reposition otoliths in patients with postural vertigo.[2] You may write a scientific paper or book. You may become an invited lecturer on a clinical topic. The odds are that you will do none of these. You will still be a credit to your profession if you provide the finest patient care you possibly can while remaining a vital member of your family and community. If you do these simple things, then the medical students and residents who follow in the years to come will, just as you did, inherit a legacy of honor, trust, and respect.

REMIND THE ASPIRING DOCTOR TO BEHAVE LIKE A PHYSICIAN

"Lord, let me be half the man my dog thinks I am." (Anon.) May you and I be half the persons our patients think we are. Years ago I was driving along a mountain road in upstate New York, and I came to a site where it was obvious that people had dumped trash down the hill beside the road. One local resident, however, had registered a protest by posting a sign that read, "Don't Dump Here. Someone Is Watching!" I can assure you that, if you are a doctor in the community, *everyone* is watching. Everyone expects you to set the standard expected of an upstanding citizen, someone who behaves in a rational and exemplary manner, a person one might encourage his or her children to emulate. And this is merely the expectation held of us as community members. Like it or not, the physician becomes a role model for young persons, a weighty responsibility that not all consider when making the "I want to be a doctor" decision.

National Basketball Association (NBA) star Charles Barkley, famously asserted, "I'm not a role model!"[3] (In fairness to Barkley, he went on to elucidate, not altogether unreasonably, "I'm not paid to be a role model. I am paid to wreak havoc on the basketball court. Parents should be role models. Just because I can dunk a basketball doesn't mean I should raise your kids.") Barkley's childrearing advice notwithstanding, like it or not, the physician *is* a role model, and society expects the physician to set a good example as a human being. To quote an individual with somewhat better role modeling credentials than any NBA star, Nobel laureate Albert Einstein (1857–1955) once remarked, "Setting an example is not the main means of influencing another, it is the only means."[4]

ENCOURAGE THOSE YOU MENTOR TO RECOGNIZE THE PRIVILEGES AND POWERS ACCORDED THE PHYSICIAN, AND TO USE THEM WISELY FOR THE BENEFIT OF SOCIETY

Rudyard Kipling offers a keen insight on the powers of a physician[5]:

You belong to the privileged classes. May I remind you of some of your privilege? You and kings are the only people whose explanation the police will accept if you exceed the legal limit in your car. On presentation of your visiting-card you can pass through the most turbulent crowd unmolested and even with applause. If fly a yellow flag over a centre of population you can turn it into a desert. If you choose to fly a Red Cross flag over a desert you can turn it into a centre of population towards which, as I have seen, men will crawl on hands and knees. You can forbid any ship to enter any port in the world. If you think it is necessary to the success of any operation in which you are interested, you can stop a 20,000-ton liner with mails in mid-ocean till the operation is concluded. You can order whole quarters of a city to be pulled down or burnt up; and you can trust to the armed co-operation of the nearest troops to see that your prescriptions are carried out

Do we physicians still hold such powers? On a trivial scale, I can attest – now that the statute of limitations for my speeding violations has expired – that on several occasions when I was driving a little too fast, returning from the hospital, I was stopped by a New York State Trooper, who then recognized me and said, "Oh, it's you, Doc, you must be rushing back to help someone in the office. Go on, but not so fast." On a more massive level, when I was in the United States Public Health Service, I served as physician on the US Coast Guard Cutter *Chincoteague*, deployed as a weather ship in the North Atlantic Ocean. While sailing up the seaway Atlantic off the Atlantic coast, we were contacted by a huge tanker – perhaps weighing 20,000 tons described by Kipling – with an ailing seaman on board. The giant tanker and our much smaller Coast Guard vessel halted in the middle of the ocean while a corpsman and I went aboard the tanker to examine the seaman. I, a neophyte doctor, indeed had the power to hold the tanker stationary in mid-ocean while I performed my examination and conveyed my recommendation as to what had to be done next. In countries around the globe, the word of a physician declaring the presence of an epidemic can trigger a panic in the population, while the arrival of a physician in a third world village can trigger an in-migration of persons seeking medical help.

REMIND THE ASPIRING PHYSICIAN THAT MEDICINE IS ABOUT HELPING OTHERS

In Chap. 1, I alluded to the Declaration of Geneva and the specific pledge we all recite: "to consecrate my life to the service of humanity," and I asserted that the art of medicine, at its core, is nothing if not service to humanity. I focused on the word *humanity*. Here I want to make a single, but important, point to young physicians about *service*: Medicine is not all about you! Medicine is not for your financial enrichment, your personal intellectual stimulation, or a means to support your true love of skiing, golfing, or playing guitar. Medicine is about *service* to others.

WARN MEDICAL STUDENTS AND RESIDENTS NEVER TO THINK OF MEDICINE AS A PATHWAY TO WEALTH

The goal of your medical practice should be to help people, and not to become rich.

Granted, almost all physicians attain a comfortable level of financial security, and yet few become truly wealthy – private-jet-riding, yacht-sailing, institution-endowing wealthy. If you crave such riches, you have chosen the wrong profession, and should have been a hedge fund manager (at least up until the year 2008), a risk-taking entrepreneur, or the only child of two doting, aged multimillionaires.

Fundamentally, what we physicians sell is a service, and not a product such as a hammer or toothbrush. If we deal with hammers or toothbrushes, we could become wealthy by building new factories and hiring others to make and sell lots of hammers or toothbrushes. But we sell services – advice, consultations, surgical procedures, and so forth. Hence, we are limited in how many services we can deliver. Yes, some physicians have tried to leverage their care by employing physician assistants and nurse practitioners, but such arrangements bring their own constellation of problems.

In medicine, if we crank up the speed on the treadmill, trying to see more and more patients in the 24 h we are allotted each day, we may augment our wealth just a little, but we pay a steep price. Borrowing some phrases from the poem by William Wordsworth (1770–1850) titled *The World is Too Much With Us; Late and Soon,* Sir William Osler offered aspiring physicians some thoughts on getting and spending: "While nothing disturbs our mental placidity more sadly than straitened means, and the lack of those things after which the Gentiles seek, I would warn you against the trials of the day soon to come to some of you – the day of large and successful practice. Engrossed late and soon in professional cares, getting and spending, you may so lay waste your powers that you may find, too late, with hearts given away, that there is no place in your habit-stricken souls for those gentler influences which make life worth living" (Osler, p. 7).

And so, as a wise physician, enjoy your practice. None of us will ever earn enough to be in the same financial league as Carl Icahn, Donald Trump or even an NBA star. If reflecting on earnings brings you joy, consider that your income is in the top 1% of all humans on earth. Just remember that your true wealth is your good health and the love of your patients and your family.

ENCOURAGE LEARNING ABOUT THE WORDS OF MEDICINE, AS VITAL TOOLS OF THE PROFESSION

Here I write about understanding the back stories of medical terms, not just by memorizing the words. I include this section in the book because I strongly feel that meandering the etymologic paths of medical history can help make one a better physician. For years our medical school, the Oregon Health & Science University of School of Medicine, has offered a Summer Observership program. In this program, sponsored by the school's Department of Family Medicine, a group of entering students come to school 8 days early. There is 1 day of orientation covering what the newly arrived students will be doing, and an introduction to clinical interviewing and physical exam skills. Then the students are sent to small communities where they will work and live in the homes of rural physicians for a week.

I tell you about this because, for the past 20 years, the Summer Observership has allowed me the honor of giving this subset of the entering school class their first medical school lecture. In this talk I discuss two key items: The first is the legacy they inherit from the best physicians of history, the imperative that they "earn it again" for themselves, and the legacy they will leave when they cease practice, all discussed above. The second point is my advice to begin now to look up and keep a notebook or a computer log of the Greek, Latin and other etymologic origins of words such as pterygium (from the word for wing) and smallpox (used originally to distinguish the disease from the "great pox" – i.e., syphilis).

Félix Martí-Ibáñez writes: "Man is the only creature able to make tools with which to make tools, and of all the tools made by him words are the most important."[6] The words of medicine are just as valuable as the stethoscope or scalpel, because they allow us – physicians in diverse specialties – to communicate with each other with both specificity and context. Sobel postulates that at the end of medical school, the graduating physician has encountered some 55,000 new words.[7] To whet your appetite, I am going to provide stories about a sample of the words found in the current 2,200+-page edition of *Dorland's Illustrated Medical Dictionary*. If you are a beginning medical student, you will spend the next decade and more attempting to master these words. Knowing their origins helps immensely. Sources for the definitions that follow include Dirckx (1983), Fortuine (2001), Haubrich (1997), Porter (1997), and Skinner (1949) – all listed in the Bibliography.

- Acetabulum: The name for the socket of the hip joint comes from a Latin word meaning vinegar cup; it was so used by Pliny, The Elder (23–79) and later entered the medical-English vocabulary in 1661 (Skinner, p. 3).
- Beriberi: The thiamine (vitamin B1) deficiency disease takes its name from the Sinhalese word for weak, and the repetition indicates intensity, i.e., "extreme weakness" (Dirckx, p. 71).
- Coccyx: In ancient Greek, the word means cuckoo. The terminal bone of the spine, with its inferior pointed shape, was so named because it resembled the beak of the bird (Dirckx, p. 61).

▓ Hunterian chancre. I should really include one eponym in this list. The primary lesion of syphilis caries the name of a famous patient – Scottish surgeon John Hunter (1728–1793) – who unwittingly infected himself with the disease. As part of his study of gonorrhea in 1767, Hunter inoculated himself with pus from a person with gonorrhea. Unknown to Hunter, the donor was also infected with syphilis.

▓ Influenza: The name of the disease causing severe malaise and fever comes from the Latin word for influence, connoting that the disease was the result of the influence of heavenly bodies – the moon, stars, and planets (Haubrich, p. 111).

▓ Innominate artery: Greco-Roman physician Claudius Galen (129–200) described the brachiocephalic trunk coming from the aorta to supply the right arm and head, but neglected to name it. Later, Italian anatomist Vesalius (1514–1564) supplied a name – the "unnamed" or innominate artery (Haubrich, p. 112).

▓ Mitral: The word comes from an ancient Greek word meaning a turban-like type of headgear. Early Hebrew high priests wore a distinctive headpiece, which was later adapted by Christian bishops, with the name miter applied to it. The miter has two parallel panels rising to a point, or cusps. Some hold that Italian anatomist Vesalius (1541–1564) first named the mitral valve of the heart (Skinner, p. 237).

▓ Myxedema: This is a word the origin of which has been traced to its source. Skinner (p. 243) states, "The name myxoedema was given to this condition by W. M. Ord (1834–1902) in 1877 on account of the 'mucous dropsy' of the skin. In an article in the British Medical Journal, May 11, 1878, p. 671, Ord writes, '... upon which I have founded the new term Myxoedema... the term myxoedema is used as an expression of the physical condition which is the true cause of the symptoms.'"

▓ Orthopedic: Herein we find a story of how a specialty name originated. First of all, the word orthopedics comes not from the Latin *pes or ped-*, referring to the foot, but from the Greek *paid*, meaning child. The word orthopedics was coined in the eighteenth century by French surgeon Nicholas André, who pioneered a surgical procedure to correct the spinal deformities of rickets, a widespread problem of children at that time. Hence a rough translation of the word is "child straightener" (Bollett, p. 195).

- Panic: From the mythologic Greek god Pan comes the word for sudden overwhelming fear. Pan was an impish being with the head and body of a man and the horns, ears, and legs of a goat. He was delighted in frightening persons who lived in rural areas. Fortuine (p. 247) suggests that Pan frightened the Persians, prompting them to flee from the 490 BCE battle of Marathon.
- Penis: This word means "tail" in Latin; early anatomists did not always get it right.
- Sacrum: The sacrum, or *os sacrum* in Latin, means holy bone. Some speculate that the "holiness" of the bone arises from the belief that, in a decomposing body, the sacrum is the last to decay, and hence represents a nidus from which a new body might arise in the afterlife (Gershen, p. 6).
- Testis: This medical term comes from a Latin word meaning "witness," in the sense of one who testifies. It seems that in early times, a man would show his forthrightness by placing his hand on his (or occasionally, someone else's) genitalia (Haubrich, p. 223). Today, we raise our right hand and swear on a Bible.
- Quarantine: From the Italian word *quaranta*, meaning 40, comes the current word for isolation of persons with or suspected of having disease. The practice seems to have begun in the port of Venice in 1374, the time of the Black Plague in Europe (Skinner, p. 297). Ships arriving in port from the Levant and other origins were detained in the harbor, first for 30 days, later increased to 40 days, *quaranta giorni*.
- Vaccine: The word comes from the Latin *vacca*, meaning cow (Fortuine, p. 99). Why does the term for immunizing agents have a bovine origin? In Chap. 2, I told how the world's first reliably effective immunization technique came from the work of country doctor Edward Jenner (1749–1823), using secretions from a dairymaid's cowpox pustule (Porter, p. 276). Today we, somewhat carelessly,

use the term "vaccine" for tetanus, diphtheria, measles, and other immunizations, but because of the origins of these other immunogenic products, such use is etymologically sloppy.

▦ Some other medical words: Tibia comes directly from the Latin word for flute; stapes means stirrup and malleus is the word that ancient Romans used for hammer; vagina means sheath; placenta means cake; and cervix is Latin for neck. Through the years, these and other word origins have helped me remember various anatomical structures (Taylor 2008, p. 71).

Standard medical dictionaries, such as *Dorland's* or *Stedman's*, provide the Greek, Latin and other less common antecedents of medical terms, but do not tell the rich history of many of the words we use today in clinical practice. I hope that the few examples provided will stimulate you to explore the fascinating world of medical etymology.

ENCOURAGE THOSE YOU MENTOR TO READ ABOUT THE HISTORY OF MEDICINE

Think of the history of medicine as a way to organize all the many bits and pieces of knowledge you learn in medical school and practice. Shortt advocates including the history of medicine in the medical curriculum. To him "it seems appropriate to introduce what might be termed a neo-Oslerian proposition: knowledge of medicine may directly contribute to the acquisition of clinical competence."[8] And here I believe that Shortt includes medical history in the "knowledge of medicine." As examples: Knowing the historical underpinnings of the word "quarantine" (see above) helps us understand the significance of the concept keeping infected persons away from those who are ill. Understanding how the innominate ("nameless") artery came to be so called (also above) may help students and surgeons recall the structure. Measles seems merely a now-preventable and previously-predictable childhood illness, until we consider the devastation caused by the introduction of the disease to previously unexposed populations in North America

and the Pacific Islands (Cartwright, pp. 131–136). One way
to recall the method of pasteurization (heating a fluid to
60°C to kill microorganisms) is to remember that Pasteur
first used the method on wine, not on milk (Firkin and
Whitworth, p. 396).

Here are some suggestions to begin the study of medical
history. I recommend that you buy or borrow one of the
following books, and try it out as bedside reading.

- Ackerknecht EH. *History and geography of the most
  important diseases*. New York: Hafner; 1972. This is a man-
  ageable book, 210 pages including the index, that traces
  the demographics of the major communicable diseases,
  plus deficiency diseases, diseases of unknown origin and
  more.
- Cartwright FF. *Disease and history: the influence of disease
  in shaping the great events of history*. New York: Crowell;
  1972. This readable book does just what the subtitle promises. It traces the influence of disease – such as typhus,
  syphilis, and the Black Death – on events in world history.
- Dirckx JH. *The language of medicine: its evolution, structure, and dynamics. 2nd edition*. New York: Praeger;
  1983. Of all the medical word origin books available, I
  prefer this one for its historical perspective and scholarly
  approach. Dirckx discusses medical words in the context
  of our classical perspectives, modern coinages, slang, and
  jargon. It is interesting to read for those who enjoy medical etymology.
- Garrison FH. *History of medicine*. Philadelphia: Saunders;
  1929. Garrison's is the traditional "Bible" of medical
  history books. In my opinion, it is still unequaled in
  scholarship. Would you believe that, in a frenzy of self-
  improvement as a young physician, I read this 996-page
  book cover to cover? As evidence, my well-worn copy
  bears the underlining.
- Gordon R. *The alarming history of medicine: amusing
  anecdotes from Hippocrates to heart transplants*. New
  York: St. Martin's Griffin; 1993. Writing in a humorous

style, Gordon explains the stone-cutters (p. 133) alluded to in the original Hippocratic Oath and how if Alexander Fleming had been a better housekeeper, he might not be remembered as the man who discovered penicillin (p. 70). I relish his quote on page 121: "Modern surgery was invented by gunpowder."

- Martí-Ibáñez F. *A prelude to medical history*. 3rd edition. New York: MD Publications: 1961. The Foreword to the book begins, "I am a lover of the spoken word. No violin rendition, no piano recital, no symphonic concert can transport me as does a well-turned lecture." The book is a collection of the author's lectures to medical students of the New York Medical College, Flower and Fifth Avenue Hospitals.

- McNeill WH. *Plagues and peoples*. New York: History Book Club; 1976. The author tells how infectious diseases have influenced events in world history.

- Osler W. *Aequanimitas with other addresses. 3rd edition.* Philadelphia: Blakiston; 1932. Although not technically a history book, Osler's collection of addresses retains its inspirational qualities a century after its initial publication in 1904.

- Porter R. *The greatest benefit to mankind*. New York: Norton; 1997. With the subtitle *"a medical history of humanity,"* this book is an ambitious, but readable, story of the human side of medicine.

- Taylor RB. *White coat tales: medicine's heroes, heritage and misadventures*. New York: Springer; 2008. Full disclosure: *White Coat Tales* is my book. It tells some of the classic tales of medical history, but attempts to present the back stories of many of these events.

- Weiss AB. *Medical odysseys: the different and sometimes unexpected pathways to 20th century medical discoveries*. New Brunswick, NJ: Rutgers Univ. Press; 1991. This book, telling stories of the often convoluted and occasionally unexpected routes to discovery, offers some lesser-known facts about key events in medical science.

SUGGEST READING SOME BOOKS ABOUT PHYSICIANS IN LITERATURE

Reading about physicians as literary figures can provide insights as to how society has viewed doctors in different settings and different times in history. Such reading can offer clues as to how noted authors, and the world in general, believe that physicians think and feel. In reading about fictional doctors, note how authors portray physicians facing life dilemmas and also notice the evolution of the physician-hero, often as a tragic figure. Lehman holds that physicians portrayed in literature "vary in their emotional devotion to patients. John Steinbeck's physicians form powerful, complicated emotional attachments to their patients. These attachments allow them to live fuller, richer lives without interfering with their proper functioning as healthcare providers. F. Scott Fitzgerald's Dr. Diver overly commits himself to a patient and suffers the consequences. The present-day physician can help modulate his own emotional connections to patients by examining these literary models."[9]

Most portrayals of physician protagonists were written by physician authors, such as William Somerset Maugham and Robin Cook. But some tales were penned by laypersons – that is, non-physicians. Here are a few selected examples of the latter group:

- *A Doctor in Spite Himself* (1666) by Jean-Baptiste Molière: In this humorous play by the French author, Sganarelle is not actually a physician, but he and his wife insist that he is a talented doctor with amazing healing powers. In this and other plays, Molière satirizes contemporary physicians whose Latin-aggrandized speech masks the fact that their remedies are worthless, or worse.

- *Middlemarch* (1871) by George Elliott (a pseudonym for female writer Mary Ann Evans): In this Victorian era story, Doctor Tertius Lydgate is depicted as a flawed hero with great potential as a physician and researcher who, following some financial challenges, eventually abandons his lofty aspirations to earn a living that will satisfy his spendthrift and socially ambitious wife, Rosamond.

▓ *The Strange Case of Dr. Jekyll and Mr. Hyde* (1886) by Robert Louis Stevenson: The Scottish author explores the contrasting urges of human nature – the good and the very bad. Dr. Henry Jekyll, of course, represents the "good" in this man with the so-called split personality. Mr. Hyde is the personification of psychopathologic evil. On a retrospective note, in her book *The Knife Man*, author Wendy Moore suggests that the description of Jekyll's home was inspired by the home of Dr. John Hunter (1728–1793), whose house had a front door for visitors and a back door through which dead bodies were delivered to be used as cadavers. An anatomist and surgeon Hunter was known to conduct studies on bodies dug up in graveyards and delivered to him by "resurrectionists."[10]

▓ *Arrowsmith* (1925) by Sinclair Lewis: The novel had a silent contributor, who assisted Lewis – microbiologist Paul de Kruif, PhD, who later wrote *Microbe Hunters* (1926) about the lives of Robert Koch, Louis Pasteur, Walter Reed, and others. Readers might even ask if the character Martin Arrowsmith is a bit of a representation of de Kruif. *Arrowsmith* is an especially noteworthy book for today's physicians, having influenced more than one generation of aspiring doctors. In 1953, my high school Latin teacher, aware that I planned a career as a physician, gave me a copy to read.

The gifted protagonist, Martin Arrowsmith, begins to question his skills as a physician following the death of a child in his care and moves from a small town practice to a lofty position in New York City research institute. When Arrowsmith's levelheaded wife Leora dies of plague where Martin fights the disease on a distant island, he loses his vision and his passion. He marries an affluent second wife, and later deserts her and resigns his post at the research institute to spend his life doing scientific research while living in rural New England.

▓ *Doctor Zhivago* (1957) by Boris Pasternak: In the midst of the 1917 Russian Revolution, physician and poet

Yuri Zhivago suffers the conflict of loving two different women amid the revolutionary brutality of the time. Readers may find an early clue to Zhivago's idealism in the face of disaster as a medical school professor notes that bacteria, although fascinating when viewed under the microscope, can cause terrible harm. Through a series of events, some horrifying, Zhivago does his best to hold firm to his sometimes-mystical ideals of loyalty, beauty, and justice.

ALERT ASPIRING PHYSICIANS TO BE AWARE OF THE HIDDEN CURRICULUM OF MEDICAL SCHOOL AND RESIDENCY TRAINING

There are things we hope that students will assimilate during their early learning years, even though there are seldom formal courses on these items. I call them the Hidden Curriculum. If I were to develop a course outline for these Hidden Curriculum topics, it would include the following:

- The role of the physician in the community
- How to deal with fellow physicians
- How to interact with others on the healthcare team
- Social issues in medicine
- The interplay of politics, money, and medicine
- Medical scholarship as a lifelong imperative
- Balancing personal and professional life
- Things doctors shouldn't do
- What to do when you encounter physician misbehavior
- Protecting one's inner self
- Deciding what medical specialty to practice

HELP THOSE YOU ADVISE TO SELECT A SPECIALTY FOR THE RIGHT REASONS

Fortunately, the twenty-plus medical specialties among which medical students will initially choose are quite diverse, not to mention all the subspecialties such as endocrinology and epispecialties such as sports medicine. Options range from the contemplative mental processing of psychiatry to the exhilaration of trauma surgery, from neonatal care to hospice and palliative care, and from hospitalist to travel medicine. With all the options, it is understandable that some young physicians make inappropriate choices. When this occurs, the problem can usually be traced to the young person focusing on the wrong reasons for making life decisions.

Gordon tells how, as a medical student in Paris, Andreas Vesalius (1514–1564) came across a dry-out skeleton of a hanged man, swinging from the gallows. The ligaments, tendons and desiccated muscles were intact. The author tells, "He hurried home his prize – any human skeleton was a *rara avis* – to found a career that culminated with a crammed anatomical amphitheater in Padua" (Gordon, p. 9). If you know your medical history, you know that Vesalius was the Renaissance pioneer of anatomical dissection; that he has been honored eponymously by a bone, a foramen and a vein; and that the amphitheater in which he taught is still present in the University of Padua, Italy.

The story of Vesalius' career choice suggests the caprice with which many of today's physicians choose their careers. Yes, it all worked out quite well for Vesalius in the sixteenth century. Today, however, I am dismayed at the number of students who enter medical school planning to become surgeons because of a brief time spent as an observer in an operating room, to become neurologists because of some research on nerve fibers done while in graduate school, or an emergency physician on the basis of what is presented in the television show "ER."

As indicated in the quotation given in the beginning of this chapter, medical training is transformative. I hope you will advise those you mentor that part of this transformation is gaining a mature recognition of whom they are, where their passions lie, and what just might be each individual's Personal Legend – which is the first step in making an informed career choice and avoiding a life practicing in the wrong specialty.

Of course, choosing a specialty for which one is temperamentally unsuited is not an ethical transgression, it is not professional misbehavior, and no medical board will sanction you for making a poor career selection. All that will happen is that one will spend the next 40 years wondering why medicine does not seem to be a truly fulfilling career, and why he or she is not truly happy as a physician. Yes, even the physician in the "wrong" specialty will enjoy a good income, and favored status in the community; the doctor will be able to afford expensive vacations, top restaurants, and club memberships. But somehow a small voice nags, "Shouldn't I be enjoying my career more than I am?"

Once upon a time, each medical graduate did a rotating internship. This was followed by a couple of years of military service, at least for men, and most medical graduates were men. During these years, young physicians had the opportunity to become emotionally mature and to sample a variety of medical specialties, before making their ultimate choice of a specialty residency or entering practice as a generalist.

Today, the rotating internship does not exist, and all residencies are specialty-specific. And because medical students must apply for residency positions in the summer preceding the fourth year of medical school, their specialty selection must be made some time during or before the third year of medical school. For all students, today's timetable means that the decision time comes before they have experienced the full spectrum of specialty rotations. Those who are able to gain experience in clerkships and preceptorships are described by Burack et al as "trying on possible selves."[11] Today students are forced to make decisions before having the opportunity to try on all possible selves.

It is remarkably easy to make a poor specialty choice. Here's why: Medical school professors, and passionate advocates for their various specialties, offer students an abundant amount of advice, usually unsolicited, that is frequently laden with bias and self-interest.

All of us in medical education strive to clone ourselves. We seek to do this by recruiting students into our specialties, and occasionally by bashing other specialties: "You're too smart to become a (surgeon, psychiatrist, family physician, and so forth)."

If the profusion of misinformation is not confusing enough, there are other opportunities to go astray in decision-making.

Here are five ways where medical students and residents make poor specialty choices:

- Choosing the same specialty as their physician father, mother, sibling or other relative – or the field that your parents favor. Family bias may be overt or subtle, but when mom or dad is a physician, some bias is there! But just because one's dad has had a successful career as a surgeon doesn't mean that the student wouldn't become a great (and happy) neurologist.
- Choosing the specialty of a compelling mentor. A favorite professor – say, everyone's favorite professor – is a radiologist. She is brilliant, she is charismatic, and she spends a lot of time with students. However, this is not a sufficient reason for anyone to become a radiologist. First of all, choosing that specialty will not magically make the student brilliant and charismatic. Secondly, and please pay attention here, the favored professor and mentor may be an outlier. That is, she or he may not be a representative of most other practitioners in the specialty. This is why, before selecting a specialty, a student or resident should spend as much time as possible with a number of physicians already in the specialty. And all this time you should be asking yourself, "Am I like these people? Would I like to spend the next 40 years practicing side by side and going to meetings with them?"
- Choosing the specialty that all the class leaders are choosing that year. Every so often at our medical school, we see a cluster of class leaders – the "cool kids" – choose early to be emergency physicians, pediatricians, or some other specialty. When this happens, a number of classmates become swayed, and there will be a large number of class graduates entering that specialty.
- Choosing a specialty for financial reasons. There is an interesting study by Kiker and Zeh that found expected relative income negatively related to the choice of an internal medical or a primary care specialty, while selection of a support or surgical specialty is positively income motivated.[12] Selecting a specialty based on projected future income can be foolish because what is well rewarded

today may not be so in the future, given the vagaries of supply and demand and the increasing involvement of government in medical policy.

■ Choosing a specialty without unbiased guidance and counseling. Today most medical schools have programs intended to offer objective advice about specialty choice. To make a career decision without making use of these resources is like beginning a cross-country drive without a road map. Yet I find that too many students fail to seek – sometimes seem to evade – the career counseling that medical schools provide.

In the end, the wise young physician studies the characteristics and values of a variety of specialties that seem appealing. Even more important, the as yet undifferentiated physician seeks to understand his or her own personal characteristics and values: "Am I really a people-person or would I be happier working quietly in a laboratory all day?" "Do I like the excitement of the emergency setting or would I prefer the relationships that come with a continuity practice?" "Do I seek a wide variety in what I see all day or would I prefer doing one thing, over and over, and becoming very good at this focused skill?" Only when a young doctor has reflected on these self-directed questions is he or she ready to make a wise career choice.

RECOMMEND THAT THE YOUNG PHYSICIAN NOT SUBSPECIALIZE TOO EARLY

Part of making a wise career choice is avoiding the trap of premature subspecialization. For some, destiny holds that they will spend their days doing retinal surgery or treating autistic children. Others will decide to be colorectal surgeons, geropsychiatrists, or specialists in aerospace medicine or physical medicine and rehabilitation. Because of the funding difficulties involved in changing specialty residencies after the first year of training, it pays to make the right decision the first time. Be aware that, once one begins a specialty residency training program, it is difficult to change careers; it can be done, but it is not easy, and may cost the resident physician a year of training in the process.

Of course, some will decide that their area of specialization will be generalism, an apparent contradiction that becomes less dissonant when we recognize that providing comprehensive and continuing care to a panel of patients whom they know well over time requires special knowledge and skills. Both Doctors William Osler and William Mayo made strong cases for specializing in generalism: Osler advised students: "Have no higher ambition than to become an all-around family doctor, whose business it is in life to know disease and how to treat it."[13] William J. Mayo (1861–1939) had this to say, "Given one well-trained physician of the highest type he will do better work for a thousand people than ten specialists" (Strauss, p. 565).

ADVISE YOUNG PHYSICIANS OF THE RISKS OF PREMATURELY LIMITING THEIR CAREER OPTIONS

In football, when you throw a forward pass, three things can happen, and two of them are not good (For those who don't watch football, the two "not good" things that can happen when the football is passed are an incomplete pass and an interception.). When you abandon one of your doctoring skills or legal rights, you gain some immediate benefit such as time to focus on activities that interests you the most , but there may be unintended and "not good" consequences.

Let's talk about specifics: Upon graduating from medical school, completing residency training, and getting a medical license and hospital privileges, you are set. You can do anything professionally. And then, at some time in your career, you will be tempted to give up some of your career prerogatives. Here is how it works, and I will use myself as an example.

Upon completing training and 2 years in the United States Public Health Service, I joined a small town family practice group. I was the fourth physician, and we moved into a new building built as a four-doctor practice. There was, however, one small problem. Although I had helped deliver a lot of babies while in the service, our group practice was 18 miles of backcountry roads from the hospital. Consequently, the group did no maternity care, and thus I gave up my obstetrical skills, a loss I would regret when I later made the move to academic medicine.

A few years later, the leaders of our practice group decided that we should all sign a restrictive covenant. Upon leaving the group, none of us could open a competing office or join a competing practice within the town limits. I later wished I had resisted signing this agreement giving away my legal rights. When I eventually resigned from the group to open a solo office, I was forced to build my new practice office in a rural site beyond the town limits, a location that lengthened the drive from my home to my office and to the hospital.

Fortunately, I maintained my hospital skills, a happy decision for which I was grateful when I eventually became an academic physician at Wake Forest University School of Medicine in 1978. Having inpatient skills allowed me to attend hospital patients and family medicine residents. Yet today I grieve to see well-trained generalist physicians graduate from residency and accept jobs that involve only outpatient work. They happily refer their patients to hospitalists, enjoying the relief from hospital responsibilities. Yet, it takes just a few years away from hospital work for a physician to find himself/herself left behind by advances in inpatient care. The office-care-only physician can become isolated from informal, but often informative, interactions with hospital-based colleagues. Furthermore, state licensing boards and hospital credentialing committees are carefully scrutinizing physicians who have eschewed hospital work, and our academic department has participated in a program to help a few of these persons regain atrophied abilities. As for me, I gave up the hospital part of my practice a few years ago as one of the steps into semi-retirement; I did so realizing that I could never go back to my previous role in hospital care.

Then there are those following non-clinical career paths, such as physician executives, often with no patient care responsibilities at all. These persons generally report a high level of satisfaction with their jobs.[14] Yet, the physician executive may have left patient care behind forever. A study by Hoff found that physician executives with graduate management degrees are especially likely not to practice medicine.[15] As a physician–educator employed by an academic medical center, I have always considered my "tenure" to be my clinical skills; if I lose my salaried job, I could always go into the community and provide care for patients.

Next, let us consider specialty recertification. Today, every specialty has some sort of recertification process. As one ages, and especially if the physician is doing chiefly administrative or research work, it is tempting to forgo periodic recertification. I have chosen to maintain my specialty certification, despite the substantial cost and the aggravation of the all-day computer-based recertification examination. I reasoned long ago that eventually hospital privileges and state license renewals would be dependent on the physician being currently board-certified. The former, hospital privileges, has become a reality, at least at our institution, and the latter, state licensure renewal, is sure to follow eventually. I am proud to report that I passed my every-7-year recertification examination last year at age 72. I may finally abandon board certification when my reexamination time comes due in 7 years, but I am reserving judgment until that time.

Finally, there is your state medical license and mine. My father died at age 96 with a valid Pennsylvania driver's license, although fortunately for local motorists and pedestrians alike, he had actually ceased driving a few years ago. Will you or I know when the time has come to surrender our medical licenses? Certainly, the step of not renewing one's medical license is the ultimate surrender of professional career options.

ALERT YOUNG DOCTORS TO BEGIN EARLY TO RESPECT PERSONAL HEALTH AS PRECIOUS

This chapter written about advising young physicians would be incomplete without an admonition to begin now to care for your body and especially your psyche. Burnout, depression, and substance misuse are common and under-reported in medical trainees. Dahlin and Runeson looked at burnout and psychiatric morbidity among medical students entering clinical training. They found that 27% of those interviewed had a psychiatric diagnosis, but only approximately a quarter of these students had sought professional help.[16] In a sample of 504 medical students, McAuliffe et al discovered that 78% of students reported using psychoactive drugs at some time in their young lives.[17]

The patterns of coping mechanisms and substance behavior established now are likely to continue into later life. Now, is a good time to establish healthy ways to deal with the stresses of medical practice and daily living. I shall return to this topic in Chap. 11 on "Caring for You, the Physician."

REMIND THOSE YOU ADVISE TO RESPECT AND HONE THEIR PHYSICAL EXAMINATION SKILLS

You will hear cynical witticisms such as "One look (i.e., an x-ray) is worth a hundred listens." Today spending much time examining the patient is sometimes considered "quaint," especially by subspecialists in imaging and laboratory testing, but in direct patient care by the best physicians, there is no substitute for a careful physical examination, repeated from time to time, with comparison to past findings.

Some physical examination skills involve clinical "tricks of the trade." Experienced doctors with these skills should share them with medical students and young physicians. Here are a few time-tested physical examination tips:

- Watch how the patient sits, moves, attends to you, and reacts to what is said. Pay attention to how the patient gets up on the examination table, especially if the chief complaint is muscle or bone pain. All these observations are part of the physical examination.
- Avoid gagging a patient with a tongue depressor by having him or her "stick out" the tongue. Then apply the tongue blade to the extended tongue, and have the patient bring the tongue (with the applied tongue blade) back into the mouth.
- When doing an ophthalmoscopic examination, use your left eye to examine the patient's left eye while holding the instrument in your left hand, and use your right eye and right hand to gaze into his or her right eye. To do otherwise may have you and the patient rubbing noses, a familiarity the patient may not appreciate.
- Especially on cold days, warm your stethoscope in your hand before applying it to bare skin of the chest.

▨ When listening to the patient's heart or examining the abdomen I always ask the patient to look to the left. Why do I do this? I always assume that I am healthy and the patient may not be. Avoiding breathing the patient's exhaled air may help keep me in a healthy state. I use the same instruction when examining a male patient for a hernia.

▨ Don't let your patient take multiple deep breaths while you listen to the chest. If you do so, the patient may become dizzy and fall from the examination table. I teach medical students to instruct, "Breathe through your mouth, just a little deeper than normal."

▨ Some physicians find that a "bearing down" Valsalva maneuver is better than the traditional cough when examining for a hernia. Compared to a cough, the Valsalva maneuver allows a few seconds of sustained intra-abdominal pressure, and it avoids the patient spraying the examiner with droplets from the cough.

▨ You can use a reflex hammer instead of your "plexor" finger in chest percussion, to save the finger that serves as "pleximeter" from bruising and damage due to fingernails.

▨ Look for hair on the toes, a generally reliable sign of adequate circulation to the feet.

▨ The tuning fork is the best instrument to detect peripheral neuropathy. Meijer et al suggest that you select a 128-Hz tuning fork, stating that others either do not work well or have not been validated.[18]

SUGGEST THAT THERE IS NO MERIT IN BEING THE SMARTEST PERSON IN THE ROOM

Recently, I asked some medical students to describe the characteristics of the best physicians. The first answer was that the best physician is "smart." Smart is what the Enron executives were called in the movie and in the book with the same name: *Enron: the Smartest Guys in the Room*. I have a slightly different opinion.

American physician and author Oliver Wendell Holmes (1809–1894) once wrote: "A man of very moderate ability may be a good physician, if he devotes himself faithfully to the work" (Brallier, p. 141). I have been in academic medicine long enough to work with hundreds of physicians in training, to know their exam scores, and then see them in practice. Based on this sample, I have a theory. I suggest that there is sometimes an inverse relationship between board scores attained and the quality of medical care delivered. Too many of the "smart people" are great test-takers, but lack what I want in a physician when I am sick. If I am ill, I want a physician who "is there" for me, who listens to my story, considers pertinent diagnostic possibilities, who follows up carefully on laboratory tests and imaging results, obtains necessary consultations, and exhibits respect for my suffering, as well as for my values and ideas about what might be wrong with me.

The young physician who consistently achieves high examination scores may believe that being "smart" is more important than attention to detail. Being over-confident as a physician can be a fatal flaw – and the fatality could be a patient.

ALERT THOSE YOU MENTOR NOT TO STRAY FROM THE PATH OF SCIENCE

Although I sometimes rail against the presumptions, the narrowness of focus, and the occasional self-interest found in the multitude of clinical guidelines available today, at least those who create them generally make an effort to make evidence-based recommendations, constructed on a reasonably firm foundation of medical science.

The history of medicine has a few chapters describing remedies that, in retrospect, were more than a little spurious. The following stories are from my book *White Coat Tales*.

While superintendent of the Battle Creek Sanitarium at Battle Creek, Michigan, John Harvey Kellogg, MD (1852–1943) and his brother Will serendipitously "cooked up" the idea that evolved into corn flakes in the early 1890s. The sanitarium was on a tight budget, and one day when the brothers had allowed some cooked wheat to become stale, they decided to produce some potentially usable long sheets of dough by forcing the material through rollers. Instead of sheets of dough, they got flakes. Sensing possibilities, they toasted the flakes and served them to patients, who seemed to like the taste and texture. They filed a patent for the product in 1894, and the American cereal industry was born.

If only Dr. Kellogg had stopped there, and built on his cereal success. However, he had other keen interests. In the sanitarium, he practiced mechanotherapy, electropathy, and radium cures. He was an advocate of a healthy bowel, and employed an enema machine that could deliver 15 gallons of water to the bowel in only a few seconds. He decried masturbation, advocating circumcision "without administering an anesthetic" for small boys and the application of carbolic acid to the clitoris of girls.[19] Those interested in seeing a humorous adaptation of Kellogg's quirky methods should view the 1994 motion picture *The Road to Wellville*, based on the 1993 novel of the same name by American author T. C. Boyle (Taylor 2008, pp. 222–223).

Following medical training at several medical schools of dubious quality, Doctor John R. Brinkley (1885–1942) was licensed to practice medicine. Brinkley is remembered today for his goat gland surgery, which began in 1918. For a fee of merely $750, Brinkley held that he could cure male impotence and infertility by surgical implantation of goat glands. By 1928, Brinkley had become a target of the American Medical Association (AMA), owing to his use of advertising to solicit patients. In 1930, his Kansas state medical license was revoked, ending his career as the "goat gland doctor."

But Brinkley was not going to quit without a fight. In an effort to gain the political power needed to appoint sympathetic members to the state board of medical examiners – members who might restore his license – Brinkley ran for governor of Kansas three times, in 1930, 1932, and 1934. He did not win any of these elections (Taylor, 2008, p. 224).

American chemist Linus Pauling (1901–1994), the only person to win two unshared Nobel Prizes, popularized the theory that high-dose vitamin C can treat cancer. Following years of consuming megadoses of the vitamin, Pauling was the victim of fate's ironic twists. Cancer claimed his wife

Ava in 1981, and then Pauling himself in 1994 (Taylor 2008, p. 226).

Then there is the laetrile tale. For a time, some American physicians administered laetrile to their cancer patients. Laetrile is the proprietary name for amygdalin, a derivative of bitter almonds, apricot pits, and some other nuts and fruits. The drug attained popularity in the 1970s as a treatment for cancer, allegedly acting by selectively killing cancer cells. As reputable physicians learned more about the drug, however, problems began to arise. First of all, laetrile turned out to be not as safe as originally claimed. In the body, the drug is metabolized to yield benzaldehyde and hydrogen cyanide. Serious side effects were reported, and a few cyanide poisoning deaths occurred.

Perhaps laetrile's side effects might have been acceptable if the drug was highly effective, but it is not. A multicenter US trial failed to show any therapeutic benefit at all (Taylor 2008, pp. 225–226). The drug is no longer used by reputable American physicians, but is still available for desperate cancer patients and can be ordered online. Just Google: "laetrile."

Today, I am just a little concerned about the enchantment of young doctors with "complementary and alternative medicine," aka CAM. Most medications recommended under this rubric are termed dietary supplements, outside the control of the US Food and Drug Administration (FDA), and they are widely used. A 2008 paper reported that 73% of US adults use dietary supplements.[20] The authors report: "Randomized, controlled, clinical trial data, which are considered the gold standard for evidence-based decision making, are lacking. Standardized guidelines for the use of dietary supplements are lacking, and dietary supplements can bear unsupported claims." Yet many physicians are recommending dietary supplements such as chondroitin, flaxseed oil, echinacea, glucosamine, St. John's wort, black cohosh, and fish oil, not to mention meditation, acupressure, and deep breathing exercises.

Pushing the boundaries of reason, shark cartilage extract has been touted as a cure for cancer, based upon an alleged absence of cancer in sharks. This practice, while failing to effect any documented cancer cures, has reportedly caused a sharp decline in the shark population.[21]

There are books on alternative medicine and herbal remedies written for physicians. There are post-graduate fellowships in integrative medicine and established physicians slanting their practices toward CAM. A generation from now will we consider today's fascination with CAM to have been prescient, as the worth of herbal remedies is confirmed by randomized, controlled trials, or a misguided enterprise that wasted money and diverted patients from legitimate therapy?

SHARE WITH YOUR ADVISEES THE TRUISM THAT WE ALL SPEND OUR PROFESSIONAL CAREERS LIVING WITH UNCERTAINTY AND GOVERNED BY THE LAWS OF PROBABILITY

"Medicine is a science of uncertainty and an art of probability." These words by Osler (Bean and Bean, p. 125) highlight that a patient's disease changes each day, if only just by virtue of the host being a day older, and may change for the better or worse. Furthermore, probability plays such a huge role in diagnosis and treatment that one could be forgiven for calling medicine a "numbers game." Almost all patients with metastatic lung cancer will be dead within a year, but not all. Most patients who smoke will eventually develop chronic obstructive lung disease, but some will not. If you have diabetes, hypertension, and hypercholesterolemia, you have a high risk of sustaining a heart attack, but one may never come. Yes, we can state the probabilities, but seldom the certainties. If you want certainty – at least the illusion of certainty become an engineer, not a physician.

SUGGEST CATALOGING THE THINGS THAT OCCUR MOST COMMONLY

One way to make peace with the tyranny of probabilities is to understand what things are common – that is, probable – and what is not. Here I want to encourage the young physician to begin one more expanding list: your list of "Most

Common Things." Knowing about what's most common in a variety of spheres will help keep you grounded when thinking about possible causes of signs and symptoms, and in formulating prognosis. Here, in no particular order, is a sampling of Most Common Things:

- The most common cause of death in the USA is cardiovascular disease.
- The most common form of cancer in the USA is skin cancer.
- The most common cause of cancer death is lung cancer.
- The most common work-related disability in the USA is low back pain.
- The most common cause of accidental death is motor vehicle crashes.
- Sudden infant death syndrome is the leading cause of death in healthy infants.
- The most common cause of visual loss in the elderly is age-related macular degeneration.
- The most common identifiable cause of skin and soft-tissue infection among patients presenting to emergency departments in 11 US cities is Methicillin-resistant *S. aureus* (MRSA).[22]
- The most common surgical emergency of the abdomen is acute appendicitis, also the most common surgical emergency during pregnancy.
- The most common neoplasm of the appendix is a carcinoid tumor.
- The most common cause of anemia is iron deficiency, whether due to deficient intake, impaired absorption, or blood loss.

As you think of more, add them to the list.

HERE IS A CHALLENGE FOR THOSE YOU MENTOR: MAKE SOCIETY GRATEFUL FOR ITS INVESTMENT IN YOU

The aspiring physician is the poster child for delayed gratification – for the individual doctor, and for everyone around – family, often including spouse and children, the community of would-be patients, and the taxpayers who underwrite the academic medicine enterprise. Surprise, young physician, you thought that your admittedly exorbitant tuition payments covered the cost of your medical education and training. Not so. Medical schools receive state and federal funding in many ways, including research and training grants. By federal law, "Section 1886(d)(5)(B) of the (Medicare) Act provides that prospective payment hospitals that have residents in an approved graduate medical education (GME) program receive an additional payment for a Medicare discharge to reflect the higher patient care costs of teaching hospitals relative to non-teaching hospitals."[23] In 2006, these payments totaled $5.6 billion dollars, more than budget dust and a noteworthy figure even in today's expansive federal budget, all spent to allow interns and residents to participate in teaching conferences and to order the extra laboratory tests that will help make them more knowledgeable practitioners.

Yes, a newly minted physician represents a major investment for many, an investment that carries a social imperative. Writing in 1942 in Timmins, Ontario, Canadian physician James B. McClinton, observed[24]:

> At thirty the doctor is a vagabond. He cost much and earned nothing. Somebody paid for his porridge, his university degree, his rented dinner jacket, his first girl's roses, his whiskey and fare as a medical missionary. Somebody also paid for his time when other lads were doing something. Economists call them wasted man-years. Unless he rewards the public for these gifts, he is a social thief

The term "social thief," may seem a little extreme, but yet what should we think of the surgeon who operates only on the wealthy or the community doctor who is "too busy to teach," or, for that matter, any physician who donates nothing to community-based charities?

THE YOUNG PHYSICIAN, AND INDEED, EVERY PHYSICIAN, SHOULD BE A PROFESSIONAL: IN THE CLASSIC SENSE OF THE WORD

From time to time throughout your training and years of practice, you will experience exhortations to be "professional" and to exhibit "professionalism." Just as the words "doctor" and "physician" have rich connotations when you know their origins, the word "professional" – the antecedent of "professionalism" – has a history worth contemplating.

My Online Etymology Dictionary tells that the word profession came into use circa 1225, originating from the Latin *professionem*, meaning "public declaration."[25] By the sixteenth century, profession had come to mean "occupation one professes to be skilled in." The word professional meaning pertaining to a profession dates from 1747, and came to represent a higher level activity than a trade, the latter meaning "specifically the process of buying and selling in the marketplace."[26] The evolutionary word, professionalism, came into use in 1856.

The words "professional" now has a variety of meanings, and we now have professional basketball players, talk show hosts, and dog-walkers. "Professionalism" has a somewhat loftier connotation. In the book's spirit of viewing medicine as service to humanity, I like the observation of Robert Moser, "Professionalism is first cousin to humanitarianism and ethical behavior. It is what we used to call 'character' (before that fine word was appropriated by actors and comics). It applies to all professions: jurisprudence, medicine, legislation, engineering."[27]

WISE WORDS TO SHARE WITH THOSE YOU MENTOR

■ *The physician is nature's assistant.* Roman physician Claudius Galen (129–200) (Porter, p. 71; Inglis, p. 39)

Galen's theories, some wise and some wildly misleading, prevailed from Greco-Roman times until the Renaissance (Taylor, pp. 8–9). In this case, his words help us advise humility in the young doctor, full of current knowledge and eager to cure.

■ *Medicine is a science in the making.* French physiologist François Magendie (1783–1855) (Strauss, p. 297)

Magendie is honored by the eponymous Foramen of Magendie. The saying highlights the opportunities open to all of us.

■ *Medicine is as old as the human race, as old as the necessity for the removal of disease.* Medical historian Heinrich Haeser (1811–1844) (Garrison, p. 14).

Haeser puts into context the origins of medicine that began when some prehistoric man or woman noted that a disease improved following the application of moss or another remedy, or perhaps after some earnest gourd-rattling.

■ *Physicians and public health officials, like soldiers, are always equipped to fight the last war.* Microbiologist René Dubos (1901–1982) (Brallier, p. 142)

Dubos seems to be describing the Maginot Line phenomena sometimes found in medicine. In the military, we always prepare for tomorrow based on past experience. The Maginot Line, a series of forts along the eastern border of France, was constructed after World War I, intended to defend against any German invasion. As World War II began, the Germans made an end run around the Maginot line, rendering it useless, but giving us a handy metaphor for endeavors that prove outmoded and ineffective. In microbiology, microorganisms seem to develop resistance to our most potent antibiotics faster than we can develop replacements. For example, The International Union against Tuberculosis and Lung Disease estimates that the median prevalence of multidrug-resistant tuberculosis is 1.1% in newly diagnosed patients, and is considerably higher (7%) in patients who have previously received anti-tuberculosis treatment.[28] On the educational front, we diligently train today's students to practice yesterday's and today's medicine – but rarely the medicine of tomorrow.

■ *The future belongs to those who shall have done the most for suffering humanity.* Louis Pasteur (1822–1895)

Pasteur's words are from an address at a dinner held at the Sorbonne in Paris on December 27, 1892 honoring his seventieth birthday.[29] In fact, Pasteur, an industrial chemist, was not a physician, even though in 1885 he successfully treated a boy bitten by a rabid dog. He did, however, advance our clinical knowledge and highlight the humanitarian side of medicine.

▓ *Whatever one sees, one must read, and whatever one reads, one must see. This is the only way to learn clinical medicine.* Indian physician T. C. Goel (Quoted in Meador, Number 159)

▓ *The aim of medicine is not to make men virtuous; it is to safeguard and rescue them from the consequences of their vices.* American writer H. L. Mencken (1880–1956) (Strauss, p. 302)

This somewhat humorous quotation, from the same man who coined the term "ecdysiast," is from Menken's book *Prejudice: Types of Men: the Physician.* Perhaps this is the author's satirical way of saying that some of medicine's greatest advances have come in the form of behavioral change – think about interventions to save us from tobacco, alcohol, drugs, and sexual promiscuity.

▓ *Medical education has been compared to teaching would-be tailors about the molecular structure of wool, how to grow cotton, and how yarn is spun in a mill. After that, they are sent out to tailor clothes.* American physician and educator Howard M. Spiro[30]

▓ *The physician educated in the liberal sense is a better physician.* American physician and ethicist Edmund D. Pellegrino (Pellegrino, p. 5)

REFERENCES

1. Klass P. *Treatment Kind and Fair: Letters to a Young Doctor.* New York: Basic Books; 2007.
2. Kohut RI. Postural vertigo. Quick relief from the postural vertigo component of vestibular diseases. *Arch Fam Med.* 1996;5(3):172–173.
3. Charles Barkley Quotes. Available at: http://www.brainyquote.com/quotes/authors/c/charles_barkley.html/ Accessed April 19, 2009.

4. Quotations on teaching, learning and education. Available at: http://www.ntlf.com/html/lib/quotes.htm/ Accessed January 8, 2009.

5. Kipling R. *A Book of Words*. New York: Doubleday, Doran; 1928:44–45.

6. Martí-Ibáñez F. To be a doctor. *MD Mag*. 1982;3:11-21.

7. Sobel RK. MSL – medicine as a second language. *N Engl J Med*. 2005;352(19):1945–1946.

8. Shortt SED. History in the medical curriculum. *JAMA*. 1982;248:79–81.

9. Lehman D. Physicians in literature: emotional approaches to patients. *J Med Humanit*. 1991;12:65–72.

10. Moore W. *The Knife Man: The Extraordinary Life and Times of John Hunter, Father of Modern Surgery*. New York: Bantam; 2006.

11. Burack JH, Irby DM, Carline JD, Ambrose DM, Elsberry KE. A study of medical students' specialty-choice pathways: trying on possible selves. *Acad Med*. 1997;72(6):534–541.

12. Kiker BF, Zeh M. Relative income expectations, expected malpractice premium costs, and other determinants of physician specialty choice. *J Health Soc Behav*. 1998;39(2):152–167.

13. Osler W. *Counsels and Ideals*. London: Oxford University Press; 1905:199.

14. Xu G, Paddock LE, O'Connor JP, Nash DB, Buehler ML, Bard M. Physician executives report high job satisfaction. Summary of findings from a survey of senior physician executives. *Physician Exec*. 2001;27(4):46–47.

15. Hoff TJ. The paradox of legitimacy: physician executives and the practice of medicine. *Health Care Manage Rev*. 1999;24(4): 54–64.

16. Dahlin ME, Runeson B. Burnout and psychiatric morbidity among medical students entering clinical training: a three year prospective questionnaire and interview-based study. *BMC Med Educ*. 2007;7:6.

17. McAuliffe WE, Rohman M, Santangelo S, et al. Psychoactive drug use among practicing physicians and medical students. *N Engl J Med*. 1986;315(13):805–810.

18. Meijer JWG, Smit AJ, Lefrandt JD, et al. Back to basics in diagnosing diabetic polyneuropathy with the tuning fork. *Diabetes Care*. 2005;28:2201–2205.

19. Kellogg JH. *Treatment for Self-Abuse and Its Effects, Plain Fact for Old and Young*. Burlington, IA: F. Segner & Co; 1888.

20. Sadovsky R, Collins N, Tighe AP, Brunton SA, Safeer R. Patient use of dietary supplements: a clinician's perspective. *Curr Med Res Opin*. 2008;24(4):1209–1216.

21. Ostrander GK, Cheng KC, Wolf JC, Wolfe MJ. Shark cartilage, cancer and the growing threat of pseudoscience. *Cancer Res.* 2004;64(1):8485–8491.

22. Goran GJ, Krishnadasan A, Gorwitz RJ, et al. Methicillin-resistant S. aureus infections among patients in the emergency department. *N Engl J Med.* 2006;355(7):666–674.

23. Centers for Medicare and Medicaid Services – Indirect medical education. Available at: http://www.cms.hhs.gov/acuteinpatientpps/07_ime.asp/ Accessed April 2, 2009.

24. McClinton JB. The doctor's own wife. *Can Med Assoc J.* 1942;47:472–476.

25. http://www.etymonline.com/ Accessed August 22, 2005.

26. King L. Medicine – trade or profession? *JAMA.* 1985;253(18): 2709–2710.

27. Moser RH. A few thoughts about professionalism. *South Med J.* 2000;93:1132–1133.

28. Sharma SK, Mohan A. Multidrug-resistant tuberculosis: a menace that threatens to destabilize tuberculosis control. *Chest.* 2006;130:261–272.

29. Vallery-Radot R. *The Life of Pasteur* [Mrs. R. L. Devonshire, Trans.]. Vol. 2. 1902;297.

30. Kravetz RE. Medical humanism: aphorisms from the bedside teachings and writings of Howard M. Spiro. *J Fam Pract.* 2008;57(10A Suppl):S27.

10

About Your Family and Community

*The doctor comes home ... whatever time that is and he or she
has to shift to "family" mode. Do you think that is an easy
shift to make? Do you think that the spouse or kids get their
doctor family member at his or her best? Or do they get the
leftover of that exhausting, long and stressful day?*
Life coach for doctors[1]

*All who are benefited by community life, especially the physician,
owe something to the community.*
American surgeon Charles H. Mayo (Mayo, p. 21)

This will not be the longest chapter in the book, but for a few
readers it will be the most meaningful, especially the thoughts
about the doctor's family. Your family can cause you more
sadness than all the no-show, heartsink and difficult patients
you will encounter in a lifetime. But there are two sides to
the coin. Your family can also bring more joy than making a
brilliant diagnosis, having a paper published in your favorite
medical journal, or receiving a national award. Do you doubt
me? Just ask any new parent or grandparent.

With the foregoing to set the stage, I will submit the thesis
that there is a world outside the medical office and hospital.
And this world is full of people and opportunities. Wise
physicians pay keen attention to these facets of their life.
Often-neglected life areas include full participation in
marriage (or other life partnership), family (however defined),
and community (which may range from neighborhood to
national involvement). This chapter will cover these three
topics, beginning with the doctor's life partnership, which is
traditionally – but currently not always – marriage.

R.B. Taylor, *Medical Wisdom and Doctoring: The Art of*
21st Century Practice, DOI 10.1007/978-1-4419-5521-0_10,
© Springer Science+Business Media, LLC 2010

BE A GOOD LIFE PARTNER

After doing a good deal of reading on the subject, I conclude that physicians do not have an enviable history of being good marital partners. The following is from a book titled *I Married a Doctor*, written by Alma Swinton, telling the story of a doctor's wife in a small Michigan town in the early 1900s. Here is how she describes arriving at their new home at the end of their honeymoon[2]:

> I walked up the dusty main street of the primitive looking small village with curious eyes. My young husband proudly pointed out the new little house tight against a store on one side, with a small open space between it and the post office on the other. The bridegroom hurried me in (I am sure he was not romantic enough to carry his bride across the threshold), and disappeared to make calls. I didn't see him again for several hours. How typical of my life as a doctor's wife this was to be! Come fire, flood, births, birthdays, parties or anniversaries, there were calls to make – they always came first. My life as a doctor's wife had begun.

Doctor Swinton may have been an excellent small town doctor, but he certainly was not a role model as a life partner. We believe that today things are different, and that physicians no longer sacrifice spouse and family to their practices, but the temptation to do so is always there.

NURTURE YOUR CLOSEST RELATIONSHIPS

If there is one key to success in life partnerships, it is the process of nurturing the relationship. This means finding ways to communicate effectively, cultivating common interests, and – most of all – spending time together.

Sounds easy, doesn't it? But the physician faces some formidable challenges in the quest for a successful intimate relationship.[3] These include:

- An acceptance of prolonged work hours, leading to fatigue, diminished family time, and a handy excuse for poor performance as a spouse and parent.

■ Smoldering hints of personal burnout, the result of heavy clinical obligations made worse by the burdens of bureaucracy and paperwork that characterize twenty-first century medicine.

■ The strategy of postponement in medical marriages, working for future goals while foregoing current enjoyable pleasures, a tactic that can result "in considerable covert marital discord," according to Gabbard and Menninger.[4]

■ The guilt-driven imperative that "patients come first"; and we can all figure out where spouse and family fit into that model.

■ The physician's perception of shame that would accompany needing help – horrors! – with personal stress or relationship problems.

I won't belabor the theme of medical marriage any further, except to say that there is a rich trove of literature on the topic. Three classic books are:

Gabbard GO, Menninger RW. *Medical marriages*. Arlington, Virginia: American Psychiatric Publishing Inc.; 1988.

Meyers M. *Doctors' marriages: A look at their problems and solutions*. New York: Plenum; 1994.

Sotile WM, Sotile MO. *The medical marriage: sustaining healthy relationships for physicians and their families*. Chicago: American Medical Association; 2000.

TAKE GOOD CARE OF YOUR FAMILY

Some of my colleagues don't marry or otherwise develop life partnerships. Some marry and don't have children. Still others divorce and shut themselves off from what had once been their families. I may be biased, but I think these physicians are missing a lot in life.

In 1983, John Callan, MD edited a book titled *The Physician: A Professional Under Stress*. Probably because of some writing my wife and I had done on the topic and because we were an intact medical family, Dr. Callan asked us to write a chapter titled "Marriage, Medicine, and the

Medical Family." We did so, with our two children, my wife, and I as co-authors. The chapter began: "Most people would consider us to be a normal medical family: a physician husband; a wife active in the community; and two daughters, both in college." I recently re-read the chapter and, the implied stereotypes of the time notwithstanding, much of its content is still relevant.[5]

Today, we would probably still be considered a normal – if no longer necessarily typical – medical family, just somewhat older. My wife and I are approaching our fiftieth wedding anniversary. Our daughters are both married and each has given us two wonderful grandchildren. We all love each other, we get together often, and we even get along – usually. Yup, we're pretty normal.

Consider that, at the time when your senses dim and your energy wanes, the people who will be there for you are your family – and maybe some especially close friends who have become "surrogate family." Not other physicians, responding to the daily demands of practice; not your contemporaries, who are busy with their own lives and families; and not your dog, whose loyalties will lie with its current food provider. Your spouse, your children, and your grandchildren are primarily the ones who will care for you when you are old and feeble, visit you in the nursing home, sit at your bedside in the hospital, and cry at your funeral.

As you age, your family – especially your grandchildren – is your reward for being a good spouse and parent, and for taking good care of your family. Do what needs to be done now to earn this reward later.

SEEK THE RIGHT BALANCE BETWEEN WORK AND FAMILY

Sotile writes, "We do not have appropriate, realistic road maps of what it means to have a lifetime partnership and what it really means in the trenches to have a reasonable balance between work and family."[6] The old guidelines to medical marriage and family life are just that – old and often outdated. What we thought was best a generation or two ago often does not necessarily apply today. Why? What has changed? I can think of several things. First of all, when I was a young physician, almost all doctors were men; today, women outnumber men in the incoming classes of most medical schools, and hence, before long most spouses are going to be men. Secondly, twenty-first century doctors are less likely to marry nurses or, as advised by Osler, "to choose a freckle-faced girl for a wife" (Osler held that such young ladies "are invariably more amiable." (Silverman, p. 229)). Today doctors are increasingly marrying other doctors, providing a handy basis for conversation, but compounding the problems of demanding work schedules.[7] I recall one resident, married to a resident in another specialty, telling how their paths seemed to rarely cross, and how they communicated using notes taped to the refrigerator door. Third, young physicians today enter practice with mountains of debt, bringing a sense of financial urgency to a time when they should be enjoying the early years of marriage and family life. And all this makes no mention of the role strains faced by many of today's women physicians, doing their best to succeed as both doctors and mothers.

WHEN HOME WITH FAMILY, BE A PERSON, NOT "THE DOCTOR"

Let's face it. We physicians tend to be perfectionistic, decisive and relentless, not exactly the characteristics most would list first if advertising for a life partner. To make things worse, early on in our careers, we are taught that one of our roles is to give orders – notably clinic and hospital chart orders for nurses and others to follow. Upon arriving home in the evening, the physician may find it hard to stop being the order-giver, and may seem to enter the front door bathed in the aura that "The Doctor is on the Floor!". If what you just read strikes a familiar chord, it may be time to acknowledge that, in the home, you are one more family member, one who must respect the equality of the spouse and the needs of the children, and whose roles may include cooking the dinner and taking out the trash.

ESTABLISH EARLY HABITS OF FINDING FAMILY TIME

I suggest that you put "family time" on your schedule. After all, we physicians tend to be both compulsive and time-oriented. For this reason, we can logically use our schedules to assure that we have adequate family time when spouse and children can have full attention. Try not to be distracted by phone calls or your Blackberry.

Here is a little trick that has helped me have regular vacations with my family. While on a family vacation, we schedule the time of the next trip. Then, as soon as I return to the office, I block out the time on my professional schedule. By doing so, vacation times don't become preempted with professional appointments.

SPEND TIME WITH YOUR CHILDREN

The penalty for failure as a parent is severe, and often not appreciated until too late to repair the damage done – when a teenage or adult child is angry, depressed, drinking too much or – even worse – suicidal or in trouble with the law. Wealth and privilege bring no warranty that children will turn out well. If that were the case, the offspring of Hollywood celebrities would be paragons of youthful virtue. We physicians can provide our families with more than our share of material advantages, but gifts, tennis clubs, and private school tuition cannot substitute for spending time with them.

HELP YOUR CHILDREN LEARN TO APPRECIATE THE VALUE OF HARD WORK AND INDEPENDENT THINKING

In 1972 I wrote a book titled *The Practical Art of Medicine*, a work in which I still take pride, even if it speaks of $7 office visits, patient account *cards*, and professional courtesy for fellow physicians and their families. Anyhow, in 1974, while I was still living in New Paltz, NY, and a full 10 years before I would think about a move to Oregon, a physician in Portland, OR named Joseph Van der Veer seems to have read my book and liked it; he sent me a book titled *The Adventures of Dr. Huckleberry*, with the inscription: "For Dr. R.B. Taylor – Because he'd like it."

Dr. Huckleberry was a general practitioner who, beginning in 1923, spent his career serving the small coastal town of Tillamook, Oregon, regionally famous for its cheese-making. Dr. Huckleberry was recruited to the job by the local physician, who "had x-ray burns on his hands and some fingers had been removed. He needed someone to serve as his hands." (Huckleberry, p. 4) For some reason, I kept the Dr. Huckleberry book and brought it with me when I moved to Portland in 1984. I tell you about this book, because I believe that this rural doctor, writing of his life, provides good insight into helping our children learn to respect the value of both honest labor and innovation. Here is what he wrote: (Huckleberry, p. 109)

During the hard times of the market crash in 1929, a lot of people had a really tough time, and we had our share of them. One group of six or eight families got together and tried to make a living cutting firewood. They built shacks of hand split shakes and bark, in the edge of a pretty scrubby patch of timber. They had no money for machinery, so they were doing everything by plain brute strength. One day when I drove past the place, my boy, then eight or nine years old, was riding with me. It was a miserable day, dark, cold, raining hard, windy, and had been for several days. These people, both men and women, were out in that rain, without proper clothing, soaked to the skin, in mud halfway to their knees, trying to man-handle poor grade logs into something salable. It was a most depressing sight, and one I have never forgotten. Just to relieve the impact of such a sight, I said the first thing that came to mind. "Son, if worse came to worst, do you think you and I could take an ax and saw and make a living for the family?"

There was no immediate reply, and I thought he considered the question too silly to answer, for I knew good and well we couldn't do it and thought he knew it too. A couple of miles down the road he said slowly, "I don't know. I guess we could do it if we had to, but it sure would be tough." Another pause, then, "But I betcha we'd find a better way to do it."

That struck me as a typical American attitude. There is a better way to do it, no matter what the problem, and we are going to find it.

TEACH YOUR CHILDREN TO BE CHARITABLE

This year my wife and I began what I think we will do for all our grandchildren as they grow old enough to understand and participate in the process. We gave our oldest grandchild a check for $25. The name of the payee was left blank for her to enter. Her assigned task was for her to complete the payee line and then give the check to her favorite charity – girl scouts, her community library, her church, or whatever she chose. It is our way of helping her learn to give back to the community.

What charity did she select? Without hesitation my granddaughter decided to give her check to the Make-A-Wish Foundation, an organization that, to quote their web site, "grants the wishes of children with life-threatening medical conditions to enrich the human experience with hope, strength, and joy."

CONSIDER INVOLVING YOUR FAMILY – SPOUSE AND CHILDREN – IN YOUR WORK

When our daughters were in their "tweens" and early teens, we lived and I practiced 18 miles from the hospital. That meant that I often needed to make a trip to the hospital on Saturday or Sunday mornings to see my hospitalized patients. Sometimes I took my daughters along, especially if my time on the hospital floors was likely to be not too lengthy. They brought books to read in the hospital waiting room while I completed my rounds. Yes, that was safe to do in the 1970s. And then we drove home together. Today, almost four decades later, my daughters fondly recall those times with their dad.

In that small town practice, my wife worked in the office and our children often helped with cleaning rooms and stocking supplies. I think this helped instill a good work ethic in the children and it gave them a sense of ownership of what was – after all – a small family business. Also, the salaries paid to the children helped lower the family taxes; my children were in a lower tax bracket than my wife and I.

YOU WILL INEVITABLY BE INVOLVED IN THE CARE OF YOUR OWN FAMILY MEMBERS

Is there a physician anywhere who does not serve as the "doctor of first resort" for his or her family members? I know I always treated the colds and stomach aches of my own children, and today, these daughters call me to consult when our grandchildren have sore throats and flu.

There is very little written about this topic, but in 2001 three of my Oregon colleagues published the results of a very interesting study.[8] They sent questionnaires to 2,014 physicians, inquiring about care they provided for their own families; there were 1,992 responses. Respondents indicated that minor prescribing, routine pediatric care, physical examinations, and minor surgery were commonly provided. Other forms of care occurred rarely, owing to complexity, severity, and privacy issues. An interesting note was that physicians were most comfortable providing care to their own children and least comfortable providing care to their grandparents.

As a physician, you will also inevitably become involved – to one degree of another – in the care of your senior family members. Chen et al conducted in-depth interview of eight physicians who reported on events that occurred when their own fathers were seriously ill.[9] The respondent physicians reported that, because of problems with their fathers' medical management such as poor communication or fragmented care, each felt compelled to intervene in the health care process.

LIVE IN THE COMMUNITY WHERE YOUR PATIENTS LIVE

Why should any physician – and his or her family – not live in the same community as his or her patients? Yet today, except in small towns, physicians and their patients often live in very different neighborhoods, if not in separate communities. Often, this separation is purposeful on the physician's part, in an effort to distance him- or herself – from patient contact outside the office.

On the contrary, I believe that the physician's life is richer and the quality of health care enhanced if doctor and patient live in the same community. Here is an example: I once treated a teenager for terrifying bouts of headache, typically occurring evenings and weekends. Extensive studies were normal, my best medication efforts were failing, and we were all puzzled. Eventually, the cause revealed itself. The key to the diagnosis lay in some serious family problems, unmentioned by the parents or patient, which came to my attention only through the community grapevine. When the family issues were resolved, the headaches miraculously ceased.

The best physicians are deeply imbedded in their communities. They shop at the local grocery stores, eat at local restaurants, and attend a local house of worship. They make house calls and funeral calls. They attend school board meetings and high school sports events. Sometimes they serve on local committees and commissions. In each of these settings, physicians learn about the lives of their patients, and they come across clues that, at some time in the future, may help explain a patient's health problems. For example, dining at a local restaurant may alert me to a patient's tendency to overeat or drink more than a single cocktail. Seeing married couples together outside the office helps me have a better understanding of their relationships. Seeing a teenager play in a basketball game or act in a play may afford insights into that young person's temperament. All this can help make us be more effective physicians.

SERVE YOUR COMMUNITY

The community looks to the physician for leadership in ways that go beyond the office and hospital. Yet, most physicians begin practice heavily in debt, debt they are earnestly striving to eliminate, and because of the long years of medical training, they are likely to join a community at an older age than some in other occupations. New physicians, if they are capable, soon have burgeoning practices that make demands on their time. The physician is also likely to be somewhat naïve as to his community responsibilities, perhaps, according again to Howe, owing to "the somewhat monastic character of medical training" (Garland, p. 19).

On the positive side, medical schools today are encouraging, even sometimes requiring, community service activities. For example, many of our Oregon medical students volunteer to help out in clinics serving the homeless of Portland. Whether a consequence of a generational shift to increased empathy for the needy in society or a perceived need to make one more competitive for medical school admission or the residency match, the trend to help others will, I hope, continue into the practice years.

In fact, even though perhaps just recently out of training and a newcomer to the area, the physician is one of the most educated persons in town. In most communities, few will have had more years of learning and hold higher degrees. With this educational endowment come obligations. For me this came, after just a few years in small town practice, as an invitation to join the local Narcotics Guidance Council. (It was, after all, the 1960s and our small town, just north of New York City, had a drug problem.) The invitation, from a member of the town council, included the observation, "Bob, you're a respected member of this community, your practice is now well established, and it's time to take on some community responsibilities." How could I say no?

The physician should lead in some local setting. In Chap. 7, I mentioned the book *Applebee's America: How Successful Political, Business, and Religious Leaders Connect with the New American Community*, in the context of seeking service-oriented employees. Authors Sosnik et al also describe how the most successful businesses strive for involvement in their communities, stressing the importance of donating time (and money) to community causes. (Sosnik et al, p. 179) Sosnik and his co-authors write about restaurant chains and other large businesses, but the lessons can be well learned by the physician engaged in making a living as a doctor. Many opportunities are available: volunteer teaching in the local school, serving the parent–teacher association (PTA), leading a scout troop, coaching a Little League team, or even running for public office.

While joining in activities with members of your community, it is perfectly okay to have some of these persons as friends. Actually, I urge you to cultivate some friends outside of medicine, that is, friends who are not physicians. Every time I visit a downtown office building or other commercial site, I reflect that there are persons by the thousands in town, doing work and following career paths quite different from mine. Getting to know a few of these people as friends can only enrich your life. In the end, some may be your patients, and some not.

WISE WORDS ABOUT YOUR FAMILY AND COMMUNITY

I have searched for aphorisms that might especially apply to today's and tomorrow's physicians. In reading the entries below, keep in mind the historical context; that is, until the past two generations, physicians were assumed to be men.

■ *Sane, intelligent physicians and surgeons with culture, science, and art are worth much in a community, and they are worth paying for in rich endowments of our medical schools and hospitals.* Sir William Osler (1849–1919) (Osler, p. 186)

Was there ever a more logical justification for generous support of our academic medical centers? If you have not recently sent a check to help support your medical school, now might be a good time.

■ *Happiness hangs around longer if the physician's (spouse) is his (or her) intellectual equal*[10]

Okay, so I updated the aphorism by adding some brackets to reflect today's gender distribution of physicians.

■ *The wife of a physician should be as different from other women as her husband is different from other men.* Canadian neurosurgeon Wilder Penfield (1891–1976)[11]

This saying can have various connotations, including the erroneous belief that a physician's spouse possesses special healing skills. Another notion is that the doctor tells the spouse *everything*. In many instances, my wife has been assumed by my patients to know about events in their private lives that they had told me about in the office. Sorry, not everything is shared with the medical spouse.

▨ *A large proportion of mankind, like pigeons and partridges, on reaching maturity, having passed through a period of playfulness and promiscuity, establish what they hope and expect will be a permanent and fertile mating relationship. This we call marriage.* English geneticist C. D. Darlington[12]

Sometimes, however, that urge for playfulness and promiscuity returns for a while at mid-life, a disruptive experience sometimes called the "hitting the air pocket."

▨ *Marriage is our last, best chance to grow up.* U.S. clergyman Joseph Barth (1932–1983)[13]

And some physicians – and others – actually do mature after marriage and become responsible adults.

▨ *The only person to whom a doctor can say exactly what he thinks about another doctor is his wife. That is why practically all doctors are married.* American author Joyce Dennys (1893–1991) (Strauss, p. 658)

Wife or husband or domestic partner, this person is still the physician's best confidant – and probably the most circumspect with regard to opinions about colleagues.

▨ *For two people in a marriage to live together day after day is unquestionably the one miracle the Vatican has overlooked.* American comedian Bill Cosby (1937–)[14]

▨ *It is a man's duty to provide moderately for his family, but anything beyond this may be a detriment to his descendants.* American surgeon William J. Mayo (1861–1939) (Mayo and Mayo, p. 52)

More than money, the wise physician gives his or her family personal involvement – which is more valuable than gold.

▨ *When the family fails, there's the community; when the community fails, there's family.*[15]

Sometimes even medical families fail, and that is when community involvement may pay off.

REFERENCES

1. Life coach for doctors. Available at: http://www.invinciblemd.com/blog/2006/11/doctors-wife.html/ Accessed December 2, 2007.
2. Swinton AW. *I Married a Doctor*. 2nd ed. Ann Arbor, MI: Edwards Brothers Inc.; 1965:4.
3. Meyers MF. Medical marriages and other intimate relationships. *Med J Aust*. 2004;181(7):392–394.
4. Gabbard GO, Menninger RW. The psychology of postponement in the medical marriage. *JAMA*. 1989;261(16):2378–2381.
5. Taylor AD, Taylor RB, Taylor DM, Taylor SJ. Marriage, medicine, and the medical family. In: Callan JP, ed. *The Physician: A Professional under Stress*. Norwalk, CT: Appleton-Century-Crofts; 1983:5–27.
6. SotileWM, Sotile MA. Success in medical marriage. Available at: Sotile.com/tips_success.htm. Accessed December 2, 2007.
7. Hall A. Medical marriage: no bed of roses. *BMJ*. 1998; 296(6616):152–153.
8. Reagan B, Reagan P, Sinclair A. Common sense and a thick hide: physicians providing care to their own family members. *Arch Fam Med*. 1994;3(7):599–604.
9. Chen FM, Rhodes LA, Green LA. Family physicians' personal experiences of their fathers' health care. *J Fam Pract*. 2001;50(11):995–996.
10. McClinton JB. The doctor's own wife. *Can Med Assoc J*. 1942;47:472–476.
11. Penfield W. *The Torch*. Boston: Little, Brown and Co; 1960:101.
12. Darlington DC. *Genetics and Man*. New York: Macmillan; 1964. Chapter 16.
13. Barth J. Quoted in Ladies Home Journal April, 1961.
14. Wisdom quotes/Bill Cosby. Available at: http://www.wisdomquotes.com/001351.html/ Accessed December 7, 2007.
15. Aphorisms by Rob Montone. Available at: http://www.jamesgeary.com/blog/?p=111/ Accessed December 7, 2007.

11

Caring for You, the Physician

The world has long ago decided that you have no working hours which anybody is bound to respect, and nothing except extreme bodily illness will excuse you in its eyes from refusing to help a man who thinks he may need your help, at any hour of the day or night. Nobody will care whether you are in your bed, or in your bath, or at the theatre. If any one of the children of men has a pain or a hurt in him you will be summoned; and, as you know, what little vitality you may have accumulated in your leisure will be dragged out of you again.

British author Rudyard Kipling (1865–1936),
writing on "A Doctor's Work."[1]

Phaenarete nodded and put a bony hand on Daphne's. "Teach him [Hippocrates] to pick the flowers," she murmured, and then in a stronger voice: "I know these ascelpiads well. I wived one and mothered one. Teacher and pupil, they've been about me, in and out of the house, ever since I married this man's grandfather. 'Work today and be happy tomorrow' – that's the physician's rule of life.'"

From Canadian neurosurgeon and author
Wilder G. Penfield (1891–1976) In: *The Torch*,
Penfield's novel about Hippocrates and
ancient Greece (Penfield, p. 136).

The grandmother of Hippocrates goes on to hope that Daphne, his bride, can "teach this grandson of mine to live a happy life." She might well also have wished him good health and longevity.

On my last airline trip, as I settled into my seat, I heard the usual recorded safety announcement which included the advice: "In event of an emergency, oxygen masks will fall from the compartment above you. Secure your mask first, before

R.B. Taylor, *Medical Wisdom and Doctoring: The Art of 21st Century Practice*, DOI 10.1007/978-1-4419-5521-0_11, © Springer Science+Business Media, LLC 2010

helping others." This is the airline oxygen mask paradox. You, as a physician, cannot help your patients unless you are fit and alert. It is not really selfish to take care of yourself first. Here is a personal example.

The year was 1968, and I was in my first few months of small town solo practice, with a wife and two young daughters to support. Would patients actually come to me as their physician? Would I be able to build a successful practice? Would I be able to pay for the new office equipment I had just bought? And then I got the flu – with fever, muscle aches, headache, and overwhelming fatigue. At one seminal moment, the telephone rang at home. One of my few patients was sick at home with a cough and low-grade fever. Would I make a house call? All I can recall is that this is what I told the patient: "I'm sick in bed with the flu – really sick! And I am only getting out of this bed to see someone who is a lot sicker than me." The patient understood and waited to see me a few days later, when I felt better. And at that moment, I resolved to try to take good care of myself, so that I could spend a good long – and happy – time with my family and my patients.

Just for the record, that patient and his family continued to be my patients for more than a decade.

TAKE YOUR OWN PULSE FROM TIME TO TIME

By this I mean this metaphorically taking stock of your happiness, your health and your life as an actual person. George Bernard Shaw once quipped that the most tragic thing in the world is a sick doctor (Brallier, p. 155). But in assessing your wellbeing, you need to look beyond your physical health status. Are you enjoying life outside the office? Is your family life fulfilling for them and for you – chock full of what the experts call "quality time?" Have you traveled recently, just for fun? What is the last good book you read? Have you been to a movie or the theater lately? Do you have occasional quiet time to reflect on your life?

THERE IS MORE TO LIFE THAN WORK

When I was an intern in 1962, I spent a 2-month obstetric rotation at Portsmouth, Virginia, Naval Hospital, during which I helped to deliver more than 120 babies. Yes, somewhere in

America today, there are that many persons in their late-40s whom I brought into the world. Anyhow, during that rotation, we interns worked every other night and every other weekend – in the navy they called this "port and starboard." When on duty, we rarely slept. The mothers in labor just kept coming, and we delivered babies in the delivery rooms, in the labor rooms, occasionally in the halls, and once in an elevator. During this time, my base was the U.S. Public Service Hospital in Norfolk, and I still recall the advice of my medical officer in charge (MOC), Dr. Zinn, as I finished the obstetrical marathon: "Bob, I hope that what you have just finished is as hard as you will ever have to work in your life. Later in your career, just be careful not to *create* a situation for yourself in which you work that hard."

AVOID THE "GROUND-DOWN," BURNOUT SITUATION

American physician and essayist Oliver Wendell Holmes, Sr. (1809–1894) once wrote:

"The longer I live, the more I am satisfied of two things: first, that the truest lives are those that are cut rose-diamond fashion, with many facets answering to the many-planed aspects of the world about them; secondly, that society is always trying in some way or other to grind us down to a single flat surface. It is hard work to resist this grinding-down action."[2]

You can drive yourself like a car that receives no maintenance until it groans to an oil-starved, rusty halt. And do you know what? Your patients and the world about you would praise you – briefly – for your dedication, and you would bask in their adulation, all the way to a premature, all-used-up retirement.

Sometime during World War II, there originated a pseudo-Latin aphorism: "Illegitimi non carborundum." The phrase "translates" to: "Don't let you let the bastards grind you down." It matters little that the phrase does not represent proper Latin. It was apparently birthed by the British early in World War II, and adopted – and thereby popularized – by American General Joseph W. (Vinegar Joe) Stilwell (1883–1946), who served in the China–Burma–India Theater. Now, we agree that your patients are not "illegitimate children," but the claims they make on your time and your well-being can certainly grind you down, if you are not careful.

As an aside, just to enlarge your knowledge of nonmedical topics, carborundum is an abrasive product derived from silicon carbide crystals. Carborundum was developed and trademarked by Edward F. Acheson in 1892 in my own hometown of Monongahela City, Pennsylvania.

Keeton et al have studied physician career satisfaction and burnout, using a questionnaire sent to a national sample of 2,000 randomly selected U.S. physicians.[3] Based on a 48% response rate, they concluded that, "Physicians can struggle with work-life balance yet remain highly satisfied with their careers. Burnout is an important predictor of career satisfaction, and control over schedule and work hours are the most important predictors of work-life balance and burnout."

DON'T SUCCUMB TO THE DELUSION OF INDISPENSABILITY

However good a physician you are, your patients will get along without you for a while. In fact, some may even improve. Or the physician covering your practice might make a diagnosis you had not considered.

Scrubbing in for surgery can offer time for reflection (washing one's hands does not command full concentration), and in one instance, I contemplated a short item that someone – perhaps a beleaguered surgical nurse – had posted above the scrub sink. As I recall it was in the form of a poem, but I can't recall the verse and so I will paraphrase here: To see just how important you are, take a bucket of water, insert your hand and arm, and churn up the water mightily. Look at the action you have caused. Then remove your hand and arm and take a look, to see just how much permanent difference you have made.

BALANCE YOUR PERSONAL AND PROFESSIONAL LIFE

One prophylaxis for burnout is to seek the personal–professional life balance that works for you and your family. I know of some couples – generally two-career couples – that maintain a firewall between work and home. By either explicit or implicit agreement, there is no discussion of work at home. For what it's worth, my family has always blended our professional and family lives. My wife has long worked in medicine, first in my private office, and now as an educator in the medical school. We both write, and sometimes do so at home on weekends. When they were younger, our children sometimes helped by doing what they could. It is often hard to tell when we're working and when we're playing. Think of how we live in this context: Turn work into play, and then play hard.

I am sure that what I just wrote will put off many physicians, who strive to keep clinical practice out of their homes. But I suspect that more than just a few wise physicians and spouses have, indeed, chosen the blended personal–professional life. If so, perhaps you will write and tell me about it.

DON'T OVERUSE ALCOHOL OR TAKE
SELF-PRESCRIBED DRUGS

Years ago, I attended a county medical society meeting. The evening followed the typical agenda of a social hour, dinner, and a speaker. For some reason, dinner was slow in coming; the bar was open and everyone, including the speaker, was having a good, old time. But when the time came for the lecture, it was apparent that the speaker had over-indulged during happy hour. He embarrassed himself mightily with slurred speech and a rambling presentation, serving as a good example of why speeches should come *before* beverages and dinner.

Osler advised physicians, "Above all things be strictly temperate" (Silverman, p. 160). I will discuss self-prescribing in Chap. 12 as an ethical issue. Here, I will focus on alcohol, which seems to be a noteworthy problem for America's physicians. Regarding alcohol use by physicians, Baldisseri tells us, "It is estimated that approximately 10–15% of all health-care professionals will misuse drugs or alcohol at some time during their career."[4] Ruben writes: "Although physicians seem generally to be reluctant to diagnose alcoholism in themselves or their colleagues, a recent AMA study indicated that 400 doctors are lost to the medical profession each year due to problem drinking." (Callen, p. 224) Callen does not specifically identify the AMA study and the figures are a little out of date, but they put the problem in perspective, and for all we know, things are even worse now.

To understand the significance of losing 400 physicians a year to alcoholism, let us consider an analogous metaphor. I have heard that each day 1,000 Americans die from the effects of cigarette smoking. A more graphic presentation of the number, however, would be to state that losing 1,000 persons each day is the same as three airliners crashing each day. Thus, given that the U.S. has 129 medical schools and that an average graduating class may be 120 persons (about the number of MD graduates of our medical school each year), we could then state that each year, we lose to alcoholism the equivalent of the graduating classes of three medical schools.

In Chap. 12, I will return to the alcohol and drugs in the context of ethical behavior and professional misconduct.

AVOID PATIENTHOOD

Some hold that every physician should be a patient from time to time, as an enrichment experience allowing us to see health care from the patient's perspective. I understand the thinking, and I know of one residency training program that even had its new interns admitted to the hospital – anonymously – just so they got a chance to enjoy patienthood, with all its depersonalization and indignities.

Nevertheless, all of us will eventually become patients, and thus I will share some long-recalled advice. The speaker at my medical school graduation hooding ceremony, a beloved infectious disease doctor whose special interest was tuberculosis, concluded his talk by offering a benediction: "May none of you ever become an interesting case." I didn't think much about his advice until, about 20 years ago, when I developed a debilitating and progressive lung disease, eventually diagnosed as a pulmonary sequestration. It required a right lower lobectomy, a huge scar on my right chest, and the opportunity to have my surgical specimen admired by colleagues at surgical grand rounds. I had become an interesting case.

EXERCISE REGULARLY

We all know that regular physical exercise can help prevent or treat many illnesses, as well as enhancing your energy level and improving your general sense of well-being. Yet too few physicians exercise regularly, citing various excuses, with being too busy high on the list. American cardiologist Paul Dudley White (1886–1973) once observed, "A man ought to have a doctor's prescription to be allowed to use a golf cart." (Brallier, p. 97)

Part of caring for you, the doctor, is finding time to exercise – if only it involves walking instead of driving short distances, climbing stairs instead of taking the elevator, and spending some spare time outdoors whenever you can.

In addition to improving your health, personal exercise might just make you a better doctor. Here's how: Abramson et al surveyed 298 primary care physicians regarding personal exercise and exercise counseling for their patient.[5] The authors concluded that physicians who exercise themselves are more likely to counsel their patients to exercise.

KEEP YOUR MIND ALIVE

Part of caring for yourself is keeping your mind active. Luckily, no matter how long you have been practicing medicine, there is always more to learn. Pity the poor gross anatomists. Gross anatomy has been described as a "completed science," no more body parts to identify and name, and today's anatomists are busily working to reinvent themselves as "cell biologists." But not so with clinical medicine, where there are new discoveries reported literally each day.

We physicians can take comfort in a passage from the *Daily Prayer of a Physician*, attributed to twelfth century physician–philosopher Moses Maimonides: "Never awaken in me the notion that I know enough, but give me strength and leisure and zeal to enlarge my knowledge and to attain ever … more. Our art is great, and the mind of man presses forward forever."[6]

LEARN A NEW SKILL, PROCEDURE OR FOCUS OF MEDICINE

Let's see: When things seem dreary, what can you do to rekindle your interest in medicine? Here is a short list of possibilities:

Teach a student in your office.

Write a medical article, perhaps reporting on an interesting case.

Attend a workshop to learn a new technique: for example, fiberoptic nasopharyngoscopy, colposcopy or medical hypnosis.

Develop a meta-specialty, such as occupational health care or travel medicine.

Volunteer to be an attending physician at a nearby residency training program.

Serve an evening a week at a local clinic providing care for the medically needy.

Join a medical team offering care in developing countries.

READ SOMETHING NONMEDICAL FOR PLEASURE EVERY DAY

Think about how much medical diagnosis is like detective work, assembling and interpreting clues that may just lead to the answer to a puzzle.[7] It seems no coincidence that a physician author created the archetypical detective in fiction, Sherlock Holmes. It is also why detective stories seem to intrigue physicians. On another theme, medicine has an extraordinarily rich history, appealing to the physician reader who yearns to be reading something that is "worthwhile."

In his book of collected addresses, titled *Aequanimitas with other Addresses* (see Bibliography), Sir William Osler ends with an oddly unnumbered page presenting his "Bedside Library for Medical Students." Here is what he wrote:

A liberal education may be had at a very slight cost of time and money. Well filled though the day be with appointed tasks, to make the best possible use of your one or of your ten talents, rest not satisfied with this professional training, but try to get the education, if not of a scholar, at least of a gentleman. Before going to sleep read for half an hour, and in the morning have a book open on the dressing table. You will be surprised to find how much can be accomplished in the course of a year. I have put down a list of ten books which you may make close friends. There are many others; studied carefully in your student days these will help in the inner education of which I speak

    I. Old and New Testament
   II. Shakespeare
  III. Montaigne
  IV. Plutarch's Lives
   V. Marcus Aurelius
  VI. Epictetus
 VII. *Religio Medici*
VIII. *Don Quixote*
  IX. Emerson
   X. Oliver Wendell Holmes – Breakfast-Table Series

In 1985, Richard C. Reynolds, then dean of the College of Medicine and Dentistry of New Jersey and coeditor of the book *On Doctoring* (see Bibliography), revisited the concept of a bedside library for medical students.[8] After a survey of 17 fellow medical educators, Reynolds offered these recommendations:

Butler, Samuel: *The Way of All Flesh*
Davies, Robertson: *Fifth Business*
Eliot, George: *Middlemarch*
Gardner, John W.: *Self-Renewal*
Kesey, Ken: *One Flew Over the Cuckoo's Nest*
Lear, Martha Weinman: *Heartsounds*
Mann, Thomas: *The Magic Mountain*
Pym, Barbara: *Quartet in Autumn*
Scott, Paul: *Staying On*
Solzhenitsyn, Alexander: *Cancer Ward*
Tolstoy, Leo: *The Death of Ivan Ilyich*
Norton Anthology of Poetry

Osler's list was compiled more than a century ago, and Reynolds' is from the mid-1980s. If you were to compile such a list today, what would be your ten top recommendations?

READ SOME OF THE GREAT PHYSICIAN–AUTHORS

There are many, which is probably no surprise given that medicine attracts many of our best minds. When physicians seek an avocation to balance the work of daily practice, some turn to writing, a fortuitous circumstance that has given us some of our finest literature. In fact, it may be true that more authors had first careers as physicians than as any other profession. Here are a few physician authors, whose works I recommend:

- François Rabelais (1494–1553). This French Renaissance physician–author is best known for his series of books telling the exploits of father and son *Gargantua and Pantagruel*.
- Oliver Wendell Holmes, Sr. (1809–1894). Recommended on Osler's list (see above), this physician author taught first at Dartmouth College, and later at Harvard, where he served as professor of anatomy and physiology. Holmes' fame came from his writing. His literary works included three series of witty essays: *The Autocrat of the Breakfast Table*, *The Professor at the Breakfast Table*, and *The Poet at the Breakfast Table*. He also wrote many poems, including some about events in the United States Civil War (1861–1865).
- Santiago Ramón y Cajal (1852–1934). This Spanish physician–scientist and Noble laureate wrote numerous scientific papers. In 1905, under the pseudonym "Dr. Bacteria," he also penned *Vacation Stories*, a collection of science fiction tales that anticipated the development of biological weapons of war. He is author of the quotation, "Like an earthquake, true senility announces itself by trembling and stammering." (Brallier, p. 120) As a tribute to his work, an asteroid – 117413 Ramonycajal – now bears his name.
- Sir Arthur Conan Doyle (1859–1930). This Scottish writer's works include nonfiction, poetry, plays, historical novels, and, of course, crime fiction. He is remembered today chiefly for his Sherlock Holmes tales. Kittle writes, "Doyle's experiences in medical school and practice served him

well and are reflected in many medical references in his stories, particularly those about Sherlock Holmes. More than any other author, he established and popularized the genre of medical fiction and, together with Poe, defined the short story as a literary entity."[9] As an interesting historical note, Sherlock Holmes' last name comes from Dr. Oliver Wendell Holmes (Reynolds and Stone, p. 34).

- Anton Chekhov (1860–1904). He has been called "Russia's most famous physician."[10] Schwartz goes on to tell that, "Chekhov's life was devoted to medicine and consumed by literature." In a letter to a friend he wrote, "Medicine is my lawful wife, and literature is my mistress" He wrote hundreds of short stories and several plays, including *The Sea Gull.*

- William Somerset Maugham (1874–1965). Maugham earned a degree in medicine, but never entered practice, instead devoting his career to writing. In *Of Human Bondage,* he tells of a young, somewhat sad, club-footed physician. His later works include *The Moon and Sixpence,* based on the life of Paul Gauguin, and *The Razor's Edge,* about a former fighter pilot seeking meaning in his life.

- William Carlos Williams (1883–1963). A generalist practitioner in Rutherford, New Jersey, from 1910 until 1951, Williams was also a poet. His best remembered poem, written in short moment of inspiration, is titled *The Red Wheelbarrow,* which begins: "so much/depends/upon/a red wheel/barrow..." (Reynolds and Stone, p. 68) Williams once wrote: "It's the humdrum, day-in, day-out, every-day work that is the real satisfaction of the practice of medicine; the million and a half patients a man has seen on his daily visits over a 40-year period of weekdays and Sundays that make up his life" (Strauss, p. 445).

- A. J. Cronin (1896–1981). After leaving a decade-long career as a practicing physician, Cronin penned novels including *The Citadel, The Keys of the Kingdom,* and *Adventures in Two Worlds,* the latter an autobiographical work.

- Ferrol Sams (b. 1922). Gifted storyteller Ferrol Sams practiced medicine in Fayetteville, North Carolina and, later in life, took up writing to pass on his stories to his descendants and also to augment his family income.

A number of his early works have autobiographical features. His prizewinning work (The Townsend Prize for Fiction) was *When All the World Was Young*, the story of a young surgical technician during the events of World War II.

■ Richard Selzer (b. 1928). Former Yale Assistant Clinical Professor of Surgery, contemporary author Selzer writes chiefly about what he knows: the human body and surgery. Among his currently available books are: *Mortal Lessons: Notes on the Art of Surgery*, *Confessions of a Knife*, and *Letters to a Young Doctor*. These should be required reading for all who plan to become physicians, and especially those who aspire to be surgeons.

■ Robert Coles (b. 1929). A child psychiatrist and a compelling and prolific story-teller, Coles has written more than 40 books, including *The Spiritual Lives of Children* and *Lives of Moral Leadership*.

■ Oliver Sacks (b. 1933). A neurologist and the child of two physicians, Sacks tells clinical anecdotes, chiefly about individuals with neurologic diseases. His book *The Man Who Mistook his Wife for a Hat* describes an instance of visual agnosia. Sacks' most famous book, *Awakenings*, telling the effects of L-dopa on patients with *encephalitis lethargica*, became a motion picture starring Robin Williams and Robert DeNiro.

■ Michael Crichton (1942–2008). This well-known contemporary author and film director, who also wrote under the pseudonyms Jeffrey Hudson and John Lange, held an MD degree from Harvard Medical School. He specialized in thrillers grounded in science and technology. On the shelves of your favorite bookstore look for: *Next, State of Fear, Prey, The Lost World, Rising Sun*, and *Jurassic Park*.

KEEP A JOURNAL

My college English professor tried to convince us all to keep journals, which we dutifully did for a while, as a requirement for the course. Over the years, I have made earnest attempts, recording thoughts, events, insights, and so forth. But I get busy and forget, and my journal pages remain blank for long periods. Perhaps my book writing, which includes many personal reflections, fills this need for me.

For you, a journal might include your record of life events, memorable quotations, instructive cases, and wise thoughts. If you make the effort to keep your journal up to date, both you and your descendents will be grateful in the future.

CREATE SOMETHING

To me, the idea of creating something evokes a favorite Einstein quotation: "Imagination is more important than knowledge." As physicians, our minds are chock full of knowledge. We need to make room for imagination. To do so, think of something you can create that does not exist today, then set out to make your vision a reality. For me, this is generally writing another book. For someone else, it may be planting a garden, painting a picture, or building a piece of furniture. What you choose is up to you and your personal preferences; what is important is that you imagine something that does not currently exist and then make it real.

JUST FOR FUN, LEARN A LITTLE ABOUT SOME OF THE CURIOUS EVENTS IN MEDICAL HISTORY

The following are just a few examples of odd chapters in the annals of medicine. If you enjoy reading these anecdotes, you will find more in my book *White Coat Tales*, listed in the bibliography.

- Ginseng, long valued in Asia for its medicinal properties and currently used as a "nutraceutical," actually played a role in American history. In his diary, George Washington described harvesting the plant and, in the 1780s Daniel Boone traded ginseng. The exportation of ginseng from America to Asia later helped open trade with China.[11]
- Robert Koch (1843–1910) was the German physician who discovered the tubercle bacillus, a discovery attributable in part to a novel culture technique that combined blood with the agar that Frau Koch used to make jam (Taylor, 2008, p. 222).
- Following the discovery of the x-ray by German physicist Wilhelm Roentgen, people began to speculate that it could allow Peeping Toms to see through women's clothing.

To combat this threat, one firm marketed a practical solution: x-ray-proof knickers (Porter, p. 606).

■ Sir William Osler (1849–1919) is known, among other accomplishments, for his epic textbook of medicine published in 1892. Less well known is that Osler had a wry sense of humor and sometimes wrote under the pen name of Egerton Yorrick Davis. One of "Dr. Davis'" articles, written to spoof a presumptuous editorial written by a colleague, was a literary hoax describing a case of *penis captivus*, an entity that almost certainly does not exist.[12]

Here is another Osler tale: While writing his now famous textbook, Osler became engaged to marry his editorial assistant Grace Revere Gross. But apparently the good lady would not marry Sir William until the book was finished. Dalrymple-Champneys tells that "on the day of its publication, February 24, 1892, Osler, with a copy of it under his arm, entered the house of mutual friends in Baltimore with whom Grace was staying and throwing the book into her lap, exclaimed, 'There, take the darn thing! Now what are you going to do with the man?'"[13]

■ American surgeon William Halsted (1852–1922) is credited with developing the prototype of surgical gloves we now use. But Halsted was an advocate of surgery using Joseph Lister's carbolic acid (Porter, 373). In fact, he developed the surgical glove for his surgical nurse, Caroline Hampton, who was also Halsted's fiancé. It seems the chemical disinfectant caused severe dermatitis of her hands, a reaction which Halsted hoped to prevent. The surgeon's use of the gloves would come later.

■ In the 1950, Colonel Robert J. Hoagland, chief medical officer at West Point Academy, observed that his cadets seemed to develop infectious mononucleosis a few days after date weekends, which were likely to include some hearty osculation. Following Hoagland's report, infectious mono acquired the sobriquet "the kissing disease."[14]

■ The antibiotic drug rifampin was, it is claimed, so named when the botanical source was discovered in an Italian forest, where the movie thriller *Rififi* was being filmed.

Drug names must be found somewhere, and it makes a great yarn, even if it strains credibility (Haubrich, p. 194).

FIND TIME FOR PERSONAL REFLECTION

Is there some time in the day when things are quiet, when distractions are minimal, and when ideas can pop into your head? For some it is during the morning tooth-brushing ritual. For others it is during the drive to and from work. Perhaps it comes in the twilight moments just before you fall asleep.

During these times, you may have fleeting glimpses of possibilities that would never occur during working hours, notions buried deep that spring into consciousness, if ever so briefly. Examples of the products of reflection might be a way to streamline something in your office or home, a better way to perform a procedure, an idea for an article to write, or even the recognition of an emerging problem that you had heretofore not noted.

CELEBRATE YOUR SUCCESSES

Despite its apparent glamour to those outside its ranks, a career in medicine is 40 years of small successes and occasional failures. Unlike the architect, you will have no grand openings of buildings your have designed. Unlike the attorney, you will win no landmark cases. Unlike the politician, you will have no stirring electoral victories. Your professional successes will be improving the health of one patient after another. Even more ethereal is the success of preventing diseases in your patients – illnesses that never begin in the first place. How in the world does one ever actually know what has been prevented? In your personal life, your successes will be – I hope – the same as those of your neighbors: your personal relationships, your first home, your financial savings for retirement, and so forth.

Pay attention to these professional and personal triumphs – and celebrate each one. Record them in the journal I recommended above. The successes you embrace will help shield you from the impact of the infrequent, but inevitable failures.

NURTURE YOUR PERSONAL SENSE OF HUMOR, YOUR "INNER CHILD"

Be able to chuckle about the funny side of medicine. Each of us has a few humorous anecdotes. For example, when I was working at the U.S. Public Health Service in Norfolk, Virginia in the early 1960s, we received a message that a Liberian freighter was headed toward us bearing a seaman with smallpox. At that time, this was entirely plausible, and would have been catastrophic if the infection spread to patients and staff in the hospital, and from there into the community. We quickly mobilized. One wing of the hospital was evacuated, isolated and made ready for the patient's arrival. Staff with up-to-date smallpox vaccinations volunteered to serve; the rest of us were hastily revaccinated. One brave young physician was sent to meet the ship. We all waited anxiously. Then after a few tense hours, the physician returned in the ambulance with the ailing seaman, who had a classic case of chicken pox.

While at the same USPHS Hospital, located in Virginia not too far from the Dismal Swamp, I was on emergency room duty one evening when a man came with a rattlesnake bite on the hand. "How did it happen?" I asked. "Well, Doc," he replied. "I was driving in my truck through the swamp in the dark. I thought I ran over something, maybe a rattlesnake. So I backed up to put it in my headlights. Sure enough, it was a snake, a big one. So I ran forward and back a few times, just to finish him off. Then, to make sure, I grabbed my tire iron and got out. That's when he bit me on the hand."

A few years later, I was a member of a group practice, working in a building with multiple exam rooms opening onto two long, parallel halls. One summer day, at the end of a busy afternoon, we all went home, unknowingly leaving two patients waiting in exam rooms behind closed doors. Eventually it seems that each of the two patients became curious and opened the exam room doors about the same time, to find themselves alone and staring at one another in a quiet, locked building.

Sometimes patients, like kids, say the funniest things. Here are some samples:

"I feel so bad I'd kill myself, except I'm afraid I'd wake the landlady."

"Getting a mammogram is like putting your breast on the driveway and letting someone drive a lawn tractor over it."

"The low cholesterol diet takes the sting out of dying."

It is even permitted for the physician to enjoy the occasional medical joke. Here is one a patient told me several years ago:

A middle aged man suffered a severe heart attack, had been hospitalized, and was ready to go home. On the day of discharge, the physician called the man's wife aside for a private conversation: "Your husband had a serious heart attack, and you need to do everything possible to reduce stress in his life: Get up early and fix him a healthy breakfast every day, don't nag him to do household chores, encourage him to play golf with his friends every weekend, and have sex with him whenever he wants. If you don't do these things, he could die"

On the drive home from the hospital, the husband asked, "What did the doctor say to you?"

She answered, "You're going to die!"

Such humor hurts no one and simply shows the human side of medicine.

SAVOR A FEW OF MURPHY'S LAWS OF MEDICINE

The classic Murphy's Law is that, "If anything can go wrong, it will." One source attributes it to Captain Edward A. Murphy, an engineer working at Edwards Air Force Base in 1949. It seems that Murphy found that a technician had crossed some wires in a device intended to test the effects of sudden deceleration, exclaiming of the unnamed technician: "If there is any way to do it wrong, he'll find it."[15] Here are a few of Murphy's Laws of Medicine, which can help provide a chuckle at the end of a long day:

- The patient always gets better just after calling for an appointment.
- Contractions always stop just after admission to the Labor and Delivery Suite.
- The doctor's family members always get the most obscure diseases.
- Your pager always sounds in the middle of your daughter's piano recital.
- The key medical report is always missing.
- Your sickest patient never speaks English.
- The patient with fever and cough whom you advise to stay home and take no specific therapy will turn out to have pneumonia requiring antibiotics.
- The lesser the indication for surgery, the greater the complication will be.
- Skin lesions removed for cosmetic reasons will result in keloid formation.
- The patient taking a new medication you prescribe will develop the one side effect you didn't mention.
- When getting directions for a home visit, the patient's use of the phrase "You can't miss it" to describe the house means only one thing: You are going to miss it.

AVOID HURTFUL HUMOR

Humorous remarks are commonly made by residents in reaction to long, stressful hours. They also desensitize physicians to suffering, and ultimately serve to dehumanize patients. Some classic examples of hurtful humor can be found in the 1978 book *The House of God*, by Samuel Shem, MD, actually the pseudonym of psychiatrist Stephen Bergman.[16] Shem popularized the term GOMER, an acronym for Get Outta My Emergency Room, indicating "a human being who has lost – often through age – what goes into being a human being." In his book, we find the Laws of the House of God (p. 420), including "GOMERs don't die." Wise, mature physicians do not engage in juvenile, hurtful medical humor.

DON'T BLAME YOURSELF WHEN GOOD DECISIONS GO WRONG

As a physician, you cannot control the outcome of the diseases you treat, you cannot predict the effects of the drugs you prescribe, you cannot foresee the complications of your procedures and, sooner or later, all your patients will die. Our goal each day is to try to help influence outcomes, minimize the mischief we cause, and hope that when our patients do die, that we have not contributed to their demise.

In medicine, we recognize that much of what we do is statistically driven. In the sense, it is "playing the odds." We advise with confidence that a person who quits smoking is less likely to develop lung cancer than one who continues to puff on cigarettes. The patient given an antibiotic for pneumonia is more likely to improve than to have an anaphylactic reaction to the drug. The child with appendicitis is more likely to recover from surgery than to suffer a complication. In most clinical settings, we do our best, and hope for the best, but must not assume too much fault when the laws of probability occasionally go against us.

LIVE LIFE TO THE FULLEST

Isaac Asimov (1920–1992), biochemist, science fiction writer, and editor or author of more than 500 books, was once asked what he would do if he had only 6 min to live. Asimov replied, "I wouldn't brood. I would type faster."[17] Asimov loved his work and lived life to the fullest. I wish this same sense of joy for you, the reader of this book.

WISE WORDS ABOUT CARING FOR YOU, THE PHYSICIAN

Hurry? Never hurry – hurry is the devil. More people are killed by hurry than by disease. Sir William Osler (1849–1919) (Silverman, p. 114)

Physicians sometimes seem to live their lives in a constant state of over-commitment, which they seek to remedy by hurrying through the day. Just consider what would happen if you worked an hour or two less each week:

You would spend more time with your family, you would have some time for hobbies or sports, you would get more rest, and you would pay less income tax. You will probably also become a better clinical communicator, diagnostician, and all-around physician.

▨ *Never have alcohol in the brain when the brain has work to do.* J.A. Lindsay (Lindsay, p. 152)
One of the vagaries of being a physician is that, at any moment, you may be called upon to make an emergency health care decision. For this reason, it is a good idea to stay away from alcohol any time when the telephone might ring or when you may be called upon to perform in a professional role.

▨ *Life is what happens when you are making other plans.* British musician John Lennon (1940–1980)
Most physicians could give lessons in delayed gratification. Why else would we spend long, austere years in medical school and residency training, while our contemporaries are moving ahead with their lives? Our mantra seems to be, "I'll defer having fun now because I have great plans for the future." But while we are earnestly planning for tomorrow, life happens day by day, even if we are not participating.

▨ *You may never diagnose a rare disease although, if you live long enough, you will probably get one*[18]
Might the lore actually be true, that the incidence of in fascinomas in physicians and their families really exceeds that of the general population?

▨ *Never go to a doctor whose office plants have died.* American comedian Erma Bombeck (1927–1996) (Brallier, p. 261)

▨ *No one on his deathbed ever wished he had spent more time at the office* (Anon.)

REFERENCES
1. Kipling R. *A Book of Words*. New York: Doubleday, Doran and Co; 1928:44–55.
2. Holmes OW. *The Professor at the Breakfast Table*. Boston: Houghton, Mifflin and Co; 1882:41.

3. Keeton K, Fenner DE, Johnson TR, Hayward RA. Predictors of physician career satisfaction, work-life balance, and burnout. *Obstet Gynecol*. 2007;109(4):949–955.
4. Baldisseri MR. Impaired healthcare professional. *Crit Care Med*. 2007;35(2 Suppl):S106–S116.
5. Abramson S, Stein J, Schauffler M, Frates E, Rogan S. Personal exercise habits and counseling practices of primary care physicians: a national survey. *Clin J Sport Med*. 2000;10(1):40–48.
6. Bogen E. The daily prayer of a physician. *JAMA*. 1929; 92:2128.
7. Nelson W, ed. *Nelson Textbook of Pediatrics*. First published as Mitchell-Nelson Textbook of Pediatrics. Philadelphia: Saunders; 1945.
8. Reynolds RC. Osler's bedside library revisited. *Pharos Alpha Omega Alpha Honor Med Soc*. 1985;48(2):34–36.
9. Kittle GF. There's more to Doyle than Holmes. *Pharos Alpha Omega Alpha Honor Med Soc*. 1997;60(1):17–20.
10. Schwartz RS. "Medicine is my lawful wife" – Anton Chekhov, 1860–1904. *N Engl J Med*. 2004;351(3):213–215.
11. Slazinski L. History of ginseng. *JAMA*. 1979;242:616.
12. Altaffer LF 3rd. Penis captivus and the mischievous Sir William Osler. *South Med J*. 1983;76(5):637–641.
13. Dalrymple-Champneys W. Wives of some famous doctors. *Proc R Soc Med*. 1959;52(11):937–946.
14. Moser RH. How "mono" made the team. *Med Opin*. 1971; August:74–78.
15. Murphy Laws Site – Origin. Available at Http://www.murphys-laws.com/Murphy/Murphy-true.html/ Accessed January 12, 2008.
16. Shem S. *The House of God*. New York: Dell; 1978.
17. Night falls for the good doctor. The Washington Science Fiction Association Journal May, 1992. Available at http://www.wsfa.org/journal/j92/5/index/htm/. Accessed January 12, 2008.
18. Bennett HJ. Humor in medicine. *J Fam Pract*. 1994;39(5): 421–422.

12

Ethics, Credibility, and Trust

> *Ethical values in medicine, such as the relationship between physician and patient, are eternal and immutable. The idea that society has regarding the patient may change, as it changed, for instance, from the ancient Babylonian concept of him as a sinner to the primitive Christian concept of the patient as a potential saint. The basic principles of medicine, however, do not vary.*
>
> Spanish-American physician and educator
> Félix Martí-Ibáñez (Martí-Ibáñez 1958, p. 70).

In Chap. 9, I told of the high regard we physicians as a group enjoy, esteem inherited from generations of honorable and trustworthy predecessors, and largely unearned by us today. Our legacy to future physicians must be to pass on the gifts we have received, by practicing medicine in an ethical manner that inspires credibility and trust.

Today too much of what is called medical ethics is bogged down in quasi-legal bickering about who can tell what to whom, whether or not we should do certain procedures such as abortion or cloning, the designation of the beginning of life, and the medical definition of death. But there is so much more. Medical ethics, credibility and trust, key ingredients of the art of clinical medicine, are really about people and the values they cherish. The three concepts have always been intrinsically linked, and are considered together in this chapter. To begin our study of these topics, I start 2,500 years ago, on the small island of Kos in the Aegean Sea, the home of Hippocrates, who is considered by many to be the "father of medicine."

R.B. Taylor, *Medical Wisdom and Doctoring: The Art of*
21st Century Practice, DOI 10.1007/978-1-4419-5521-0_12,
© Springer Science+Business Media, LLC 2010

OUR CURRENT ETHICAL CODE IS ROOTED
IN THE HIPPOCRATIC OATH

What began as the *Oath of Hippocrates* has been tweaked over the years, but the fundamental principles endure. Granted, like *Aphorisms* and other works attributed to Hippocrates, the *Oath* may well have been written by one of more of his disciples, based on teachings of the master. The identity of the actual scribe or even scribes matters little. What matters about the Hippocratic Oath is described by Rapport and Wright, who write that, "Its greatest significance lies in the ethical standard, the moral code which is established, and which no reputable physician will transgress. It has inspired physicians in a way which is itself inspiring. Surely no other art of business or profession can boast such record of devotion to human welfare" (Rapport and Wright, p. 1952).

Here is a translation of the classical version of the Hippocratic Oath:

> I swear by Apollo the Physician, and Asclepius, and Hygeia and Panacea, and all the gods and goddesses, that according to my ability and judgment, I will keep this oath and its stipulation:
>
> To hold him who taught me this Art as equally dear to me as my parents, to live my life in partnership with him, and if he is in need of money to give him a share of mine; and to regard his offspring in the same footing as my own brothers, and to teach them this Art if they desire to learn it, without fee or stipulation; and that by precept, lecture, and every other mode of instruction, I will impart a knowledge of the Art to my own sons, and to the sons of my teachers, and to disciples bound by a stipulation and oath according to the law of medicine, but to none other.
>
> I will follow that system of regimen which, according to my ability and judgment, I consider for the benefit of my patients, and will abstain from whatever is deleterious and mischievous.
>
> I will give no deadly drug to anybody if asked, nor suggest any such counsel. Similarly I will not give to a woman a pessary to produce abortion.
>
> With purity and with holiness I will pass my life and practice my art.

I will not cut persons laboring under the stone, but will leave this to be done by men who are practitioners of this work.

Whatever houses I may visit, I go into them for the benefit of the sick, and I will abstain from every voluntary act of mischief and corruption; and, further from the seduction of females or males, of freemen and slaves.

Whatever, in connection with my professional practice, or not in connection with it, which ought not to be spoken abroad, I will not divulge, holding that all such should be kept secret.

While I continue to keep this Oath faithfully, may it be granted to me to enjoy life and the practice of this Art, respected by all men, in all times. But should I transgress it and violate this Oath, may the reverse be my lot.

Over two and a half millennia, things changed and, bit-by-bit, phrases in the classic Hippocratic Oath became inappropriate or irrelevant. Here are some items that don't fit with today's medical education and practice:

- Assuming that the physician is male. Today about half of all medical students are women.
- Giving money to one's teacher "if he is in need." I think we do so still, but it is now called medical school tuition, and is routed through the institution to pay the salaries of professors.
- Teaching the children of one's instructors, which today might be regarded as affording preferential treatment to certain medical school applicants.
- Not teaching medical knowledge to non-physicians. But what about the many physician–authors who write for the lay audience and the health experts who appear on television talk shows?
- Not giving a "deadly drug to anyone if asked." This prohibition is challenged in debates about "death with dignity," notably in my home state of Oregon, where physician assisted suicide is legal, albeit with stringent legal safeguards.
- Not inducing an abortion in a pregnant woman; abortion as a surgical procedure is currently legal in the USA.

▓ Not "cutting persons laboring under the stone." In early days before we had life-saving drugs, medical therapy involved chiefly dietetic recommendations, herbal remedies, and other health-promoting activities. Those who performed surgical procedures were held in low regard. This is not the case today.

▓ Keeping secret "that which ought not to be spoken abroad." Today confidentiality is compromised in many subtle ways as patient information is widely shared, as discussed below.

In order to preserve the tradition of commitment upon beginning a career in medicine, and to side-step the anachronisms in the traditional Hippocratic Oath, the General Assembly of the World Medical Association adopted the Declaration of Geneva in 1948. There have been subsequent minor revisions, the latest in 2006. Although a few medical schools use their own unique versions, the Declaration of Geneva is recited by most U.S. medical school students as part of their graduation ceremonies.

Here is today's Declaration of Geneva:

> At the time of being admitted as a member of the medical profession:
>
> I solemnly pledge to consecrate my life to the service of humanity;
>
> I will give to my teachers the respect and gratitude that is their due;
>
> I will practice my profession with conscience and dignity;
>
> The health of my patient will be my first consideration;
>
> I will respect the secrets that are confided in me, even after the patient has died;
>
> I will maintain by all the means in my power, the honor and the noble traditions of the medical profession;
>
> My colleagues will be my sisters and brothers;
>
> I will not permit considerations of age, disease or disability, creed, ethnic origin, gender, nationality, political affiliation, race, sexual orientation, social standing or any other factor to intervene between my duty and my patient;

I will maintain the utmost respect for human life;

I will not use my medical knowledge to violate human rights and civil liberties, even under threat;

I make these promises solemnly, freely and upon my honor.

Note that the pledge is a "declaration," and no longer an oath. Women have been included, in the phrase "sisters and brothers." Surgeons seem to have been welcomed to the house of medicine, with no prohibition on "cutting for the stone" or for anything else. The Declaration is silent on abortion, and there is a curious absence of the Hippocratic imperative to teach the art of medicine to the next generation of physicians.

These pledges are the foundation of ethical medical practice, and the physician is distinguished by professing an oath like no other. Recall from Chap. 9 that the word "profession" comes from the Latin *professionem*, meaning public declaration. Its meaning in medieval times related to vows taken upon entering a religious order. The moral imperatives of the Oath, and probably also the Declaration, can be interpreted as having religious – that is, moral – underpinnings. Whether you subscribe to the original Hippocratic Oath or the more up-to-date, and more politically correct, Declaration of Geneva, it is important to recognize that both offer some guidance regarding many of today's ethical dilemmas. If only the issues were as clear as the counsel offered.

RECOGNIZE THE UNDERPINNINGS OF TODAY'S MEDICAL ETHICS

Ethics is about values – moral principles to which we believe that any reasonable person would subscribe. There following are the main ones we physicians face from time to time:

Beneficence

The word beneficence comes from two Latin words, *bene* and *facere*, together meaning to "do good." Medical care is, at its core, a transaction between patient and physician. In this context, the transaction is a little atypical in that the doctor's chief concern is (ideally) to "do good" for the patient.

This differs from other transactions such as, for example, between a car salesman and customer, in which the fundamental goal of the salesman is to sell the customer a car – any car – today. Yet, in Chap. 1, I discussed the commercialization of medicine, a trend that threatens to replace the ethics of medicine with the code of commerce, whatever that may be.

Non-malfeasance

Primum non nocere, translated as "do no harm," is often attributed to Hippocrates, not unreasonably so since the phrase is found in Epidemics (Book I, Section XI). "Do no harm" can also be inferred from the Hippocratic Oath in the admonitions to not give deadly drugs and to avoid mischief when attending patients. In fact, "do the sick no harm" can be found in the Oath of Hindu Physicians, which predates the Hippocratic Oath by a millennium. (Strauss, p. 325) Whatever the source, "do no harm" has been and continues to be a fundamental precept of ethical medical practice.

Autonomy

Loosely defined as freedom from external influence or control, autonomy is a cherished ethical value of both physicians and the patients they serve, but can become a bit of problem in the medical encounter as the patient looks to the physician for unbiased advice on whether to take an antihypertensive medication that may cause side effects, have surgery on a painful lumbar disc, or sign an advance directive form. Is the physician, working under institutional and governmental rules and regulations, truly autonomous? Can the patient have autonomy in a setting when the physician clearly has an advantage in knowledge and power? Following a qualitative study looking at patient autonomy and paternalism, Woodward states, "Respect for patient autonomy is identified as an essential element of individualized patient-centered and ethical care but conversely, it is suggested that overemphasis may confuse and suppress beneficent intervention."[1]

Confidentiality

What is told behind the door of the examination room is to remain between patient and physician – except, of course, for the receptionist, the case manager, all the consultants, all the nurses, the physical therapist, medical students, residents in training, insurance clerks, the billing coder and anyone else with access to the medical record. I am not sure that my ability to access patient records from my home computer has advanced medical confidentiality. Despite my cynicism about the current status of not repeating secrets told by patients, I believe that most doctors today are careful about what they directly reveal about patients and to whom they reveal confidential facts. The medical information system may be another story.

Truth-Telling

My mother was fond of saying, "Always tell the truth; that way you don't have to remember what you told someone." Of course, you need not tell everything you know at every visit, an affliction common to third year medical students, proud to display their newly-acquired knowledge of disease. I was taught early to always tell the truth, but sometimes in measured doses, according to the patient's readiness to hear. An example was a middle-aged man for whom I was performing a pre-employment physical examination in my rural practice office in upstate New York. In this office, I had my own x-ray machine and, as requested by the prospective employer, I did a chest x-ray. Following a "wet reading," I could see that the patient had a large tumor, one that was probably advanced lung cancer, and thus very likely a death sentence. Other than being a long-time cigarette smoker with a "smoker's cough," the patient considered himself healthy. I did not share all this new information and my personal speculation with the patient. What I told him was that he had a lung mass, that I did not know for sure what it was, that a prompt diagnosis was imperative, and that I would arrange the appropriate diagnostic studies and consultations needed to get the answers he and I needed. In not revealing the full truth about what I believed, did I violate medical ethics?

Justice

Justice in medicine comes into play as fairness. If there is only one donated kidney and two potential recipients, would it be just and fair to give the kidney to the patient who had insurance and to do so only for that reason? Should age make a difference in who gets the only available kidney? What about the relative contributions to society of the two potential recipients? Or should we be totally fair and flip a coin to see who lives and who dies?

RECOGNIZE THE GENESIS OF ETHICAL DISAGREEMENTS IN MEDICINE

An ethical conflict begins when each side believes that one value takes precedence over another. In fact each side may subscribe to both values, yet hold that one must supersede the other. For example, let us take the cost of bariatric surgery for a very obese patient. The operation may be life-changing, even life saving, but for the cost of that surgery, dozens of pregnant patients could receive prenatal care or hundreds of children receive immunizations. But with only so many health care dollars in the system shall we respect the obese patient's autonomous and beneficial "right" to potentially life-saving bariatric surgery or use the money in what seems a fairer way on prenatal care and immunizations that help far more individuals? Does it make a difference if the patient is on Medicaid, has "Cadillac" insurance, or is a wealthy self-pay individual?

Here is another example of a similar ethical dilemma: A dying patient could be kept alive for a while by using repeated transfusions, but she was depleting the blood bank's stock of Rh-negative blood. Some thought this blood should be reserved for persons whose lives might be saved. Others disagreed. The ethical dilemma was: Should the patient receive the blood? Or should she be denied the blood – saving it for some future patient who might need a transfusion of this blood type – and be permitted to die? If so, then whatever happened to non-malfeasance?

The dying patient requiring use of a scarce resource in order to sustain life a little longer highlights how the physician, like it or not, sometimes is forced into the role of "double agent," attempting to protect the interests of both the individual and society. In 1950, Dean of Harvard Divinity School Willard R. Sperry (1882–1954) wrote a book on medical ethics.[2] His work was prompted by questions raised by young physicians. In Chap. 8 of book Sperry tells his opinion, "Once a doctor subordinated the claims of an individual patient under his care to the abstract claims of society in general, or the hypothetical claims of some possible alternative patient, he has sold his pass." But would we agree with Sperry today, a half-century later, at a time when we are all sensitive to the fair use of scarce resources? At the end of the day, physicians would champion both ethical values – beneficence for one patient and do no harm to another – but are forced to choose.

ACKNOWLEDGE THE ETHICAL ISSUES IN DAILY PRACTICE

Ethical issues don't just arise in public policy debates or in the critical care units of hospitals. In fact, we face small ethical dilemmas every day as we make decisions about ordering laboratory tests, prescribing increasingly expensive medications, selecting primary diagnoses that will determine billing codes, and telling patients our true opinions.

Not all daily practice decisions are minor. Here are some examples of troublesome issues I have faced over four decades of practice, with my best analysis of why the events seemed to present an ethical challenge.

Deciding What to Tell to Whom

The patient is a 91-year-old woman with congestive heart failure. She also has laboratory evidence of past infection with syphilis. Her mental status has become a little clouded, and she has signed no advance directive. She and I, her physician, have never discussed who should be told what. Her family, headed by a 59-year-old son who is both smart and keenly interested in his mother's health, asks for a full update about her condition. My sense is that he and the rest of the family are just trying to help by becoming engaged in the care process. Thus bringing them into the information loop would be doing the right thing for the patient, i.e., beneficence. But what about confidentiality? Is not the patient entitled to privacy of information concerning her health status? A 2005 study conducted in Spain surveyed 227 physicians about confidentiality in the doctor–patient relationship. The investigators found that of the respondents, 95% had shared a patient's medical information with a family member and 35% had provided information to others – all without the patient's consent.[3] Presumably these physicians who shared medical information believe that beneficence trumps confidentiality.

Easing Pain but Perhaps Doing More

The patient was a 62-year-old man, dying at home of metastatic prostate cancer with painful bone metastasis. His chief caregiver was his wife, who has been taught to administer morphine injections for pain. I became aware that she was requesting prescriptions for increasing doses of morphine, representing huge amounts of the drug. Was she overmedicating her husband, and thus hastening his death? Was it even possible that their son, whom I knew had had some brushes with the law, was selling part of the patient's drug supply on the street? Or was the patient's tolerance to the drug simply calling for increasing doses to control pain. Were doses even being stockpiled for use as a single lethal injection? To me this seemed to be a case of doing good (relieving pain) while being careful to do no harm, an issue we physicians face daily. Or was I enabling malfeasance?

Flying the Risky Skies

Another patient was a 52-year-old regional airlines pilot, whose job each day involved flying passenger jets. He presented in my office with a history of chest pain, probably angina pectoris, and with a request: "Please don't tell my employer – the airline." Now here is a serious quandary. What is the doctor's responsibility here? As far as the patient is concerned, the ethical value seems to be confidentiality, but does the doctor have a greater duty to tell the truth to those who control the safety of passengers trusting in their pilot? Would informing the airline simply be an issue of fairness? When it comes to confidentiality, is the physician's chief obligation to the individual or to faceless individuals who may be affected if the patient goes on to have a sudden fatal heart attack while flying a plane, a possible but admittedly not very likely event? Even for experts, this issue has no clear-cut answer. Bird, writing about fitness to operate a motor vehicle, holds that physicians "may need to consider breaching their patient's confidentiality and notifying the Driver Licensing Authority that a patient is unfit to drive."[4] On the other hand, Kipnis, writing in the American Journal of Bioethics, holds the following: "Though doctors have a professional obligation to prevent public peril, they do not honor it by breaching confidentiality." He goes on to make the case that "the protective purpose to be furthered by reporting is defeated by the practice of reporting." Although the logic leading to the conclusion presented in the previous sentence seems a little convoluted, the author does make a strong plea for unqualified medical confidentiality.[5]

SOME EVERYDAY ETHICAL ISSUES ARE COMPLEX AND MAY EVEN CALL FOR COURAGE

How many times in the last few months have you seen a patient's well-being compromised by recommendations or even mandates by insurance company representatives or by case managers employed by your own hospital? For example, you are informed that your abdominal surgery patient, age 76, must go home on post-operative day 4 even though there is no one at home to see to her needs. In this setting, I think the conflict involves beneficence, truth-telling, and fairness. Are we as physicians willing to speak up to insurance companies – even though it will take time and effort, and with repeated objections may risk our being "delisted?" Or, by remaining silent are we allowing unfair treatment of our patients?

Here is another ethical quandary a physician may encounter. Your patient is in the hospital near death and may have some salvageable organs. According to a New England Journal of Medicine article by Truog, a problem arises in how regulations from the Centers for Medicare and Medicaid Services are being interpreted and implemented. "These require hospitals to notify the local OPO [Organ Procurement Organization] 'of individuals whose death is imminent or who have died in the hospital' and to ensure that the person who initiates the request to the family is a representative of the OPO or a 'designated requestor.'" Now, you and I as everyday practicing physicians are unlikely to be "designated requestors." In fact the organ procurement coordinators "are encouraged to introduce themselves to families as members of the 'medical team' or as 'grief counselors,' without necessarily disclosing that their role is explicitly one of dual advocacy, since – operating under the assumption that organ donation is simply 'the right thing to do' – they simultaneously represent the interests of the patient or potential donor and the pool of potential recipients." In some cases, the donor patient's dying is prolonged to permit optimum perfusion of transplantable organs. Truog goes on to cite the words of a critical care physician in Chicago: "I have seen these guys come in and almost browbeat families into submission to get them to donate organs."[6] In citing Dr. Truog's article, I have used several quotes because I wanted to get the wording correct. I find the described behavior of the "designated requestors" to be highly objectionable. Whatever happened to non-malfeasance, truth-telling, and justice? What would be the fate of the attending physician who questions the methods of the OPO?

Even our relationships with pharmaceutical sales representatives have come under ethical scrutiny. Wall and Brown describe a program in which physicians provide pharmaceutical sales representatives with a preceptorship experience, observing the physician during daily patient care. The physician, of course, receives an honorarium for the service. Presumably this was a truly beneficial educational experience for the pharmaceutical representatives, one that could improve future communication with physicians.[7]

We should note that this report is published in the journal *Obstetrics and Gynecology,* and hence did the drug representatives observe the elicitation of women's personal histories, gynecologic examinations, pelvic surgery, and obstetrical deliveries? This practice seems to challenge a wide spectrum of ethical issues, including confidentiality, patient autonomy, beneficence, non-malfeasance, and truth-telling (Are patients told about the honorarium?).

BE AWARE OF HOW PATIENT CARE DECISIONS ARE MADE IN YOUR DAILY PRACTICE

No matter how much we value patient autonomy and eschew paternalism, there may be a place for what I will call the *informed opinion imperative.* After all, the physician presumably knows more about disease, treatment, and prognosis than the patient or family, and is considered the "expert" in the encounter. When I am a patient and a decision must be made regarding the next step in my own health care, I like to look my physician in the eye and ask, "Doctor, if you were the patient, what would you do?" Facts are important, and as a physician–patient I am certainly more medically knowledgeable than the average patient. Nevertheless, when faced with an important decision, as I was last year when an area of high grade dysplasia was found in my colon during routine colonoscopy – I want my doctor to tell me the facts, lay out the options, and then give me his *informed opinion* as to what should be done.

Writing in the *Journal of Medical Ethics*, Savulescu, at the University of Oxford, describes the drawbacks of the physician acting chiefly as a "fact-provider." The author writes, "If doctors are properly to respect patient autonomy and to function as moral agents, they must make evaluation of what their patients ought to do, all things considered." He advocates for *rational non-interventional paternalism* – "a practice in which doctors form conceptions of what is best for their patients and argue rationally with them."[8]

Let us frame this issue in the jargon of medical ethics: On one hand, we want the patient to have the freedom to make personal healthcare decisions, even if he or she will never have attended a single medical school lecture. We will stand up and defend the patient's right to autonomy. On the other hand, we want the right thing done (beneficence) and not allow harm to happen (non-malfeasance), and to achieve these values, we may inject a little subtle paternalism.

Whatever happens in your next encounter in which there seems to be a conflict between patient autonomy and rational non-interventional paternalism, I think that the most important thing is to recognize which side of the issue you have espoused that day.

DO IN PRACTICE ONLY THAT WHICH YOU CAN BE PROUD OF DOING

American writer Mark Twain (1835–1910) once said: "Always do right. This will gratify some people and astonish the rest." Perhaps this dictum is a key to ethical and moral practice. For example, there are ways to double your income – by doing things you wouldn't want described in your local newspaper. These include procedures you really shouldn't be performing, using billing methods that your accountant would not approve, and seeking ways to pyramid charges rather than acting in the patient's best interest. For example, if you perform a lab test in your office, are you doing so because it enhances the quality of your care, is convenient for the patient, and can be done for equal or less cost when compared to a clinical laboratory? Or are you performing the test because you *can* – and chiefly because it boosts your bottom line at the end of the month? Never do anything in practice if you would hesitate to explain your motives to your mother.

MAINTAIN CONFIDENTIALITY EVERYWHERE

Patient information is not only divulged systematically by easy access to the electronic medical record and other system problems. We are also sometimes simply careless. "Loose lips sink ships," was a slogan during World War II, implying that revealing confidential information might cause serious harm to someone, somewhere.

' Working as I do in a large academic medical center with hundreds of medical students, nurses, and young physicians around, I am often appalled as what I hear during discussions held in elevators. At our medical center, originally built on a high hill (And yes, it is called "Pill Hill.") with a new clinic building below at the river level, we physicians and patients travel between the two sites on an aerial tram. The 3-min ride, with 20–30 people standing in a quiet cable car, invites "tram talk." On any given day you might hear how a colectomy patient has turned septic or how "We need to get a genetics consult for the funny looking kid on the 8th floor," as if not actually naming the patient makes the comment less offensive. Any time two physicians are discussing a patient in an elevator – or a tram or in a cafeteria line – you can be sure a relative is within earshot. It is one more of Murphy's Laws of Medicine. I was once in a crowded elevator in which two senior medical students were discussing a patient, to the quiet amusement of the other passengers standing nearby. As it happened, also in the elevator, standing in the rear of the car, was the dean of the medical school. When the elevator door next opened, I watched as the dean stepped to the doorway, pointed at the two students, and said, "You and you: Get off with me now!" The elevator door closed, the rest of us continued our descent quietly, and thus I can't tell you what happened to the two students. I certainly would not have wanted to be in their shoes.

KEEP PERSONAL POLITICS OUT OF YOUR PRACTICE

I don't care if you are liberal, conservative, prohibitionist, or vegetarian. Imposing your political views on patients and their families abuses your power in the physician–patient relationship. Napoleon Bonaparte once said, "A physician and a priest ought not to belong to any particular nation, and be divested of all political opinions." (Brallier, p. 151). I would not go to that extreme. After all, what happens to medicine today and tomorrow is significantly affected by political decisions. Because of this, physicians may reasonably be involved in politics, and even a few of us should serve as political leaders. But there should be a firewall between the physicians' political opinions and the medical practice. This means, for instance, no candidate signs on the office lawn or in the waiting room, and no political haranguing in the exam room. To use the power of the physician in the doctor–patient relationship to advance a political cause would be an unfair use of the physician's power and thus unethical.

HOW WE DEAL WITH ERRORS IS AN ETHICAL ISSUE

Medical errors, especially those that actually cause harm to patients, can present challenging ethical choices. Writing in the early twentieth century, Sir William Osler observed, "Errors in judgment must occur in the practice of an art which consists largely of balancing probabilities." (Silverman, p. 45) Today, with the explosion of new therapeutic options and the advent of innovative technologic interventions, the potential for errors – and for resultant injury – is even greater than in Osler's day.

Dovey et al have provided a good overview of medical errors in family medicine, with a taxonomy that seems applicable to all areas of clinical practice.[9] The authors use a very functional definition of a medical error: something that occurred, that was not anticipated and that makes you say, "That should not happen in my practice, and I don't want it to happen again." With this preface, and after reviewing 344 reports submitted by 42 physicians, they found the following clusters of errors:

- Administrative failures (30.9%): These involved bungled appointments, lost or unavailable information, errant messages, and similar system problems.
- Investigation failures (24.8%): Here we find wrong tests ordered, errors in processing specimens, and inappropriate response to an abnormal report.
- Miscommunication (5.8%): These errors include diverse communications among physicians, staff, and patients.
- Mistakes in execution of clinical tasks (5.8%): These errors, such as unrecognized crossed leads on an electrocardiogram, reflected lack of clinical knowledge and skills.

More serious is the "tenfold error," described by Kozer et al, which often occurs in calculation of pediatric drug doses.[10] The tenfold error, in which a recommended dose of 10 mg may become administered as 100 mg, "may be especially high in resuscitation situations and is underestimated by spontaneous reporting."

- Treatment decision errors (4.2%): An obvious example would be prescribing penicillin for a patient with an allergy to the drug. Less obvious is prescribing mefloquine as malaria prophylaxis for a patient with a history of psychosis and then sending him off into the jungles of Africa.

- Misdiagnosis (3.9%): This number is consistent with the findings of Neale et al who found that approximately 6% of admitting diagnose in British hospitals were incorrect.[11] Think of diagnosing sleep apnea when the patient actually has paroxysmal nocturnal dyspnea caused by congestive heart failure. Another example is the patient with an impending stroke misdiagnosed as migraine headache.

- Payment system problems (1.2%): A colleague once told me how he and his wife had a new baby girl, and shortly after arriving home from the hospital, they received the hospital bill that included a charge for infant circumcision. Whoops!

In reading the study by Dovey et al, I was a little surprised to see how relatively few errors involved misdiagnosis and poor treatment decisions. In a study by Burroughs et al of patients seeking care in emergency departments, the most common concern was misdiagnosis.[12] Of course, we tend to hear of catastrophic misadventures – such as amputating the wrong leg – because these are the errors that might result in litigation.

So now that we have described the spectrum of medical errors, what are the ethical issues involved? In this realm, the most common value conflict is truth-telling versus beneficence. When the hospitalized patient fails to receive a medication dose on time, generally no great harm is done. Will the patient benefit by being told of the error?

If the laboratory technician stumbles and drops a specimen bottle on the floor, necessitating another blood draw, is it ethically necessary to share the details of the mishap with the patient? The postoperative patient receives ibuprofen instead of the ordered naproxen, and the legion of lawyers employed by your hospital insists on full disclosure of all errors, including this one. Most reasonable physicians would agree that this was a "no harm-no foul" incident. Institutional policy mandates disclosure, but will the knowledge make the patient feel better – or worse? Will trust be compromised unnecessarily? Should common sense or legal policy prevail?

DO NOT BECOME THE "SECOND VICTIM" OF A MEDICAL ERROR

Let not your soul be troubled by the honest errors you have made. American physician and educator Sherwin Nuland has published an intriguing book titled *The Soul of Medicine,* in which he and 16 colleagues describe their most memorable patients. In the book, several of the physicians, choosing among a lifetime of clinical encounters, chose to tell about an error or a clinical failure.[13]

I think that a clinical error, along with raising issues of physician credibility and trust, also can shake the physician's self-confidence. Upon reflecting on Nuland's charge to his authors – to tell about their most memorable patients – I pondered my 50+ years of practice and the thousands of patient encounters I have experienced. Some I recall because of the relationships with the patients, some because of zebra diagnoses, a few because of happy and memorable events, but some because of disastrous outcomes. I think, as physicians, we never forget this latter group.

What we must not do, however, is become the "second victim" of a bad medical outcome. To do so would be a breach of the confidence that society has placed in us. To fail to deal with your feelings about an actual or perceived error and allowing such feelings to affect your practice would be letting down your patients and your colleagues. And so, if you find yourself perseverating over a perceived error or unfortunate outcome, take action. Talk to a trusted colleague, talk to your spouse, or seek counseling. Sometimes it helps to talk to the patient or family, if that seems appropriate. As evidence I cite a study by Mazor et al, who studied the responses of 407 individuals to medical errors and disclosure. The authors concluded, "This study provides evidence that full disclosure is likely to have a positive effect or no effect on how patients respond to medical errors."[14]

Of course, for we who tend to intellectualize emotion-laden situations, one approach would be to seek a lesson to be learned from the experience, using the misstep as a teachable moment.

A CLINICAL ERROR CAN BRING PROMPT USEFUL CHANGE

News item: A Bavarian surgical team operated on a woman who needed a leg operation; somehow, however, she ended up with surgical reconstruction of her anal sphincter. The surgical team has been suspended, and changes in operating room procedures are sure to come. There will be new rules for doctors and nurses to follow.

Rules are the scar tissue of past errors. Buses stop at railroad crossings, even if there is no train visible within 20 miles. Surgical sites are identified with *Sharpie* markers before patients enter the operating room. Hospital identification bracelets are checked before each medication injection. Whenever an error occurs, after dealing with the issues surrounding disclosure, the health care team looks at ways to prevent the misstep from happening again.

Sometimes clinical misjudgments result in profound policy changes. All doctors should know the name Libby Zion, who at age 18 was admitted to a New York City Hospital in March, 1984 with a presumptive diagnosis of "viral syndrome with hysterical symptoms." Under psychiatric treatment prior her arrival at the hospital, she was taking phenelzine, a monoamine oxidase inhibitor. Following admission, she received meperidine intramuscularly for restlessness. She went on to develop serotonin syndrome as a complication of the coadministration of phenelzine and meperidine. The response of a tired intern to the crisis was inadequate at best, and the patient died. Libby's father, an attorney and *New York Times* columnist, complained vocally, citing poor care from an overtired house staff, leading to a grand jury investigation and eventually to the enactment of rules limiting the hours that interns and residents can work.[15]

DO NOT LIGHTLY CRITICIZE JUDGMENT DECISIONS MADE BY ANOTHER PHYSICIAN

Someday you will encounter a patient for which things have turned out terribly: The operation failed; complications occurred; things went from bad to worse; and the patient is sure that his or her treating physician is to blame. In fact, from what you hear today, maybe the patient, who is seeking your concurrence, is correct. Regarding such circumstances, Sir William Osler wrote, "Never let your tongue say a slighting word of a colleague." (Silverman, p. 27) This is just the time to take a deep breath and think of Osler's words. The events that led to today's findings happened at another time, when the patient's disease was at a different stage then it is right now, and when the context of clinical decisions may have been quite different that they are currently. The physician you are tempted to censure went to medical school and completed post-graduate training, just as you did, and almost certainly did his or her best to provide good medical care. What's more, you are probably only hearing one side of the story. When tempted to criticize, begin by pondering what you just might have done if faced with the same circumstances; that is, start by offering the benefit of the doubt.

Remember also that someday one of your patients may present to another doctor, criticizing your care. You can only hope that hypothetical physician accords you the same benefit of the doubt that you would afford others.

PROTECT YOUR CREDIBILITY AS A PROFESSIONAL

Like it or not, physicians are held to a higher level of conduct – just as is a school teacher or judge. When all is said and done, the only thing that any of us can control is our behavior, and behaving like a professional is at the core of what it is to be a physician.

Behaving like a professional is essential to maintaining your credibility in the community. Patients want their physicians to be honest, thoughtful, and serious. Without such attributes the physician begins to lose the trust of the patient. Lebanese-American writer Kahlil Gibran (1893–1931) advised, "Therefore trust the physician and drink his remedy in silence and tranquility." Such trust can only be accorded the credible physician.

RESOLVE TO AVOID THE CLINICIAN'S DUMBER ETHICAL MISADVENTURES

Sad to say, physicians are capable of doing some stupefyingly unintelligent things. Here, let me mention four egregious ethical transgressions, acts that can stain your reputation forever:

- Inflating your academic credentials. If you did not complete an accredited psychiatric residency, then you are not a psychiatrist, no matter how amazing your counseling skills may be. A physician whose board certification has lapsed is no longer board-certified. If you were co-investigator on a grant, then you were not the "primary investigator" (PI), and thus probably not the author of the grant proposal. Changing the order of contributors listed on a published paper doesn't make you the lead author.
- Concealing errors. If you nicked an artery during surgery, be sure to describe it in the operative note, even if you believe that you were able to tie it off securely, just in case the patient suffers a delayed bleed when you cannot be readily consulted. If a patient receives a wrong injection dose, be sure to record what happened and let the patient know even if you believe that no harm will result.
- Falsifying medical records. This ethical blunder often follows the filing of a professional liability suit, which is just the wrong time to be making changes in the medical record. There is, of course, a proper way to correct clerical errors – striking through the wrong information, adding the revision, and then appending your initials and date. But the time to do this is before – not after – problems arise.

■ Self-prescribing controlled substances. Such actions can cost you your license. If you need a controlled substance, for pain or even to induce sleep on a long flight, see your personal physician, and resist the temptation to write and fill your own prescription.

NEVER CLAIM KNOWLEDGE AND SKILLS BEYOND YOUR TRAINING AND EXPERTISE

I am licensed by the State of Oregon to practice "medicine and surgery" – including, apparently, brain surgery. Fortunately for the unsuspecting public, the hospitals in which I work prohibit me from performing craniotomies. As physicians, we all must learn our limits, and have the humility to seek consultation when presented with a problem outside our sphere of expertise. I cringe at generalists administering botulinum toxin injections without a single hour of instruction, just as I am appalled when a surgeon attempts to manage a post-operative patient's soaring blood pressure or sudden, severe headache.

One might ask, "Do reputable physicians really ever profess knowledge and skills beyond their training and experience?" Let us consider one well-documented instance that had wide-ranging consequences. When Franklin Delano Roosevelt became the president of the United States in 1933, he suffered, in addition to his well-known polio, severe chronic sinusitis. Roosevelt appointed as his personal physician Admiral Ross McIntire, MD, an otorhinolaryngologist, who attended his presidential patient with "regal sycophancy." (Gordon, p. 34) But Roosevelt's chief medical problem would not turn out to be sinusitis or even polio, but cardiovascular disease, retrospectively evident even when he assumed the presidency at age 51 (Gordon, p. 34).

In time Roosevelt's blood pressure reached alarming heights, his heart began to fail, and he was admitted to Bethesda Naval Hospital in March, 1944. Hospital records from that time document paroxysmal nocturnal dyspnea, cyanosis of the lips, left ventricular enlargement, and a blood pressure of 186/108. Following evaluation of the presidential patient, however, McIntire reported reassuringly, "I can say to you that the checkup is satisfactory. When we got through, we decided that for a man of 62 we had very little to argue about, with the exception that we have had to combat the influenza plus the respiratory complications that come along afterward." (Post and Robins, p. 27). Certainly Roosevelt's grave condition should have prohibited him from running for a fourth term in 1944, but the nation and even Roosevelt himself were kept in the dark.

As physicians with charity toward our colleagues, we may conclude that Dr. McIntire was guilty of over-reaching the limits of his professional expertise and did not understand the implications of Roosevelt's severe cardiovascular disease. To believe otherwise is to agree with the conclusion of biographer Jim Bishop who concluded, "McIntire was lying – not only to the world but to the president himself."[16]

Sometimes, even though practicing within the boundaries of their own specialties, physicians just don't have the skills that they – and sometimes their colleagues – believe they possess. In Kent, England, a gynecologist performed a hysterectomy on a 48-year-old woman. For reasons unknown, he also removed her ovaries, which he had described to the patient as healthy and functioning a few weeks before. During surgery he damaged her left ureter, and went home without checking to see if the patient was bleeding. Later he returned to the hospital, finding that she had lost two liters of blood into her pelvis. In a report to the patient's personal physician, the gynecologist described the surgery and post-operative course as "uncomplicated."[17]

NEVER JEOPARDIZE CREDIBILITY AND TRUST BY ENGAGING IN ANY TYPE OF PROFESSIONAL MISCONDUCT

Professional misconduct is a somewhat general heading that includes diverse acts such as violation of physical boundaries, physical or emotional abuse of a patient, exploitation of a patient, sexual harassment, and substance misuse. There are more we could identify. A few especially dim-witted types of professional misconduct are highlighted below.

Grant and Alfred remind us that the definition of "unprofessional conduct" varies across America, as defined by each state's medical practice act. In addition to the examples mentioned above, they add inadequate record keeping and not recognizing or acting on common symptoms. The authors opine, "The most significant finding is that there are a very large number of repeat offenders upon physicians who have received medical board sanction, indicating a possible need for greater monitoring of disciplined physicians or less reliance upon rehabilitative sanctions."[18] These repeat offenders may be examples of what Crow et al have termed the "rogue doctor," one who exhibits unacceptable patterns of behavior.[19]

Who are the medical practitioners who are ultimately disciplined by state medical boards? In a study of 890 physicians disciplined by the Medical Board of California, Kohatsu et al. found that four factors were associated with an increased risk for disciplinary action: male sex; lack of board certification; increasing age; and international medical school education. The specialties at increased risk for discipline were: family medicine; general practice; obstetrics and gynecology; and psychiatry.[20]

What are the specific behaviors that lead to disciplinary action for unprofessional behavior? Papadakis et al. categorized 740 violations among 235 physicians in 40 states that led to disciplinary action by state medical boards.[21] From their long list of bad behaviors, here are top ten:

- Use of drugs or alcohol
- Unprofessional conduct
- Conviction of a crime
- Negligence
- Inappropriate prescribing or acquisition of controlled substances
- Violation of a law or order of the board, of a consent or rehabilitation order, or of probation
- Failure to conform to minimal standards of acceptable medical practice
- Sexual misconduct
- Failure to meet requirements for continuing medical education or other requirements
- Fraud or inappropriate billing practices (e.g., Medicare billing irregularities)

The Papadakis et al study was done to determine if there is a way to predict which doctors will exhibit unprofessional conduct resulting in disciplinary action. In fact, there are some early warning signs, beginning in medical school. Students most likely to exhibit unprofessional behavior during their practice years were those described earlier in medical school as being irresponsible and as having diminished ability to improve their behavior.[21]

At this point, I will discuss four especially egregious examples of doctors acting badly: Alcohol and drug misuse, practitioner sex abuse, unprofessional romantic entanglements, and dishonesty.

Alcohol and Drug Misuse

Substance misuse can be harmful not only to the physician but also to the patient. Now, many of us use alcohol socially (although I hope that none of us use illicit drugs.) An old saying holds that an alcoholic is one who drinks more than his doctor. A study by Hughes et al found that physicians were actually more likely to use alcohol than their age and gender counterparts, although the authors suggest that this finding may reflect socioeconomic class rather than profession.[22] For whatever the significance may be, Kenna and Wood report that dentists consume alcohol more than doctors or nurses.[23] Nevertheless, the wise physician never, ever uses alcohol when all one's wits may be needed – as in seeing a sick patient or driving a car.

The Hughes et al study may not have provoked concern about physician alcohol use, but it does raise questions about doctors using drugs. No, we generally don't use the "hard stuff." Physicians were less likely than age and gender counterparts to use marijuana, cocaine or heroin, or for that matter, cigarettes. However, it seems that we have a higher prevalence than age and gender controls to use minor opiates and benzodiazepine tranquilizers, a worrisome tendency to self-medicate that raises the specter of dependence.[22]

Why do doctors use prescription drugs so freely? First of all, they are readily available, although less so now that indiscriminate sampling is a thing of the past. Secondly, physician and other health professionals may feel that they know all about the drugs and are immune to their addictive effects, what Kenna and Lewis call "pharmaceutical invincibility."[24]

It's too bad that physicians Sir Arthur Conan Doyle, Sigmund Freud, and iconic surgeon William S. Halsted – cocaine users one and all – didn't heed the risks of physician drug use. The creator of the fictional detective Sherlock Holmes, Sir Arthur was a cocaine user. So was Sigmund Freud, who described the drug as a "magical substance" that could cure fatigue, asthma, headache, depression, and impotence. William Halsted, who promoted the use of surgical gloves in America, became a proponent of the topical effects of cocaine. Eventually he became habituated to the drug, a condition well known to colleagues at Johns Hopkins University School of Medicine. He endured treatment, suffered relapses, and lived a life of "controlled addiction" for 36 years. (Taylor, 2008, p. 217)[25] If these heroes of medical history can fall victim to drug misuse, are we today any less vulnerable?

Sexual Abuse of Patients

This brings us to sexual abuse of patients and others who put trust in physicians. During my academic medicine career, I have worked with seven medical school deans (a fact which tells a little about the life expectancy of academic medical center administrators). The wisest of these six men and one woman, an endocrinologist by specialty, coined a phrase: "testosterone storm." The appellation, borrowed from the phrase "thyroid storm," describes what happens when an otherwise respectable male professor acts on his sexual fantasies about a patient, colleague, student, or a member of his staff. In the medical school setting, these problems land on the desk of the dean. In private practice, they end up with the State Board of Medical Examiners or even in court.

The world-wide-web and the popular press tell many examples of testosterone storm. In Illinois, an internal medicine specialist was disciplined by the state medical board because of his "unprofessional and dishonorable conduct in his interactions with several female staff members. Specifically, the physician would touch them in a manner suggesting sexual overtones and make sexual propositions."[26] In Massachusetts, a well-regarded pediatrician was accused of sexually abusing at least seven boys in his practice. The legal complaint alleged "numerous acts of genital fondling, masturbation, and other attempted and threatened acts of assault."[27]

One health professional in California – a dentist – is accused of fondling the breasts of 27 female patients, claiming that massage of this type is a splendid method of treating temporomandibular joint syndrome.[28] One woman reported repeat treatments – six massages over 2 years – which made me wonder if we physicians are ignorant of a ground-breaking therapeutic breakthrough. In March 2009, I searched PubMed in vain for clinical evidence to support the merits of this inventive treatment.

The literature does, however, discuss the incidence of sex abuse. One study puts the incidence of sex abuse – with a spectrum ranging from inappropriate meddling in patients' sexual lives to inappropriate touching and even rape – for male practitioners at approximately 10%.[29] Perpetrators are most likely to be psychiatrists, general practitioners, or obstetrician–gynecologists, ages 45–64, suffering from a mental disorder or in the midst of a life crisis.

Becoming romantically involved with patients (or anyone else who would logically be considered an inappropriate love interest for a physician or, for that matter, any upstanding member of the community)

The spark of romance can inspire even the most apparently prudent physician to consider overstepping boundaries. Actually there are several gray areas worthy of discussion here. First of all, the ethical codes all medical professional bodies prohibit sexual relationships between a doctor and a current patient.[30] This prohibition is quite clear and such a relationship is considered sexual misconduct. Yet in a survey of 1,891 family physicians, internists, surgeons, and obstetrician–gynecologists, 9% reported having had sexual contact with one or more patients.[31] The 9% strikes me as an egregiously high number for such foolish behavior.

The issue of romantic involvement with former patients is a bit less clear. If, for example, a young emergency physician treats a patient or even a friend for a fracture, may he or she never have a date with that individual? On a policy basis, the American Medical Association has offered guidance: A romantic or sexual relationship with a former patient is unethical "if the physician uses or exploits trust, knowledge, emotions, or influence derived from the previous professional relationship."[32] Psychiatry seems, not illogically, to be a special case. The American Psychiatric Association prohibits – forever – sexual contact between a psychiatrist and a former patient.[33]

This brings me to the murky area of sexual risks no wise physician would undertake. Even if there were neither codes of ethical behavior nor state laws, common sense generally tells us what is and is not proper. One physician serves as the poster child for inappropriate romantic antics. Here is the story.

The physician, a successful, married, medical school professor, began to have paid sex with a prostitute much younger than himself. In time the relationship became more than "professional," and the doctor bought her expensive gifts and helped pay her college tuition. The young woman became pregnant, had the baby, and things began to deteriorate. He took out a stalking order against her, and she accused him of failing to help support their child.

Then the doctor, against all reason, sued her for allegedly accessing his e-mail accounts, asking $24,000 in damages. In response, she sued the doctor, alleging infliction of emotional distress, and the entire mess ended up in the local newspapers, for all his patients to read.

Dishonesty and Dishonorable Behavior

The imperative to preserve your integrity begins on first day of medical school and continues as long as you have MD after your name.

Medicine, and today's society, offer abundant opportunities to sacrifice your integrity. For example, just recently in one of our practices, the temperature in the refrigerator containing vaccines somehow rose above the critical point. In this refrigerator was thousands of dollars worth of vaccines. What should be done? The doctor learning of the problem could have quietly ignored the transient temperature rise, assuming that no real harm would result. Yet, I'm proud to report that my colleagues destroyed the vaccines in question, rather than risk patient safety.

Then there are instances of less than honorable behavior. The New York Times tells of a Harvard Medical School professor lecturing first-year students about cholesterol-lowering drugs who "seemed to belittle a student who asked about side effects"[34] Not content to having his comments dismissed in class, the student did some research, revealing that the full-time Harvard professor was also a consultant on the payroll of five companies making anti-cholesterol drugs.

Another New York Times article describes the plans of federal health officials and prosecutors to file civil and criminal charges against a number of surgeons, alleging that they insisted upon lucrative consulting contracts with surgical device manufacturers in return for using their prostheses, stents, and other items.[35]

From Australia comes the tale of two pediatric cardiac surgeons involved in 29 deaths and four survivors with brain damage in 53 pediatric heart operations. As unskillful as the surgeons seemed to be, the act that compromised their integrity (aside from continuing to operate in the face of such dismal mortality rates) was "not communicating to the parents the correct risk of death for these operations in their hands."[36]

Fred has written a thoughtful article titled *Dishonesty in Medicine Revisited*, in which he discusses many types of dishonesty, which he describes as "an embarrassment that pervades our profession and undermines its core values of truth, integrity, philanthropy, and altruism."[37] Here are some examples of dishonorable behavior:

Medical school
▪ Copying from another student during an examination
▪ Signing an attendance sheet for another student

- "Dry-labbing" a laboratory experiment
- Recording false information on a medical history or physical exam
- Using someone else's words on a homework assignment

Postgraduate training
- Listing an item in the medical history, such as the Past Medical History, as "non-contributory" when this information has never been elicited at all
- Recording spurious physical findings, e.g., "Cranial nerves intact" and "PERRLA" (pupils equal, round, and reactive to light and accommodation) when not everything on the list has actually been checked
- Using data from another's recorded history and physical to create one's own clinical note
- Blaming technology ("My pager didn't beep.") for one's personal failures
- Failing to own a patient care error that one has made

Medical practice
- Entering false data on one's curriculum vitae
- Accepting payments from industry for enrolling patients in clinical trials
- Altering medical records in the face of peer review or litigation
- Billing for services not actually performed
- Manipulating data on a research study
- Serving as an expert witness whose opinion can be bought

It seems to me that the list above shows how early acts of questionable integrity make subsequent ones all that much easier. Is it really so difficult to go from "fudging" physical findings as a student to modifying medical records after a lawsuit has been filed?

ALWAYS PRACTICE IN WAYS THAT INSPIRE TRUST

Throughout history, the medical profession's commitment to high ethical standards has helped promote patient trust in the individual physician. On a philosophical basis the trustworthiness of physicians comes, in part, from the doctor's unwavering quest for beneficence in dealing with patients. That is, a patient coming to a physician with pain or fever can reasonably expect that the physician will put the patient's needs first, and not mistreat, cheat or abandon him or her. By virtue of such trust, the patient can put aside the sick role, abandon any affectation, and join the physician in seeking the best road to health.[38]

Of course, in the twenty-first century there are identifiable and even researchable aspects of perceived physician trustworthiness. Attire can be a factor. Rehman et al queried 400 persons about physician attire, trust, and confidence. They concluded: "Respondents overwhelmingly favor physicians in professional attire with a white coat. Wearing professional dress (i.e., a white coat with more professional attire) while providing patient care by physicians may favorably influence trust and confidence-building in the medical encounter."[39]

A study by Bonds et al found greater patient trust when there was gender concordance between patient and physician.[40] On the other hand, race can be a factor. Gordon et al studied 103 lung cancer patients, both black and white. They found that black patients had lower trust in physicians, concluding: "Perceptions that physician communication was less supportive, less partnering and less informative accounted for black patients' lower trust in physicians."[41]

Other factors influencing trust are time spent with the patient and the physician's communication abilities. In a study using standardized patients (SP) making unannounced visits to the offices of 100 community-based physicians, the authors discovered, "Each additional minute spent in SP visits was associated with 0.01 SD increase in patient trust."[42] Another study of patients with rheumatologic disease led the authors to conclude, "Trust in physicians can be improved by using a patient-centered approach, being sensitive to patient concerns, and providing adequate clinical information."[43] It is reassuring that these studies seem to add scientific credibility to what we have long believed intuitively.

BE WORTHY OF THE TRUST PATIENTS PLACE IN YOU

In the previous section, I alluded to trust. The very act of a patient scheduling an appointment, braving traffic, showing up at your office, offering you a medical history and submitting to a physical examination altogether represent an expression of trust in your abilities and your diligence. When I had surgery last year, I trusted that my anesthesiologist and my surgeon had the requisite training and experience, had both given thought to the procedure I would undergo, and would arrive in the operating room rested and focused. Throughout my career, whenever I saw a patient with a headache or abdominal pain, I think that some small part of my brain reminded me that the patient was showing confidence in my diagnostic and therapeutic abilities, a confidence that may somehow even include an unspoken agenda that would become revealed sometime later in our relationship. Just as an example, the patient with abdominal pain, without actually articulating the concern, might trust that I will rule out the possibility of an ovarian cancer, the type of malignancy that killed her cousin in Detroit.

British surgeon Sir Berkeley Moynihan (1865–1936) has this to say about the trust patients place in us[44]:

> A patient can offer you no higher tribute than to entrust you with his life and his health, and, by implication, with the happiness of all his family. To be worthy of this trust we must submit for a lifetime to the constant discipline of unwearied effort in the search of knowledge, and of the most reverent devotion to every detail in every operation we perform.

I admire the author's use of the phrase "reverent devotion," which must not be limited to surgical procedures. Whether you are examining a sore throat, counseling a depressed middle-age person, or evaluating a patient with chest pain, our patients trust that you will do your job, however mundane the encounter may seem, with reverent devotion. After all, as American physician and author Oliver Wendell Holmes, Sr. (1809–1894) wrote: "The best a physician can give is never too good for the patient."[45]

WISE WORDS ABOUT ETHICS, CREDIBILITY, AND TRUST

■ *The medical profession is the only one in which anybody professing to be a physician is at once trusted, although nowhere else is an untruth more dangerous.* Roman philosopher Pliny the Elder (23–79) (Strauss, p. 377)

Pliny's cynicism may arise from the fact, now well recognized, that the physicians of the first century CE had virtually nothing in their tool box that could actually help combat disease.

■ *The physician strives for the good as the artist strives for the beautiful, each pushed on by that admirable feeling we call virtue.* French novelist Honoré de Balzac (1799–1850) (Strauss, p. 380)

Balzac has a keen appreciation of the physician's sense of beneficence, and the literary skill to frame the concept with an engaging simile.

■ *It is curious that physical courage should be so common in the world and moral courage so rare.* American author Mark Twain (1835–1910)[46]

Perhaps the reason is that moral courage requires us to "dig deeper" than does physical courage.

■ *The best doctor, like the successful general, is the one who makes the fewest errors.* Sir William Osler (1849–1919) (Silverman, p. 57)

If you have ever played Texas Hold-Em poker, you know that the best way to be a winner at the end of the night is to avoid losing too many hands.

■ *Commercialism in medicine never leads to true satisfaction, and to maintain our self-respect is more precious than gold.* Doctor William J. Mayo (1861–1939) (Quoted in Willius, p. 51.)

■ *My old man used to say that he guessed the percentage of scoundrels was less among doctors than any other class of men, professional or otherwise, in the world.* American author Damon Runyon (1880–1946) (Quoted in Strauss, p. 178)

High praise, indeed, from a down-to-earth guy. Despite the few practitioners that go astray, by far most physicians are honorable persons.

▪ *In a time of universal deceit, telling the truth is a remarkable act.*

This is from a bumper sticker I saw last week in downtown Portland, Oregon. As my mind moved beyond the cynicism and the political overtones, I thought about physicians and how we hold truth-telling to be a core value we all embrace.

▪ *A person's work is part of a person's life, and the two combined as lifework must be seen as constantly responsive to the moral decisions that we never stop making, day in and day out.* American physician and author Robert Coles (b. 1929) (Reynolds and Stone, p. 277)

▪ *Professionalism is the single most important of the clinical competencies.* Patrick Duff[47]

And the first imperative under professionalism must be personal integrity.

REFERENCES

1. Woodward VM. Caring, patient autonomy and the stigma of paternalism. *J Adv Nurs*. 1998;28(5):1046–1052.
2. Sperry WL. *The Ethical Basis of Medical Practice*. New York: Hoeber; 1950.
3. Perez-Carceles MD, Pereniguez JE, Osuna I. Balancing confidentiality and the information provided to families of patients in primary care. *J Med Ethics*. 2005;31(9):531–535.
4. Bird S. Epilepsy, driving and confidentiality. *Aust Fam Phys*. 2005;34(12):1057–1058.
5. Kipnis K. A defense of unqualified medical confidentiality. *Am J Bioeth*. 2006;6(2):7–18.
6. Truog RD. Consent for organ donations – balancing conflicting ethical obligations. N Engl J Med 2008 358: 12:1209–1211.
7. Wall LL, Brown D. Pharmaceutical representatives and the doctor/patient relationship. *Obstet Gynecol*. 2002;100(3):594–599.
8. Savulescu J. Rational non-interventional paternalism: why doctors ought to make judgments of what is best for their patients. *J Med Ethics*. 1995;21(6):327–331.

9. Dovey SM, Meyers DS, Phillips RL Jr, et al. A preliminary taxonomy of medical errors in family medicine. *Qual Saf Health Care*. 2002;11:233–238.

10. Kozer E, Scolnik D, Jarvis AD, Kozer G. The effect of detection approaches on the reported incidence of tenfold errors. *Drug Saf*. 2006;29(2):169–174.

11. Neale G, Woloschynowych J, Vincent D. Exploring the causes of adverse events in NHS hospital practice. *J R Soc Med*. 2001;94:322–330.

12. Burroughs TE, Waterman AD, Gallagher TH, et al. Patient concerns about medical errors in emergency departments. *Acad Emerg Med*. 2005;23:57–64.

13. Nuland SB. *The Soul of Medicine*. New York: Kaplan; 2009.

14. Mazor KM, Reed GW, Yood RA, Fischer MA, Baril J, Gurwitz JH. Disclosure of medical errors: what factors influence how patients respond? *J Gen Intern Med*. 2006;21(7):704–710.

15. Boyer EW, Shannon M. The serotonin syndrome. *N Engl J Med*. 2005;352:1112–1120.

16. Bishop J. *FDR's Last Year: April 1944-April 1945*. New York: Hart-Davis MacGibbon; 1975:201–202.

17. Dyer C. Obstetrician accused of committing a series of surgical blunders. *BMJ*. 1998;317(7161):767–768.

18. Grant D, Alfred KC. Sanctions and recidivism: an evaluation of physician discipline by state medical boards. *J Health Polit Policy Law*. 2007;32(5):867–885.

19. Crow SM, Hartman SJ, Nolan TE, Zembo M. A prescription for the rogue doctor: part I – begin with diagnosis. *Clin Orthop Relat Res*. 2003;411:334–339.

20. Kohatsu ND, Gould D, Ross LK, Fox PJ. Characteristics associated with physician discipline: a case-control study. *Arch Intern Med*. 2004;164(6):653–658.

21. Papadakis MA, Teherani A, Banach MA, et al. Disciplinary action by medical boards and prior behavior in medical school. *N Engl J Med*. 2005;353(25):2673–2682.

22. Hughes PH, Brandenburg N, Baldin DC, et al. Prevalence of substance use among US physicians. *JAMA*. 1992;267(17):2333–2339.

23. Kenna GA, Wood MD. Alcohol use by healthcare professionals. *Drug Alcohol Depend*. 2004;75(1):107–116.

24. Kenna GA, Lewis DC. Risk factors for alcohol and other drug use by health care professionals. *Subst Abuse Treat Prev Policy*. 2008;3:3–5.

25. Spirling LI, Daniels IR. William Stewart Halsted – surgeon extraordinaire: a story of drugs, gloves and romance. *J R Soc Health*. 2002;122(2):122–124.
26. Physician profile. Available at: http://www.healthgraded.com/directory_search/physician/profiles/dr-md-reports/ Accessed March 7, 2009.
27. Physician accused of sex abuse of children. Available at: http://www.boston.com/news/local/articles/2008/04/01/physician_accused_of_sex_abuse_of_children/ Accessed March 7, 2009.
28. Dentist claims breast rubs appropriate. Available at: http://www.msnbc.msn.com/id/21325760/ Accessed March 7, 2009.
29. Jousset N, Gaudin A, Penneau M, Rouge-Maillart C. Practitioner sex abuse: occurrence, prevention and disciplinary sanction. *Med Sci Law*. 2008;48(3):203–210.
30. Hall KH. Sexualization of the doctor-patient relationship: is it ever ethically permissible? *Fam Pract*. 2001;18:511–515.
31. Gartrell NK, Milliken N, Goodson WH 3rd, Thiemann S, Lo B. Physician-patient sexual contact: prevalence and problems. *West J Med*. 1992;157(2):139–143.
32. American Medical Association. *Policy Compendium*. Chicago: American Medical Association; 1997.
33. American Psychiatric Association. *The Principles of Medical Ethics with Annotations Especially Applicable to Psychiatry*. Washington, DC: APA; 2001.
34. Harvard Medical School in Ethics Quandary. Available at: http://www.nytimes.com/2009/03/03/business/03medschool.html. Accessed March 7, 2009.
35. Crackdown on doctors who take kickbacks. Available at: http://www.nytimes.com/2009/03/04/health/policy/04doctors.html?_r=1&ref=health/Accessed March 8, 2009.
36. Bolsin SN. Professional misconduct: the Bristol case. *Med J Aust*. 1998;169(7):351–352.
37. Fred HL. Dishonesty in medicine revisited. *Tex Heart Inst J*. 2008;35(1):6–15.
38. Parsons T. Some theoretical considerations on the field of medical sociology. In: Parsons T, ed. *Social Structure and Personality*. London: The Free Press, Collier-Macmillan; 1964:325–358.
39. Rehman SU, Nietert PJ, Cope DW, Kirkpatrick AO. What to wear today? Effect of doctor's attire on the trust and confidence of patients. *Am J Med*. 2005;118(11):1279–1286.
40. Bonds DE, Foley KL, Dugan E, Hall MA, Extrom P. An exploration of patients' trust in physicians in training. *J Health Care Poor Underserved*. 2004;15(2):294–306.

41. Gordon HS, Street RL, Sharf BF, Kelly PA, Souchek J. Racial differences in trust and lung cancer patients' perceptions of physician communication. *J Clin Oncol.* 2006;24(6):904–909.
42. Fiscella K, Meldrum S, Franks P, et al. Patient trust: is it related to patient-centered behavior of primary care physicians? *Med Care.* 2004;42(11):1049–1055.
43. Berrios-Rivera JP, Street RL, Garcia Popa-Lisseanu MG. Trust in physicians and elements of the medical interaction in patients with rheumatoid arthritis and systemic lupus erythematosus. *Arthritis Rheum.* 2006;55(3):385–393.
44. Moynihan B. Abdominal Operations. Vol I, Revised. Preface to the 4th edition. Philadelphia: Saunders; 1926:11–12.
45. Holmes OW Sr. *Medical Essays.* Boston: Houghton Mifflin; 1891.
46. Mark Twain aphorisms. Available at: http://www.faculty.rsu.edu/~felwell/HomePage/aphorisms.htm/ Accessed April 10, 2009.
47. Duff P. Teaching and assessing professionalism in medicine. *Obstet Gynecol.* 2004;104(6):1362–1366.

13

Planning for Tomorrow

Tomorrow, tomorrow ... You're only a day away.
Lyrics of a song in the Broadway musical Annie
(adapted from the comic strip Little Orphan Annie)

The wise clinician, like the astute leader, always looks ahead to tomorrow – and the day after that. In patient care, envisioning tomorrow means trying to anticipate the course of the patient's illness and the outcome of recommended therapy, discussed in Chap. 5 on *Disease Treatment and Prevention* and even in Chap. 6 on *Caring for Dying Patients and Their Families*. In the practice of delivering top quality health care to our patients, planning for tomorrow involves staying current with the advances in clinical care and the new developments in health policy and economics (Chap. 7 on *Making a Living as a Clinician* and Chap. 8 on *Staying Up to Date*). And, there is also the consideration of what to anticipate in your own life and that of your family. In this chapter, we will touch on a few of these topics, but the emphasis will be on your personal preparation for some life changes that may lie ahead.

TOMORROW CAN BE DIFFICULT TO PREDICT

Planning for tomorrow connotes a small amount of predicting the future, a risky endeavor, at best. We are humbled by the uncertainty as to what lies ahead for each of us and for medicine, in general. As an example of the hazards of forecasting what will come, I quote Spanish physician and author Félix Martí-Ibáñez (1912–1972). In 1958, he expressed his thoughts on diseases of the future: "The profound change

R.B. Taylor, *Medical Wisdom and Doctoring: The Art of 21st Century Practice*, DOI 10.1007/978-1-4419-5521-0_13,
© Springer Science+Business Media, LLC 2010

taking place in the natural history of infections warrants the prophecy that by the year 2000 the diseases caused by bacteria, protozoa, and perhaps viruses will be considered by the medical student as exotic curiosities of mere historical interest, as is the case today with tertiary syphilis, gout, and smallpox." (Martí-Ibáñez 1958, p. 20) Even sage Doctor Martí-Ibáñez could not anticipate the human immunodeficiency virus, methicillin resistant *Staphylococcus aureus* (MRSA), and the resurgence of tuberculosis in the world.

Just in case you might suspect that Dr. Martí-Ibáñez and medicine stand alone in failed prognostications, here are a few more, plucked from a web site listing famous quotations.[1]

■ *"Everything that can be invented has been invented"*
    Charles H. Duell, Commissioner, US Office of Patents, 1899

■ *"Who the hell wants to hear actors talk?"*
    H. M. Warner, Warner Brothers, 1927

■ *"We don't like their sound and guitar music is on the way out."*
    Decca records, upon rejecting the Beatles, 1962

■ *"There is no reason in the world anyone would want a computer in their home. No reason."*
    Ken Olsen, Chairman, DEC, 1977

RECOGNIZE THE LIFE CHANGES THAT LIE AHEAD

Unless our careers or health are truncated by some major catastrophe – loss of one's medical license, dementia, debilitating injury or illness, or something equally disastrous – most of us will experience surprisingly similar events in our jobs and our lives. There are five more-or-less predictable stages of medical professional life (MPL):

Stage 1. Medical Education and Training. These are the medical school and residency years, spent gaining knowledge and skills, while accumulating a little wisdom and a ton of debt. The knowledge, skills, and wisdom will be your foundation for future practice and learning. The student debt will influence personal and professional decisions until it is finally wiped off the books.

Stage 2. Early Practice Years. At this time, there are the paired challenges of establishing a practice while paying down student loan debt. For many, these are also the years of early family life. Activities undertaken during the early practice years are often energizing ventures (except, of course, for the paying down debt part). Many senior physicians reflect that these times, when life was lived in a simple manner and spending was frugal, were the best of all.

Stage 3. Maximum Career Demands. By this stage, most physicians have successfully established their practices, and many are busier than they wish. On balance, however, financial strain is likely to be behind them, and a little cash can be saved for future college tuition and retirement.

Stage 4. Career Plateau. Accepting no new patients, cutting back on night call, and taking more vacations characterize the career plateau. The family's financial future appears to be more or less secure, and new ventures may seem not worth the effort. It is during this career stage, however, that some physicians experience the "Is-this-all-there-is-midlife-crisis air pocket" and set out to undermine all they have achieved.

Stage 5. Winding Down and Retirement. In this stage of professional life, lots of things seem less compelling than before. These include evening and weekend office hours, hospital committee meetings, and out of town professional meetings. Also at this time, physicians tend to cut some "meat" from their practices, which I'll discuss below under the topic of adjusting your practice to your tolerance. Then, at the end of the stage, comes retirement – the eventual cessation of direct patient care – although, as described below, many physicians maintain their identity as physicians in creative ways.

RECOGNIZE THE STAGES AND THE TRANSITIONS IN YOUR OWN PROFESSIONAL LIFE

The preceding describes just some of the challenges faced during each professional life stage. In this chapter, I want to emphasize the inevitability of transitions and the need for anticipatory preparation. Here I will add some detail to my life story, briefly summarized on page xv, in the context of the stages and transitions in MPL.

In 1964, as I completed my training and service with the United States Public Health Service, ending Stage 1, I placed an ad in the *Journal of the American Medical Association* (JAMA), indicating that I was a general practitioner (Remember: there was no family medicine specialty until 1969), and that I sought to join an established community practice. From more than 100 replies, I selected the five most promising sites, and traveled to visit each one of them. On that journey, I learned a great deal about the practice of medicine in a community setting, and also about myself. In the end, satisfied that I had performed conscientious research, I joined a 4-physician practice in New Paltz, New York, beginning MLP Stage 2 – the Early Practice Years – in a pleasant setting supported by three more senior colleagues.

After 4 years, I left the partnership in an acrimonious separation and opened my own solo practice – a practice setting which suited my temperament quite well at the time. And the shift to private solo practice soon propelled me into MPL Stage 3 – Maximum Career Demands.

In 1978, to the dismay of my parents and my patients, I left my highly successful practice in rural New York and entered academic medicine at Wake Forest University School of Medicine in Winston-Salem, North Carolina. Keenly perceptive readers might suspect this represented a mid-life air pocket.

In 1984, my wife and I moved across the country to Oregon, where I became the Chairman of a medical school clinical department, a role that no one (including me) would ever have predicted when I began my career. I held this position until 1998, when I declared that I was at my career plateau, MPL Stage 4, and I resigned to become "chairman emeritus."

I am now, almost 50 years after receiving my MD degree, in MPL Stage 5 – winding down to retirement. I have done my best to prepare for each transition to a new stage in professional life. With each change, I have become aware that I could have or should have planned a little better for the last. Even in my careful search for my first practice, I now reflect that, during my interviews, I should have attended to small clues (some tell-tale practice management peculiarities and a slight hint of personal cognitive dissonance). Perhaps as I grow older, I will gain greater skills in recognizing clues, what Coelho calls *omens*. (Coelho, p. 62.)

PREPARE TODAY FOR TOMORROW'S PRACTICE OF MEDICINE

Whatever the stage of one's professional life (and yes, even if in semi-retirement), the wise physician looks ahead to the future of medical practice. At the dawn of the current millennium Murtha et al wrote a paper titled *Medical Practice 2010: How We Get There*.[2] As they sought to look ahead, the authors humbly observed, "Predicting the future is a tricky business. Futurists note that we typically overestimate the effects of change in the short run and underestimate its effects in the long run. By focusing on the fundamental forces already in place that will shape the practice of future physicians, we can better estimate their likely effects." The authors go on to cite as one of the changes the shift of physicians from independent practice to working in health care systems. This, they assert, has enabled the development of "systems thinking," disease management programs, and decision support systems. The authors predicted, "By 2010, physicians will be increasingly linked – functionally, financially, electronically, and psychologically – to and within organizations."

The Murtha et al paper was published in 2000 and as I read it today it is interesting to note how many of their prognostications are becoming reality: changes in patient interactions such as open access scheduling; new models for patient visits including group visits; and the ascendency of evidence-based care.

At this point, I will inject some of my own ideas into the Murtha et al template. The authors write of "fundamental forces already in place" and their "effects in the long run."

I believe that there are three fundamental forces that will shape medicine in the long term.

The first of these is *economics*. By this I do not mean the microeconomics of your practice or mine. Rather I refer to the larger issues of who pays for care, where the funds come from, and how they are distributed to those who actually provide healthcare services. Underlying these economic issues are the considerations of who is entitled to which health services and what happens when we recognize that we cannot afford all possible healthcare – preventive, elective, cosmetic, therapeutic, and palliative – for everyone. When funds run short, as they have with my state's well-regarded Oregon Health Plan, will the last dollars go for immunizations and prenatal care or for organ transplants with doubtful outcomes or care of the elderly in the last months of life? The economics of healthcare is not an abstract issue, because how you and I are paid for our work strongly influences how we interact with patients. For example, I have visited countries in which the government-run health system pays each doctor a small amount per patient visit, regardless of the complexity of the problem or length of the visit. The effect: Doctors may see one hundred or more patients daily.

The second fundamental force is *government*. Those of us who practiced before 1966, when Medicare and Medicaid became reality, recall a world when patients actually paid us for our services and physicians each did our share to care for the "medically needy." Over the past four decades, government has become increasingly involved in healthcare. What the future will bring is never clear, but government intrusion into medicine seems unlikely to abate.

The third fundamental force effecting long term change is *information technology*. As transformative as robotic surgery and gene therapy may be, in the long term the greater changes will come with information technology – our ability to find, record, organize, and transmit data, thanks to the marvels of microchips. I will discuss this paradigm-changing topic next.

**LEARN THE INFORMATION TECHNOLOGY SKILLS
YOU WILL NEED IN YOUR FUTURE PRACTICE YEARS
AND IN RETIREMENT**

In the coming decades, medicine and life in general will change rapidly, driven by technologic innovation. The key items, at least as far as we can see today, will be the computer, the Internet, and the cell phone.

The computer, together with systems thinking of larger medical practices, has allowed the universal implementation of the electronic medical record (EMR). Your graduation from high school was called a "commencement," not because you were ending your secondary school education, but because you were "commencing" your next stage of life. In a somewhat similar fashion, the EMR is not an end in itself, but the platform that helps us offer a number of innovative services to patients and colleagues, including the disease management and decision support programs described by Murtha et al. Medical records can easily be flagged to alert patients with diseases such as diabetes or heart failure to advances in managing their diseases. And researchers are salivating at the possibilities for population based research brought by the widespread use of the EMR.

Add the Internet to the desktop computer and possibilities expand. One fairly recent application is communication between patients and physicians using secure Internet links. In my case, working in an academic medical center where my e-mail address is easily discovered, a few of my savvy academician patients took the lead and began to send me – their physician – updates and questions via our university's internal email system. Today asynchronous patient–physician communication is widely used, prompting Stone to write: "The 'laying on of hands' will increasingly include the pressing of keys."[3] Email communication between patient and clinician was only the beginning. Today we offer virtual office visits, virtual home visits, and virtual group visits. We have teleradiology, and radiologists in the United States can now sleep peacefully through the night, knowing that the 2 A.M. emergency radiograph is being read by a colleague in Spain or India. The distant radiologist, awake when the US colleague is asleep, has been called a "nighthawk," and if you think this a great idea you can invest in *Nighthawk Radiology* stock. It is listed on the NASDAQ under the symbol NHWK.

Norman writes of telepsychiatric services in the UK, concluding that "the use of video conferencing can enhance psychiatric services within the UK especially for those patients who live in rural areas."[4]

On another front, patients are currently seeking second opinions on line. A service called Partners Online Specialty Consultations, affiliated with Harvard Medical School and other prestigious institutions, advised patients: "Getting the answers you need is only a few steps away. After you and your doctor register and send all your case material, your doctor will get the consultation back about a week later."[5]

What about the cell phone? Yes, the telephone has come a long way since the days of the 1876 Western Union internal memo that opined: "This 'telephone' has too many shortcomings to be seriously considered as a means of communication. The device is inherently of no value to us." As significant an innovation as the computer has been, wireless technology, with today's cell phone as the prototype, seems to be subsuming many of the computer's function. My 11-year-old granddaughter sends me text messages from her cellphone. Consider that worldwide, many more persons have cell phones than computers. They are smaller, lighter, and cheaper than computers. As we learn to pack more and more chips into smaller and smaller packages, and as we learn to use these devices in medical practice, the possibilities are endless. Today in some settings, physicians have laboratory tests beamed to their cell phones. In the future, we will increasingly use these portable devices for communicating with patients, managing disease, and monitoring progress.

All of this and more has been called telemedicine, and it has, admittedly, a few challenges. In Japan, Liu and colleagues compared doctor–patient communications in clinical consultations via telemedicine technology to doctor–patient communications in face-to-face clinical consultations.[6] Among their findings were the following: Telemedicine consultations took much longer than face-to-face visits, and were less likely to include facilitation and empathy utterances.

Although patients reported satisfaction with the telemedicine encounters, doctors were dissatisfied, citing "communication barriers."

Of course, in the end we need to be paid for what we do. What about private payer reimbursement for telemedicine services in the US? Whitten and Buis studied this issue, finding that "the US is progressing toward expanded private reimbursement for telemedicine services with 58% of responding organizations who provide potentially billable telemedicine services receiving private reimbursement (up 5% from 2003)." While they find modest improvements on reimbursement for telemedicine services, "the change appears to lag behind a pace needed to optimize telemedicine deployment."[7] Eventually, and to paraphrase Sir Winston Churchill, we Americans will do the right thing about paying doctors for their telemedicine efforts, after we have tried everything else.

PIONEER TOMORROW'S PRACTICE

To continue with the subject of tomorrow, let us consider the future role of wise physicians in trailblazing best practice methods. If wisest physicians don't do so, who else will? The answer to that rhetorical question is chilling. In a world where the wise physicians don't lead and innovate, the less-than-wisest physicians or – even worse – administrators, bureaucrats, and politicians will create the future.

American computer scientist Alan C. Kay has written, "The best way to predict the future is to invent it."[8] Note that this aphorism was created by a computer scientist, not a clinical scientist or medical scholar, and was first published in an engineering journal. Today the future of medicine is being invented, built on bedrock of silicon. Interactive computing, light years beyond today's promising but still somewhat challenging electronic medical records, will involve analysis of scientific data, compilation and retrieval of clinical information, and active learning. Here is a current and evolving example: the Human Genome Project was completed in 2003; the Phase I HapMap Project was completed in 2005; and the Encyclopedia of DNA Elements (ENCODE) project finished in 2007. Today we can envision personal genomic sequencing to detect genetic risk factors for diabetes, heart disease, and cancer.[9] None of these advances would have been possible without computers, and future applications of genomics to individual patients will be limited only by the speed of advances in computer science.

Now, to be clear, I don't advocate that you or I become computer wizards. In order to invent our future, the future of medicine, however, we need to do three things. First of all, we must resolve to make information science an integral part of our professional lives, being sure to keep current on our computer use skills; just as in clinical medicine, once you get behind with advances in medical informatics, it is hard to catch up.

The second job for physicians inventing tomorrow is to assure that innovation is tempered with reason. Just because we *can* do something – such as electronic fetal monitoring of normal labor in healthy young women today or cloning humans tomorrow – doesn't mean that we *should* do it.

Thirdly, physicians must assure that medicine's future – and especially our e-medicine future – remains morally grounded. This means, for example, that technologic advances must be used to benefit humanity, not individual entrepreneurs. A heartwarming precedent was set with the release of the Human Genome Map. The paper, listing scores of participants in the process, states that "all data were released without restriction into the public domain."[10] It also means that we must do our best to see that the coming advances are simply, as all of medicine should be, as accessible and affordable as possible.

PREPARE FOR THE FUTURE BY ASSURING THAT YOU CAN AFFORD THE OPTION OF RETIREMENT

In my personal library is a wonderful little book titled *The True Physician: the Modern "Doctor of the Old School,"* written in 1936 by Dr. Wingate Johnson. At one point in his book, Johnson states: "Far be it from a humble practitioner of medicine to offer advice about the purchase of stocks and bonds – except this dearly bought counsel ..." He then goes on to relate his opinions on the topic of investing. (Johnson, p. 83.) Here I will do a little of the same.

The topic of investment may seem slightly out of place in a book about medical wisdom, but I don't think it is. In life we encounter some unexpected realities, and one of these occurred shortly after I began private practice in the early 1960s. I met a venerated physician colleague in Kingston, New York at the end of his career who couldn't afford to retire. He had worked hard all his life, and been a good husband and father; he had just neglected to save for retirement. These were, of course, the days before the individual retirement plan (IRA) and the 401k. And so he continued working, long after he should have quit practice owing to both failing health and fading medical knowledge. Then he died, and his widow was left to survive on her meager social security payments and the kindness of friends and family.

Luckily for many doctors, one of the benefits of the corporatization of American medicine is that, by being employed by a healthcare system of some type, the physician is virtually forced to undertake some sort of retirement planning. That is the good news, meaning that the risk of you or I ending up like my Kingston colleague is quite low. The bad news is that we can still make uninformed and even foolish decisions.

Here is a potpourri of things that you, as a relatively high-income professional with an advanced degree, should be able to explain to your teenage child. (The answers are below.)

1. Why is a dollar of investment income generally more valuable than a dollar of practice earnings?
2. What is the S&P 500?
3. What is the "rule of 72?"
4. What happens to the interest rate when a bond's price rises?
5. What is a 529 plan?
6. What is a "required minimum distribution?"
7. What is your current asset allocation of stocks, bonds, and cash?

If you don't understand the items on this list, you should not leave the house with a checkbook and you are at risk of becoming shark bait.

Here Are the Answers to the Questions Above

1. The Internal Revenue Service (IRS) taxes investment income – dividends and capital gains – at a lower rate than earned income. Some states, however, are not so enlightened.
2. The S&P 500 is a stock market index containing the stocks of 500 very large corporations. Some mutual funds and exchange traded funds (ETFs) hold stocks that mimic the index and thus turn its ups and downs into profit or loss.
3. The rule of 72 is a way to calculate how long it takes the value of an investment to double, given a fixed income rate. Take, for example, a fixed income investment with an 8% interest rate. Divide 8 into 72. The answer tells that an investment paying a fixed interest rate of 8% will double in value in 9 years.
4. Interest rates fall when bond prices rise. The two move in opposite directions.
5. The 529 Plan, named for a section of the IRS tax code, allows parents and grandparents to save money, tax-sheltered, for a child's education, a very good program if for no other reason that it removes the funds from your taxable estate.
6. All persons with Individual Retirement Accounts (IRAs) are required to begin withdrawing some funds each year beginning at age 70.
7. This is a figure you should calculate yourself. Experts disagree on specifics, as experts tend to do, but generally one should have more stocks when younger and more bonds or cash when older, although there is much more to it than that simple generality.

What can the young (and typically debt-encumbered) physician do to begin learning the skill of investing? First of all, begin reading about investing. Books by or about Benjamin Graham, Peter Lynch, Warren Buffet, John Bogle, and Jeremy Siegel are good introductions to investing. Amazon has a list of "Best Investment Books" that may be helpful. One book not on that list, but one that I think all neophyte investors might profitably read is *Mugged on Wall Street: An Insider Shows You How to Protect Yourself and Your Money from the*

Financial Pros, by C. David Chase (New York: Simon and Schuster, 1987), telling how the financial professionals make a living with your money. Chase gives a sobering account of what goes on inside brokerage firms, including teaching new recruits more about selling than about investment theory.

The second thing you can do early in your professional life is open a self-directed brokerage account with a discount brokerage firm such as Fidelity or Schwab. Then carefully research a few stocks, mutual funds or ETFs, and actually make purchases. Start small; the idea is not to get rich in the first year, but to learn how you can actually manage your own finances, without being dependent on money managers and financial planners. I personally followed this advice: When in medical school I opened a brokerage account with about $200. Since then I have bought and sold stocks, bonds, mutual funds, and more, allowing me to accumulate sufficient funds for a reasonable stream of income in retirement.

MAKE PEACE WITH THE LIMITATIONS THAT COME WITH AGING

At about this moment, the perceptive reader will note that I am easing into the topics of maturity and retirement. Wise physicians recognize that, specific health problems notwithstanding, older persons just don't have the vigor of younger persons. I think we all accept this reality, which is why I no longer believe that basketball is a life sport and that I will never be an Olympic skier. Today I seek no job that would entail the long workdays and the on-call responsibilities that characterized my early practice years.

What is even more annoying is the effect of aging on cognitive functioning. Sadowsky and Kunzel studied the effect of age and age-related professional characteristics in dentists.[11] Specifically, they assessed dentists in various age groups as to their knowledge with regard to prevention of infective endocarditis. They found, "Age had a profoundly negative effect on knowledge level, i.e., the level progressively declines as clinicians grow older." Note that this study looked at practicing dentists; it was not a study of dementia in the elderly.

Sir William Osler had some strong feelings about older physicians. Here is what he wrote in a discussion of some of his firmly held beliefs: "My second fixed idea is the uselessness of men above 60 years of age, and the incalculable benefit it would be in commercial, political, and in professional life if, as a matter of course, men stopped work at this age ... That incalculable benefits might follow such a scheme is apparent to anyone who, like me, is nearing the limit, and who has made a careful study of the calamities which may befall men during the seventh and eight decades." (Osler, p. 382.) Now, in rebuttal, I could cite the examples of Colonel Sanders, who founded Kentucky Fried Chicken in his sixties Grandma Moses, who began painting in her seventies and Harry Bernstein, author whose first book *The Invisible Wall*, was published in 2007 when he was age 96. Perhaps if, as has been said, age 60 is the new 40, then we could update the numbers in Osler's admonition, and some of our gifted senior clinicians could remain on the job a few years longer.

ADJUST YOUR PRACTICE TO YOUR TOLERANCE AT EACH STAGE OF LIFE

Pediatrician Béla Schick (1877–1967), who developed the Schick test for diphtheria, is quoted as saying, "It is very difficult to slow down. The practice of medicine is like the heart muscle's contraction. It's all or none." (Strauss, p. 445.) But Dr. Schick's simile notwithstanding, many physicians succeed in actually cutting back progressively. They do so by two maneuvers: cutting out what they really don't like doing any more and emphasizing what they like to do that is compatible with a career slowdown.

First, I will discuss the "cutting out" process. With humility, I will use myself as an example. I am a general practitioner who became a family physician when the specialty was born in 1969. I think family medicine is a good example to consider because family physicians do so many things: office and hospital practice, home care, surgical procedures, maternity care, geriatric, and nursing home care. In the beginning, that is, while in training, I did it all.

Gradually, as my practice became busier, I began to give up a few things. First to go was maternity care, a reluctant move since I really liked delivering babies, but the time commitment, an 18 mile drive to the hospital, and the sleepless nights convinced me that obstetrics must go. Then I abandoned hospital surgery. I had always enjoyed being first assistant on major surgery. But the pay as a surgical assistant was poor and operating room delays played havoc with my office schedule. I also did my best to limit home visits, but never really eliminated them.

Such was my professional life through mid-career. Then in my early sixties, by now working in an academic medical center, I gave up inpatient care, which also took me off the night call schedule. I must admit that I do not grieve the absence of telephone calls at 2 A.M. I focused on office care of my private patients and helping residents see patients in the clinic. A few years ago, in my late sixties, I found that my professional travels were interfering with continuity in my office practice, and I transferred my private patients to other doctors in our clinic. Today, in my seventies, my clinical care is limited to assisting the residents in the clinic, a task made possible by good computer skills and wise, supportive colleagues close at hand.

Cutting back occurs in all specialties. I have seen middle-aged obstetrician–gynecologists give up delivering babies and have known neurosurgeons who have abandoned the operating room to focus on pain management or second opinions.

Eliminating the unsustainable should be linked with decisions about where to focus energy in retirement. For me, this has meant teaching students and residents, leading continuing medical education programs, and writing books and papers – options open to academic physicians, some of whom have truly elevated "cutting back" to an art form. Both community-based and academic physicians can choose among a variety of options:

- *Administration.* Look for a focused position in your clinic or hospital.
- *School health.* There are often part-time positions in local schools and colleges.

■ *Nursing home care.* Consider a job as medical director of a nursing home.

■ *Insurance examinations.* There are various opportunities in the insurance industry, including workers' compensation, disability evaluations, and medical examinations of applicants.

■ *Travel medicine.* Being the physician for a travel clinic offers fixed hours and a limited clinical focus. Or you could become a cruise ship doctor and travel the world.

■ *Volunteer teaching faculty.* There is no salary for volunteer teaching faculty at an academic medical center, but the stimulation of working with medical students and residents may well make the absent paycheck seem unimportant. Below on page 328 I have quoted one physician, Dr. Henry Siedel, who has walked this trail.

DON'T CONTINUE PRACTICE AFTER YOUR SKILLS HAVE WANED

It all happened decades ago, and some of my information at the time was second-hand. With that disclaimer, here's what happened. For many years, Doctor Vincent (not his real name) had been the town doctor. The only source of medical care for miles around, he had made the house calls, delivered the babies, cared for the sick, and comforted the dying. All over the county there were little boys and young men named Vincent, after the doctor who had helped bring them into the world. A local civic building bore his name. The doctor no longer went to the hospital, but he continued to make home visits to some of his long-term patients. And then aging began to take its toll.

Dr. Vincent developed some sort of age-related neurological deterioration. You could see it in hands and in his walk. Then the local pharmacist noted some errors on his prescriptions. When referring patients, he made a few comments to specialists that suggested to them that his medical knowledge was, to be kind, becoming slightly muddled. The crucial event occurred when one patient of Dr. Vincent's was treated at home too long, and admitted to the hospital with advanced disease. Fortunately, the patient did well once hospitalized and suffered no permanent harm. There were no formal complaints and hence no official sanctions. One could argue that Dr. Vincent held a valid medical license, and was acting within his scope of practice.

One day some county medical leaders caucused informally. A venerable senior physician was chosen to speak with Dr. Vincent. Fortunately all went well, and shortly thereafter, Dr. Vincent was honored at a retirement dinner attended by several hundred patients and family members. Looking back, I think we can conclude that collective wisdom prevailed and the non-system of the time actually worked to protect both patient and physician.

How old is too old to practice medicine? Certainly there is no magic age, no chronologic based definition of physician competence, but, as noted above, we know that the incidence of being disciplined by state medical boards for some sort of professional misconduct increases with age.

Surgeons come under special scrutiny, although objectively assessing a physician's procedural skills is notoriously difficult.[12] Currently 5% of orthopaedists in active practice are age 70 or older.[13] But there can be cognitive as well as technical errors, and physical harm to patients is a legitimate worry as medical knowledge and skills decline. Today we cannot count on the informal system that came to the rescue of Dr. Vincent. The wise physician, regardless of specialty, does not ignore signs that the time has come to retire and perhaps, in making this important life decision, seeks the counsel of one or more trusted colleagues.

LEARN THE ART OF RETIREMENT

The time to learn about the art and skills of retirement is when you are still professionally active, not the month following your retirement party. Happily, I can report that there have been some studies of physician retirement. A study by Virshup and Coombs a few years ago yielded encouraging findings: Their survey of retired physicians living in California revealed that, following retirement, most enjoyed a standard of living that was "comfortable" or better. Respondents also described improvement in both their personal health and in their relationships with spouses and children. Most described their lives as active and happy, and there were few emotional problems reported. Concerns about boredom were reported as "unfounded."[14]

Just to confirm that the physicians studied by Virshup and Coombs were not happily retired solely because they lived in sunny California, Seim and Mitchell surveyed a large group of retired Minnesota physicians.[15] Their findings echoed those of Virshup and Coombs, in that their respondents were living comfortable lives and, in general, enjoying good health. The authors go on to report that the retired physicians studied spent most of their time in non-medical activities, notably visiting family, reading and travel. Furthermore, and quite interesting to me, "The study also showed that retired physicians consider nonmedical activities much more important than medical activities."

Guerriero et al have studied life satisfaction in retired physicians and their spouses.[16] In this study, both physicians and spouses reported "high levels of life satisfaction." For physicians, the factors associated with better life satisfaction were good health, a sense of optimism, confidence in financial security, interests in hobbies and other activities, and a good sexual relationship. That is what the physicians reported. What about their spouses? For the spouses, higher levels of life satisfaction were related to having a husband (the authors' gender identifier, not mine) willing to help with chores, satisfying personal relationships including sexual relationships, and getting out to the theater and other activities.

RESOLVE TO LEAVE MEDICINE WHEN THE TIME IS RIGHT FOR YOU

It is a matter of not staying too long at the party. We physicians all wish to leave practice well before the time when someone might use the dreaded adjective "impaired." In Australia, Peisah and Wilhelm studied a cohort of doctors age 60 and older enrolled in the Impaired Registrants Program of the New South Wales Medical Board.[17] Here is what they found. Of the practicing but allegedly impaired physicians studied, there were two work patterns: One was the "dabbler," practicing just enough to cause mischief, but not enough to maintain skills. The other work pattern was the "workhorse," seemingly determined never to slow down. The impaired physicians had more health problems than retired physicians in the same age group. The authors conclude, "Older doctors are prone to suffer 'the four Ds:' dementia, drugs, drink, and depression. We need to encourage mature doctors to adapt to age-related changes and illness and validate their right to timely and appropriate retirement."

The trick, of course, is to recognize when to keep working full steam, when to begin to cut back, and when to quit. Or in American country music singer Kenny Rogers' tuneful metaphor: "You got to know when to hold 'em', know when to fold 'em'." And sometimes you walk away. When thinking about retirement, it is truly best not to need to run.

PLAN WHAT YOU WILL DO WHEN YOU AREN'T PRACTICING AT ALL

"Millions long for immortality who do not know what to do with themselves on a rainy Sunday afternoon," wrote British author Susan Ertz (1894–1985).[18] Find the avocation that will sustain you when you don't go to the office every day. There are many possibilities. For example, did you know that Peter Roget, creator of the Thesaurus we all use, was a physician?[19] I describe a number of physician–authors in Chap. 11, including A.J. Cronin, Oliver Sacks, Michael Crichton, and Richard Selzer.

Other opportunities in retirement include charitable work, woodworking, gardening, and managing investments. Your choice really doesn't matter, but you must do *something*! I heard a recent remark attributed to comedian Jerry Seinfeld, who retired in early middle age. He was recently asked what he was doing in retirement. He replied, "Nothing. And it's harder than it sounds." Seinfeld's personal epiphany regarding the difficulty of filling idle time may explain why he is once again doing performances on stage.

STAY INVOLVED WITH MEDICINE AND OTHER PHYSICIANS IN RETIREMENT

Do you recall the Declaration of Geneva, based on the Hippocratic Oath, discussed in Chap. 12? When we recited the Declaration, we pledged that, "My colleagues will be my sisters and brothers." Throughout our professional lives, our fellow physicians, those who have shared our training and our experiences, have been persons we could count on for support when things went wrong professionally. They have cheered our successes, knowing the extent of our efforts. When in a social setting, conversation is somehow more open when the group is just physicians and spouses, rather than a group of friends who are not physicians. Is this something you or I want to give up in retirement?

I grew up in southwestern Pennsylvania, an area of steel mills and coal mines where the accepted life plan was as follows: Work hard, save your money, and then, as soon as you can, leave your friends, your community, and the harsh winters behind. Retire to Florida, sail a boat or play shuffleboard, and never work again. But for most physicians, medicine is a way of life, and not a job, and we will maintain our physician contacts and our medical interests as long as our faculties permit.

Writing in JAMA, pediatrician Henry Seidel tells of his retirement in 1990 at age 68.[20] He describes his last day at work: "It was not suffused with pleasure." Not wishing to give up learning and relationships with colleagues, he promptly volunteered to serve in the pediatrics department of his local teaching hospital. His roles included attending in the clinic, serving on committees, and participating in various learning activities. He reports: "That's how I got started. It has been almost 17 years. I'm approaching 85, still feeling whole; still a pediatrician; still teaching."

On the other hand, above I described the study by Seim and Mitchell, which found that retired physicians in their cohort valued nonmedical activities greater than medical activities.[15] For those who choose not to make formal professional commitments following retirement, there are other ways to maintain contact with colleagues. Our hospital has a Senior Physicians' Forum that meets quarterly to discuss health policy and ethical issues. I am a member of the Portland, Oregon Society of Physicians for Wine and Health. I confess that my wife and I are not dedicated oenophiles, but we do enjoy the company of the physicians and spouses that attend the dinners and bus trips to wineries. Throughout my professional life, I have attended the annual meeting of my state and national specialty societies, and see no reason not to do so in retirement. There are friends I see at these meetings that I have known for three or four decades. Why should I give up these relationships just because I am retired?

DON'T SPEND SOME OF YOUR BEST YEARS WAITING FOR DEATH

In doing research for this chapter, I came upon a wonderful quotation in my Strauss book on *Familiar Medical Quotations*. (Strauss, p. 85) It is attributed to Dr. William M. Beaumont (1851–1928). This is not the US army surgeon William Beaumont (1785–1853), who is famous for studying the digestive system of his patient Alexis St. Martin, the victim of a gunshot wound providing an open window to his stomach, and I have been unable to further identify the "other" Dr. Beaumont. No matter. It is the quote that is important. According to Strauss (p. 85), the following is a passage from the will of Dr. William M. Beaumont:

> The one object of most doctors seems to be to make a competence (SIC) and then retire, after which they patiently wait on the platform for the train to bear them into eternity. When my time comes, may I rush into the ticket station without time to think of the ticket or where I am going and jump onto the Express as it is on the move.

In the end, Dr. Beaumont died suddenly just as he finished a visit with a patient.

WISE WORDS ABOUT PLANNING FOR THE FUTURE

▓ *Don't think of retiring from the world until the world will be sorry that you retire.* British author Samuel Johnson (1709–1784) (Strauss, p. 512)

I decided to include Dr. Johnson's comment on retiring after writing above about the dangers of continuing to practice too long. There is a golden moment to retire – or at least limit your activities to something like writing, in which you are in no danger of hurting someone. The trick is to recognize that moment – when the world will grieve your retirement and when you risk becoming less than you should be for your patient.

■ *The speed of life is not the same for all.* English surgeon Sir James Paget (1814–1899) (Lindsay, p. 4)

We thank the namesake of Paget disease, Paget cells, and Paget-von Schrötter syndrome for this observation, which I interpret to mean that some of us, as physicians, will seem to cram more into their lifetimes than others, and some will remain intellectually vigorous into late life, while others may not.

■ *Growing old is like being increasingly penalized for a crime you haven't committed.* British author Anthony Powell (1905–2000). (McDonald, p. 81)

Of course there are also rewards for many: financial security, grandchildren, and opportunities to explore new horizons, just to name a few.

■ *The danger in … a man's life comes with prosperity. He is safe in the hard-working day, when he is climbing the hill, but once success is reached, with it comes the temptations to which many succumb.* Sir William Osler (1849–1919) (Osler, pp. 416–417)

Recall that, as described above, two of the "four Ds" of impaired older physicians are actually temptations: drugs and drink.

■ *It is strange how the memory of a man may float to posterity on what he would have himself regarded as the most trifling of his works.* Sir William Osler (1849–1919) (Silverman, p. 239)

Sadly, the enduring memory about an individual might also be about his or her mistakes. Think of Roy "Wrong Way" Riegels, University of California football player who, in the 1929 Rose Bowl, scooped up a fumble and ran 65 yards toward the wrong goal. With an 8–7 final score, Riegels' blunder cost his team the game, but it earned him a place in football history.

■ *A man is as old as his arteries.* Anon. (Lindsay, p. 54) Today we may give thanks for the benefits of good genes, exercise, statins, and an occasional glass of red wine.

■ *To live with the full consciousness of living is to recall the past and to dream of the future.* Spanish novelist Benito Pérez Galdós (1843–1920)

REFERENCES

1. BizRules Blog: (<http://www. bizrules.info/weblog/2005/07/ famous_quotes_about_resistence.html/> Accessed April 23, 2008).
2. Murtha S, Norman G, O'Neil E. Medical practice 2010: how we get there. *West J Med.* 2000;172(4):274–277.
3. Stone JH. Communication between physicians and patients in the era of E-medicine. *N Engl J Med.* 2007;356(24):2451–2453.
4. Norman S. The use of telemedicine in psychiatry. *J Psychiatr Ment Health Nurs.* 2006;13(6):771–777.
5. Partners online specialty consultations. <https://www.econsults.partners.org/v2/(bbhrdi45xzi1vynjginwm43y)/adgoogle. aspx?adid=22/> Accessed August 26, 2008.
6. Liu X, Sawada Y, Takizawa T, et al. Doctor–patient communication: a comparison between telemedicine consultation and face-to-face consultation. *Intern Med.* 2007;46(5):227–232.
7. Whitten P, Buis L. Private payer reimbursement for telemedicine services in the United States. *Telemed J E Health.* 2007;13(1):15–23.
8. Kay AC. Predicting the future. *Stanford Eng.* 1989;1(1):1–6.
9. Feero WG, Guttmacher AE, Collins FS. The genome gets personal – almost. *JAMA.* 2008;299(11):1351–1353.
10. International HapMap Consortium. A haplotype map of the human genome. *Nature.* 2005;437:1229–1320.
11. Sadowsky D, Kunzel C. Professional life cycle changes and their effect on knowledge level of dental practitioners. *Soc Sci Med.* 1989;29(6):753–760.
12. Leopold SS, Morgan HD, Kadel NJ, Gardner GC, Schaad DC, Wolf FM. Impact of educational intervention on confidence and competence in the performance of a simple surgical task. *J Bone Joint Surg Am.* 2005;87:1031–1037.

13. Watkins-Castillo S. *Orthopaedic Practice in the United States 2005–2006*. Rosemont, IL: American Academy of Orthopaedic Surgeons; 2006.
14. Virshup B, Coombs RH. Physicians' adjustment to retirement. *West J Med.* 1993;158(2):142–144.
15. Seim HC, Mitchell JE. Life after medical practice: a retirement profile of Minnesota physicians. *Minn Med.* 1995;78(12):27–30.
16. Guerriero AM, Perkins AJ, Damush TM, Hendrie HC. Predictors of life satisfaction in retired physicians and spouses. *Soc Psychiatr Epidemiol.* 2003;38(3):134–141.
17. Peisah C, Wilhelm K. Physician, don't heal thyself: a descriptive study of impaired older doctors. *Int Psychogeriatr.* 2007;19(5):974–984.
18. On life, aging, and death. <http://www.easydiagnosis.com/secondopinions/newsletter12.html/> Accessed September 27, 2007.
19. Kendall J. *The Man Who Made Lists.* New York: Putnam; 2008.
20. Seidel HM. On retirement. *JAMA.* 2007;298(2):147–148.

14

Wise Physicians, Twenty-First Century Challenges, and Doctoring

> *There is one thing in this world that you must never forget to do. If you forget everything else and not this, there is nothing to worry about; but if you remember everything else and forget this, then you will have done nothing in your life. It is as if a king has sent you to some country to do a task, and you perform a hundred other services, but not the one he sent you to do. So human beings come to this world to do particular work. That work is the purpose, and each is specific to the person. If you do not do it, it is as though a priceless Indian sword were used to slice rotten meat. It is a golden bowl being used to cook turnips, when one filing from the bowl could buy a hundred suitable bowls. It is a knife of the finest tempering nailed into a wall to hang things on.*
>
> From "The Real Work," by Persian poet and
> mystic Jalāl ad-Dīn Muhammad Rūmī,
> aka Rumi (1207–1273)[1]

Are you and I doing what Rumi called our "Real Work?" Before beginning this chapter, you and I should pause to reflect that we are a self-selected group. I don't mean to seem elitist, but not every physician would pick up a book on *Medical Wisdom and Doctoring*, much less read it as far as page 333. But you have done so. Applause! Your attention to the thoughts expressed this book suggests that, as a physician, you aspire to make your work meaningful, perhaps even spiritual, and certainly more than the mechanical effort of passing a colonoscope or reading an X-ray over and over each day.

R.B. Taylor, *Medical Wisdom and Doctoring: The Art of 21st Century Practice*, DOI 10.1007/978-1-4419-5521-0_14, © Springer Science+Business Media, LLC 2010

So far we have shared a bountiful harvest of medical wisdom, largely thanks to seeds planted by those who have gone before us. In these final pages, I shall present some thoughts about how we can integrate the best medical wisdom into our clinical practices and into our daily lives, with particular attention to the challenges facing the twenty-first century physician and the joys that make the struggle worthwhile.

RECOGNIZE THE CHALLENGES OF TWENTY-FIRST CENTURY PRACTICE

Becoming aware of our treasury of medical wisdom is the first step; next comes imbedding these wise concepts in our lives and practices, an endeavor not without some difficulty. Here are five of the trials – and perhaps opportunities faced by the aspiring wise physician in today's practice.

Managing the Evolution of Technology in Medicine

In prior chapters, I have written about the growing use of technology, especially web-based communication, in medicine. And all this is well and good, as long as it enhances both patient care and the ability of patient and physician to communicate more effectively, email messaging between doctor and patient being a prime example of web-based enhanced communication. There can, however, be a dark side which we must beware. I have already given you some hints of the so-called advances that concern me – the "nighthawk" enterprise in which an X-ray taken in a Kansas hospital at midnight may be read by a wide-awake radiologist in India. And in Chap. 1, I mentioned the little robot with an interactive television monitor, cruising around the hospital from patient to patient. But what has really caught my attention is the telemedical intensive care unit (ICU).

The telemedical ICU allows a physician sitting in a workstation surrounded by monitors to direct a small team of nurses and doctors caring for a large number of very sick patients in geographically dispersed hospitals. Writing in his book, *The Edge of Medicine*, Hanson calls the workstation physician a "doc-in-a-box."[2] The literature extolls the many benefits of ICU telemedicine, and tells how many hospitals are embracing the technology.[3] As a physician who has always advocated patient-centered medical care, and as a senior citizen who will inevitably be a patient some day, the depersonalization of ICU telemedicine gives me pause. Are we truly improving health care, at the expense of the bedside presence of physicians, or is there some other reason, such as some economic advantage? Breslow et al suggest an answer to the question, writing that multiple site ICU telemedicine programs "may provide a means for hospitals to achieve quality improvements associated with intensivist care using fewer intensivists."[4] This hint of favorable economic outcomes resulting from healthcare decisions brings me to our second challenge.

Being Sensitive to the Pervasive Influence of Financial Considerations in Healthcare Delivery

So far in this book, I have written little about healthcare macroeconomics. Nevertheless, money considerations have an impact on what patients you see, how long you can spend with them, what services you can provide for them, what referrals you can make, what drugs they may receive, and how long they can stay in the hospital – even in the telemedical ICU – when they are sick. Financial realities even control what patients we do not see, generally the uninsured and underinsured, although these persons may escape our consciousness on a busy day. In short, money – or lack thereof can trump the physician's best intentions.

What are some of the many financial forces out there that influence practice decisions? One example is the "pay for performance" (P4P) initiative, in which physicians receive quality-related payments for reaching targets such as glycosylated hemoglobin or blood pressure levels in a panel of patients. There is also the National Institute for Health and Clinical Excellence, with the tortured acronym NICE, struggling to "reach consensus concerning principles for healthcare distribution in the face of resource constraints."[5] The phrase "resource constraints," of course, always connotes cost considerations. Then there is the emerging field of pharmacoeconomics, wading in the murky waters of treatment costs for specific drugs and diseases, in a setting in which some biotech drugs can cost more than $100,000 per treatment course.[6]

What a wise physician can do is to recognize the impact of macroeconomic decisions on patient care, speak out on issues when our elected leaders are debating heathcare proposals, and advocate fair treatment for individual patients in one's practice and in society. Caring physicians champion reasonable distributive justice, including fair access to fundamental human necessities, and are willing to work to see that all receive the basic healthcare they need, although not necessarily all care they might desire, in a setting of reasonable limits on costs.

Recognizing Your Epiphanous Moments When They Occur

From time to time, a sage mentor has shared an insight and you have thought: "Wow! Now I see things differently." That, for you, was an epiphanous moment – a time when you experienced a sudden, perceptive look into the heart of an issue or a clinical dilemma. Other epiphanous experiences come upon noticing something that seems, well, simply curious. In the 1670s microscopist Anton van Leeuwenhoek (1632–1723) certainly had such a moment when he first saw "many thousands of living creatures in one small drop of water," and he named the organisms "animalcules."[7] Such a moment was also, I presume, experienced in 1895 by Wilhelm Roentgen (1845–1922), when he discovered that his cathode ray emissions could pass through his wife's hand, leaving the outline of the bones on a screen beyond. For those of us who deal not in microscopes or mysterious rays, but in direct patient care, most of our flashes of insight occur when we encounter an idea that expands our horizons. I hope that you, the reader, have had a few such moments when reading this book.

As I think about my life, I can recall times when I learned concepts that changed my thinking. I shall share some with you, recognizing that what might be an epiphanous event or fact for one person may be "old news" for someone else.

For example, as an academician who gives lectures, I remember the first PowerPoint presentation I ever saw, thinking at the time, "This is game-changing technology that I need to master, and soon." With that preface, here are a few of "eureka" moments I have experienced (and which are described elsewhere in this book):

- I remember the patient who taught me the importance of "being there." (Chap. 2)
- I can visualize the patient who taught me about the "ticket of admission" – the softball widow described in Chap. 3.
- I recall when, as a medical student, I heard my medicine professor list the diseases that can be suspected by shaking hands with the patient. (Chap. 4)
- I recall when I first learned the concept that sometimes the doctor is the drug. (Chap. 5)
- I can remember the experience that taught me to listen very carefully when a patient begins to talk of death. (Chap. 6)

Perhaps for some the experiences mentioned above would not seem transcendent, and yet, for you there may have been other events that expanded your understanding, based on your education and life experiences. Your charge for the future is to be alert for the epiphanous moment, recall and cherish it, and perhaps share it with a colleague.

Seeking Personal Simplicity in an Increasingly Complex World

Few physicians have ever matched the literary skills of Doctor Félix Martí-Ibáñez (1911–1972), whom I have quoted many times in this book. This fact is all the more remarkable considering that he lived in Spain until age 25, when he fled the Franco regime to America, and thus English was his second language. He subsequently became the founder of MD magazine and Professor of the History of Medicine at New York Medical College.[8] Here is what Martí-Ibáñez wrote about greatness and simplicity:

> Remember that the important thing in life is to be great, not
> big, a *great* man, not a big man. Let your actions be great but
> preserve your personal modesty and humility. What counts
> in a man and in a physician is his greatness. By greatness
> I mean grandeur in the things we do and simplicity in the
> way we do them, doing things that influence the lives of many
> people, but preserving always the greatest personal simplicity.
> For greatness is simplicity. (Martí-Ibáñez, 1961, p. 195)

Simplicity is at the core of being a great, and a wise physician.
To me simplicity is seeking the beauty of the commonplace –
the adoration of young parents for their newborn, the bonds
of young siblings, the day-by-day achievements of young
adults, and the loving care provided by an adult for an aging
parent. We physicians have more than a front-row seat to all
of this; in some ways we are actors in the play, because all
these persons trust their health to us. To find the simplicity of
greatness, we just need to acknowledge that medicine is not
about medical politics, receipt of awards, or even published
papers and books. It is about serving our patients each day,
finding grandeur in what both William Carlos Williams and
Sir William Osler have both called the "humdrum" routine
of everyday work.

Remembering That, Even in the Most Troubled Times, We Are Privileged to Practice Medicine

Ours is the most noble profession. As Sir William Osler wrote
to young physicians: "You enter a noble heritage, made so by
no efforts of your own, but by generations of men who have
unselfishly sought to do the best they could for suffering
mankind." (Silverman et al p. 67.) It is a humbling honor to
be a physician.

I think medicine is an even better job than being a
National Basketball Association player, better than being a
movie star, better than being the president of the USA. Of
course, I have never been any of these, but I am nevertheless
convinced that my opinion is correct. After all, I will not be
"too old to play" at age 35, I am not hounded by paparazzi
and the weight of the world's security is not on my shoulders. I probably could have been a successful executive at

Coca-Cola or Kraft foods, but then I would have spent my life making sugar water or peanut butter. You and I have the best jobs in the world. We recognize that we will never be faultless and will never practice perfectly. We just need to be the wisest physicians we can be.

SOME MUSINGS UPON COMPLETING THE MANUSCRIPT FOR THIS BOOK

Writing this book has been a 2-year adventure involving excavation into medical history, meanderings through the current clinical literature, and personal recollections and self-searching. Here, as I work on the final pages of the manuscript, and at the risk of seeming repetitive, I offer some conclusions. The following is a distillation of my thoughts about medical wisdom and doctoring, and because all this ground has been plowed earlier in the book, the selected insights are offered without annotation.

1. Medicine is, first and foremost, about helping others achieve the best health possible.
2. The immutable truth of one era may seem ludicrous in the next.
3. Studenthood never ends.
4. Our tools can enable us as healers or imperil our humanity.
5. We physicians are far from infallible.
6. Teaching is part of doctoring.
7. Medicine is an optimistic profession.
8. Being a physician demands the highest ethical and moral behavior.
9. Becoming a wise physician is a process and not an end.
10. Striving each day to be the wisest physicians and best persons we can be is both energizing and ennobling.

WISE WORDS ABOUT WISE PHYSICIANS AND DOCTORING

▩ *The physician should possess the following qualities: learning, wisdom, humanity, and probity.* Hippocrates (ca. 460 BC–370 BC). (Quoted in Lindsay, p. i.)

▨ *The practice of medicine is an art, not a trade; a calling, not a business; a calling in which your heart will be exercised equally with your head.* Sir William Osler (1849–1919) (Osler, p. 368)

And sometimes your gut – your instincts – will play a key role.

▨ *Since the beginning of history, the physician has been the man who heals. This he did in primitive times through magic and sorcery; later, through natural resources based on a healthy Hippocratic criterion; today, through scientific medicine.* (Martí-Ibáñez F, 1961, p. 45)

Yes, and today's healing art also involves some personal doctoring skills, along with the magic of current scientific medicine.

▨ *The growth of the professional as a person depends on the concurrent development of both the societal and individual functions of the intellect. In the physician, their relationship is indissoluble.* American physician and humanist Edmund D. Pellegrino (Pellegrino, p. 213)

As I type these words, I wonder how many of our current medical students would truly comprehend these two sentences, and how many will *ever* "get it." Certainly recognizing and understanding the indissoluble relationship of the two functions of the intellect – the societal and the individual – is fundamental to becoming a true healer.

▨ *Medicine is the best of all the professions, the most hopeful.* American surgeon William J. Mayo (1861–1939) (Willius, p. 1988.)

In fact, sometimes hope is all we have to offer, and yet hope can be a powerful therapeutic weapon.

▨ *It is indeed curious that in an age when every human value is up for a second opinion, the expectation for physicians to be compassionate remains unchanged.* American physician Ralph Crawshaw.[9]

▨ *It might be illusory to imagine that we can learn from the mistakes of others, but the alternative is to make them all ourselves.* American family physician and educator G. Gayle Stephens[10]

Stephens' word reminds me of one of life's humorous pranks:

What makes a successful physician?
Good judgment
How do you get good judgment?
Experience
How do you get experience?
Making mistakes

I adapted this favorite witticism for the Preface of my book *Academic Medicine: a Guide for Clinicians,* written to help young physicians embarking upon academic medicine careers.[11] For academicians, physicians and patients alike, it is truly better to learn from the mistakes of others.

If a doctor really and sincerely cares to help his fellow man his results are almost always at least moderately good. The doctor who feels this intangible bond linking him to mankind has a firm basis on which to build his art. Such a man is almost certain to grow in medical knowledge and in personal stature. On him or her the future of our profession must rest. American general practitioner and medical author Paul Williamson (Williamson, p. 4)

Written in 1961, the year I graduated from medical school, this observation continues to ring true today, regardless of all the new antimicrobials, imaging modalities, professional societies, malpractice problems, health insurance schemes, and government programs that have emerged over the past half century.

Good doctoring entails the humanistic act of delivering appropriate medical knowledge to a patient by a determined and responsible physician who cares about and understands the patient as a person. American cardiologist J. Willis Hurst.[12]

It is a wonderful thing to be a physician. American endocrinologist A. H. Rubenstein, as part of the graduation address, University of Witwatersrand, Johannesburg, South Africa, December 5, 2001.[13]

REFERENCES

1. Harvey A, ed. *Jalāl ad-Dīn Muhammad Rūmī, aka Rumi. The real work. From the teachings of Rumi.* Boston: Shambhala Publications; 1999.
2. Hanson W. *The edge of medicine: the technology that will change our lives.* New York: Palgrave Macmillan; 2008:23.
3. Lawrence D. Telemedicine: with limited specialists, more areas to cover, and better reimbursement models, many hospitals are embracing telemedicine. *Healthc Inform.* 2009;25(14):42-44.
4. Breslow MJ, Rosenfeld BA, Doerfler M. Effect of a multiple-site intensive care unit telemedicine program on clinical and economic outcomes: an alternative paradigm for intensivist staffing. *Crit Care Med.* 2004;32(1):31-38.
5. Schlander M. The use of cost-effectiveness by the National Institute for Health and Clinical Excellence (NICE): no(t yet an) exemplar of a deliberative process. *J Med Ethics.* 2008; 34(7):534-539.
6. Hay JW. Using pharmacoeconomics to value pharmacotherapy. *Clin Pharmacol Ther.* 2008;84(2):197-200.
7. Hanson W. *The edge of medicine: the technology that will change our lives.* New York: Palgrave Macmillan; 2008:131.
8. Bogdan HA. Félix Martí-Ibáñez Daedalus: the man behind the essays. *J Royal Soc Med.* 1993;86:593-595.
9. Crawshaw R. Humanitarianism in medicine. In: Smith MEC, (ed). *Living with medicine: a family guide.* Washington, DC American Psychiatric Association Auxiliary; 1987.
10. Stephens GG. A family doctor's rules for clinical conversations. *J Am Board Fam Pract.* 1994;7(2):179-181.
11. Taylor RB. *Academic medicine: a guide for clinicians.* New York: Springer; 2006.
12. Hurst JW. What do good doctors *try* to do? *Arch Intern Med.* 2003;163:2681-2686.
13. Rubenstein AH. A way of life. Graduation address, University of Witwatersrand, Johannesburg, South Africa, December 5, 2001. Available at: http://www.gradnet.wits.ac.za/archive/GradSpeeches/051201.asp/; Accessed August 8, 2007.

15

Epilogue

TO REALIZE ONE'S DESTINY IS A PERSON'S ONLY OBLIGATION

On the quotation page at the beginning of this book, we began our journey with the words of Paulo Coelho, from his haunting fable, *The Alchemist*. The Andalusian shepherd boy named Santiago – with the encouragement of the Gypsy woman, the man who says he is a king, and the Alchemist – risks everything as he leaves Spain to seek his Personal Legend and his promised treasure among the Egyptian pyramids. Along the way, the boy learns to listen to sage counsel, to attend to clues (which Coelho calls *omens*), and to trust his own judgment. In the end, he finds his treasure in a most unlikely place and, more important, he catches a glimpse of his Personal Legend, the core purpose of his quest. (Coelho, p. 22)

Andalusian shepherds, twenty-first century physicians and, indeed, all of us seek our destinies in the context of the life paths we have chosen. We work to define who we are, and how we see ourselves in the mirror. Professionally, do you see yourself as a healer, a teacher, an administrator, a scholar, or a researcher? All play important roles on the medical stage, but each is quite different from the others. Thus, the quest involves finding two related things: your true role, that secret vision of yourself that sustains you on difficult days, and also what the Persian poet Jalāl ad-Dīn Muhammad Rūmī, aka Rumi (1207–1273) calls your Real Work.[1] (See Chap. 14)

Examining some of these journeys, Rabow et al surveyed personal mission statements of a national cohort of medical students, young persons seeking their identity – their

R.B. Taylor, *Medical Wisdom and Doctoring: The Art of 21st Century Practice*, DOI 10.1007/978-1-4419-5521-0_15,
© Springer Science+Business Media, LLC 2010

Personal Legends – as physicians, based on values they hold in high regard. The study had as its foundation the *Healer's Art* professional course taught in 59 medical schools in the United States and internationally. As part of this course, students – chiefly in the first and second years of medical school – are asked to write a medical mission statement telling their ideal professional life, based on their highest values.

The authors randomly selected 100 statements from students in ten schools, and analyzed them, seeking a "thematic catalog of individual mission statements." Three major themes emerged: (1) professional skills, including dealing with the negatives of training, listening and presence, and empathy; (2) personal qualities, such as constancy, wholeness, integrity, and self-respect; and (3) professional identity, including relationships and service. Representative comments included: "Show me how best to learn, how best to use my experiences to help me grow"; "Show me how to look every person I see in the eyes and connect at a basic human level"; and "May I stay true to honest service for others." What I found heart-warming was that, unlike so many dry "professionalism" statements, the students wrote about courage, balance, love, self-care, fears, healing, and awe.[2]

We should all, throughout our lives, continue to cherish the values expressed by these students. And among these, I especially hope that we can maintain our sense of awe regarding the privilege of being a physician. As one student wrote, "May I retain and nurture the humility essential to this noble calling."

As I close this book, I leave you with seven tasks, my assignments to you as a physician and as a person:

1. Do not put this book on a shelf to gather dust. Instead, take it down from time to time and reread the parts that inspired you, and recommend it to a young person seeking his or her own Personal Legend.
2. Do your best to see each patient as a reasoning, feeling person, someone who may have a broken story that needs to be mended, and not simply as a reservoir of pathology.
3. Teach and mentor the next generation of physicians, unselfishly sharing your knowledge, skills, and wisdom.

4. Cherish your family and tell them often how much you care for them.
5. Protect your own physical and emotional health. After all, when it comes to providing medical care, *you* are your most important instrument.
6. Leave the House of Medicine a little better than you found it. Maybe somehow, this will help bring better health care for all in the future.
7. Never stop seeking your own destiny – your Personal Legend. May it be to become a Wise Physician.

REFERENCES

1. Harvey A, ed. *Jal l ad-D n Muhammad R m , aka Rumi. The real work. From the teachings of Rumi.* Boston: Shambhala Publications; 1999.
2. Rabow MW, Wrubel J, Remen RN. Promise of professionalism: personal mission statements of a national cohort of medical students. *Ann Fam Med*. 2009;7:336–342.

Glossary

Aphorism A pithy saying conveying a useful truth in a memorable way. A classic medical aphorism (whose original author is unknown) is as follows: The doctor who makes the correct diagnosis will be the one who sees the patient last. Here is another, this one an Oslerism: The doctor who treats himself has a fool for a patient. See Chap. 1.

Argot In general, the word *argot* refers to an idiomatic vocabulary. In medicine, it indicates words and phrases we use that we think patients don't understand, such as "high serum porcelain level" (suggesting a "crock," or hypochondriac) or "flick" (the pronunciation of the acronym FLK for "funny looking kid"). For many reasons, medical argot should not be used. See Chap. 3.

Bedside doctor A physician who avoids physical barriers – such as footboards of hospital beds or exam room desks – between doctor and patient. See Chap. 5.

Beneficence Ethical jargon referring to "doing good" for the patient, and the opposite of malfeasance. See Chap. 12.

Closeted anarchism What Francis S. Collins describes as the hope held by many scientists and practicing physicians that someday they will turn up an unexpected fact that will force a disruption of the framework of the day. See Chap. 8.

Collusion of anonymity A state described by Balint in which, with many physicians and other providers, making decisions, writing orders, and offering advice to patient and family, no one is really in charge, resulting in a dilution of responsibility that can compromise patient care. See Chap. 5.

Consultation The act of sharing care with another physician, generally resulting in improved outcomes and offering valuable learning opportunities. See Chap. 5.

Declaration of Geneva An adaptation of the Oath of Hippocrates, intended to avoid some Hippocratic anachronisms, currently recited by graduates of most American medical schools. See Chap. 12.

Delusion of indispensability The erroneous belief that your patients cannot get along without you, even for a short while. See Chap. 2.

Designated requestor One whose job is to seek organ donations from family members at the time of a death. See Chap. 12

Disease denial and rationalization syndrome A medical *pas de deux* in which both patient and physician enter into an unspoken pact to ignore the need for action in a clinical setting. See Chap. 2.

Distributive justice An ethical principle describing the fair allocation of goods and services. See Chap. 14.

Doctor as the drug An allusion to the healing power of the physician's presence, often more potent than any medication available. See Chap. 5.

Doctoring The art and science of providing healthcare to patients – one person at a time. See Chap. 1.

Etiquette-based medicine The process of integrating good manners into the clinical method. Examples include introducing yourself, shaking hands with the patient, sitting down to talk, and explaining your role. See Chap. 3.

Evidence-based medicine (EBM) Highly valued by today's clinician, EBM is defined by Sackett as the conscientious, explicit, and judicious use of current best evidence in making clinical decisions about the care of an individual patient. See Chap. 8.

Executive function The ability to plan, initiate, sequence, monitor, and inhibit goal-directed activities. See Chap. 2.

Experience What we acquire as we age, and what we sometimes call our mistakes. See Chap. 8.

Furor therapeuticus A tongue-in-cheek, mock-Latin phrase describing the frantic urge to prescribe something – anything – to treat a disease. See Chap. 5.

GOBSAT An acronym for "good old boys sat around a table," usually used to describe a clinical guideline that is short on evidence and long on opinion and "experience" (See definition of Experience, noted earlier).

Health literacy The patient's ability – or inability--to comprehend printed handouts, instructions on prescription labels, and all the other written material presented to patients in the course of receiving healthcare. See Chap. 5.

Heartsink patient Someone whose name on the appointment schedule makes your heart sink just a little. See Chap. 7.

Hidden curriculum What you might learn in medical school along with diagnostic techniques, drugs and doses, and technical skills. Examples are how to relate to other physicians and how to nurture your inner self. See Chap. 9.

Hierarchy of natural systems A theoretical model of systems ranging from sub-atomic particles to the biosphere, based on the principle that any change (called a perturbation) at any level in the hierarchy has an impact throughout all systems. See Chap. 5.

Illness A concept that includes not only disease, but also the patient's experience in regard to the disease, including pain or other type of suffering, the economic impact, and its influence on his or her life and that of the family and close friends. See Chap. 2.

Impact factor A measurement used by medical editors and publishers to describe how often an article published in a specific journal is cited in other journals. See Chap. 8.

Improvisation In a clinical sense, and especially in the setting of eliciting a medical history, improvisation refers to the physician's unscripted ability to respond to cues provided during the dialogue with the patient, allowing the narrative to meander in a meaningful way – analogous to the manner in which some jazz musicians communicate while playing music. See Chap. 3.

Information mastery The art of conquering the huge amounts of scientific data the physician encounters each day via journals, books, continuing educations programs and, of course, the Internet. See Chap. 8.

Informed opinion imperative This is my term for what I consider the physician's duty, when a decision must be made and after explaining all the choices, to give the patient guidance as to the best option. See Chap. 12.

Malingering by animal proxy A term applied to situations in which pet owners bring animals to veterinarians, describing non-existent ailments in an effort to obtain controlled substances for their own (human) use. See Chap. 3.

Medical professional life Five more-or-less predictable stages, beginning with *medical education and training* and ending with *winding down and retirement* that most of us experience during our years as physicians. See Chap. 13.

Narrative-based medicine The clinical act of helping the patient tell a part of his or her life narrative, and helping that person "fix the broken parts of the story." See Chap. 3.

Narrative competence The ability to acknowledge, absorb, interpret, and sometimes even act on the stories of others. See Chap. 3.

Nighthawk A type of teleradiology in which a radiologist, wide-awake in Spain or India, reads a diagnostic film taken in, for example, Ketchum, Idaho, in the middle of the night. See Chap. 13.

Non-malfeasance Ethical jargon roughly equivalent to the maxim: "Do no harm." The dictum especially applies to eschewing intentional harm, such as assisting suicide. See Chap. 12.

Nutraceutical A neologism combining the words *nutrient* and *pharmaceutical*, indicating a food or food supplement used for medicinal purposes. Examples include ginseng and green tea. See Chap. 11.

Open-ended question A query that cannot be answered "yes" or "no." See Chap. 3.

Pareto principle Named for the Italian economist who first advanced the concept, the Pareto 80/20 principle holds that 20 percent of a set is responsible for 80 percent of a related outcome. See Chap. 7.

Pathognomonic A pathognomonic clinical finding is a symptom, physical sign, laboratory or imaging result that is unique to a specific disease; its presence confirms a diagnosis. The finding of Koplik spots of measles is an example of a pathognomonic sign. See Chap. 4.

Pathologic grief Describing a situation in which a person, following a death of a loved one or some other type of loss, becomes bogged down in one of the first four stages of grief: denial, anger, bargaining or depression. See Chap. 6.

Pearl Also called a clinical pearl or diagnostic pearl (since most have to do with diagnosis), a pearl is a little known, clinically valid factoid stated in a way that is easy to remember. For example: The patient with appendicitis is unlikely to be hungry. See Chap. 4.

Personal legend According to the man who calls himself king, one's Personal Legend is "what you have always wanted to accomplish." (Coelho, p. 21.) See Epilogue.

Pharmaceutical invincibility The notion, not altogether rare among physicians, that just because we know about drugs and their actions, we are immune to their addictive effects. See Chap. 12.

Plastic pearl These are seemingly clever gems of wisdom that have not turned out to be exactly true. An example is the widespread misconception that administering narcotics to a patient with acute abdominal pain makes it subsequently difficult to determine the diagnosis. See Chap. 4.

POEMs An acronym for "Problem Oriented Evidence that Matters," an effort to use EMB to answer key clinical questions. See Chap. 8.

Polypharmacy The pharmacologic Wild West of multiple drug use, ruled by the dictum, "If one drug is good, then three must be even better." See Chap. 5.

Premature declaration of death The phenomenon of being avoided that is sometimes reported by persons with cancer or other potentially fatal diseases, leading to a sense of isolation and abandonment. See Chap. 6.

Quiz-Doc A Doctor Seuss neologism, a Quiz-Doc is a physician who is good at asking many questions, but not necessarily good at listening. See Chap. 3.

Rational non-interventional paternalism A practice described by Savulescu in which doctors form conclusions as to what is best for their patients and argue rationally to convince them to make what the physician sees as the best choice. See Chap. 12.

Red flag Clinical "red flags" are danger signs indicating the possible presence of "must-never-miss" diagnoses. An example is painless gross hematuria, which may be the first sign of a tumor of the urinary tract. See Chap. 4.

Rogue doctor The professional misconduct frequent flier, who exhibits repeated evidence of unacceptable behavior. See Chap. 12.

Second victim What happens when there is a medical error harming a patient and then the physician suffers a subsequent crisis of self-confidence that undermines future practice decisions. See Chap. 12.

Systems-based medicine A healthcare concept that embraces thinking of systems both "above" (such as the person, family, and community) and "below" (such as tissues and cells) a diseased organ such as the heart. See Chap. 5.

Telemedicine The rapidly evolving fusion of healthcare with many applications of computerization, including electronic medical records, telecommunications, and the World Wide Web. See Chap. 13.

Tenfold error A clinical misadventure involving medication use in which, for example, a recommended dose of 10 mgm may become administered as 100 mgm. See Chap. 12.

Testosterone storm A whimsically named condition, describing what happens when an otherwise respectable male physician acts on his sexual fantasies about a patient, colleague, student, or a member of his staff. See Chap. 12.

Third ear An anatomical improbability usually stated as "listing with the third ear," the concept describes the ability, when eliciting a medical history, to attend to how things are expressed, body language and emotion, and what is carefully not stated. See Chap. 3.

Ticket of admission A complaint offered by a one who believes in it, rightly or wrongly, instead of what really brings the patient to the physician. An example might be a complaint of vague upper abdominal pain when the real problem lies with the patient's job, marriage, finances, or family. See Chap. 3.

Virtual E-learning On-line learning based on a virtual practice with virtual patients, peer-to-peer learning, and "ask-the-experts" opportunities, customized to the needs of the individual physician. See Chap. 8.

WHIM An acronym for "What have I missed?" Physicians should ask themselves the WHIM question at the end of any clinical encounter, especially if anything seems a little unsettled. See Chap. 4.

Wise physicians Doctors who provide excellent, up-to-date care for their patients while taking good care of their own families, their communities, and themselves. See Chap. 1.

Zebra A metaphor for the unusual diagnosis, especially one that may pop up among a herd of ordinary "horses." Someday, among all the patients reporting fatigue, you will find a person with myasthenia gravis. See Chap. 4.

Bibliography

Ackerknecht EH. *History and Geography of the Most Important Diseases*. New York: Hafner; 1972.

Balint M. *The Doctor, His Patient, and the Illness*. 2nd ed. London: Churchill Livingstone; 2000.

Bean RB, Bean WB. *Aphorisms by Sir William Osler*: New York: Henry Schuman; 1950.

Birnholz JC. *Clinical Diagnostic Pearls*. Flushing, NY: Medical Examination Publishing Co.; 1971.

Bloomfield RL, Chandler ET. *Pocket Mnemonics for Practitioners*. Winston-Salem, NC: Harbinger Medical Press; 1983.

Bollett AJ. *Plagues and Poxes: the Impact of Human History on Epidemic Disease*. New York: Demos; 2004.

Bordley J, Harvey A McG. *Two Centuries of American Medicine*. Philadelphia: Saunders; 1976.

Brallier JM. *Medical Wit and Wisdom*. Philadelphia: Running Press; 1994.

Breighton P, Breighton G. *The Man Behind the Syndrome*. Heidelberg: Springer; 1986.

Brody H. *Stories of Sickness*. New Haven: Yale University Press; 1987.

Callan JP. *The Physician: a Professional Under Stress*. Norwalk, CT: Appleton-Century-Crofts; 1983.

Cartwright FF. *Disease and History: the Influence of Disease in Shaping the Great Events of History*. New York: Crowell; 1972.

Cassell EJ. *Doctoring: the Nature of Primary Care*. New York: Oxford; 1997.

Coelho P. *The Alchemist*. New York: HarperCollins; 1993.

Collins FS. *The Language of God*. New York: Free Press/Simon and Schuster; 2006.

Dirckx JH. *The Language of Medicine: its Evolution, Structure, and Dynamics*. 2nd ed. New York: Praeger; 1983.

Dorland's Illustrated Medical Dictionary. 31st ed. Philadelphia: Saunders; 2007.

Durham RH. *Encyclopedia of Medical Syndromes*. New York: Harper and Brothers; 1960.

Ellerin TB, Diaz LA. *Evidence-Based Medicine: 500 Clues to Diagnosis & Treatment*. Philadelphia: Lippincott, Williams & Wilkins; 2001.

Evans B, Evans C. *A Dictionary of Contemporary American Usage*. New York: Random House; 1957.

Evans IH. *Brewer's Dictionary of Phrase and Fable*. New York: Harper & Row; 1970.

Firkin BG, Whitworth JA. *Dictionary of Medical Eponyms*. Park Ridge, NJ: Parthenon; 1987.

Fortuine R. *The Words of Medicine: Sources, Meanings, and Delights*. Springfield, IL: Charles C. Thomas; 2001.

Fowler HW. In: Gowers E, ed. *A Dictionary Of Modern English Usage*. 2nd ed. New York: Oxford; 1965.

Garland J. *The Physician and his Practice*. Boston: Little, Brown and Co.; 1954.

Garrison FH. *History of Medicine*. 4th ed. Philadelphia: Saunders; 1929.

Gershen BJ. *Word Rounds*. Glen Echo, MD: Flower Valley Press; 2001.

Gordon R. *The Alarming History of Medicine: Amusing Anecdotes from Hippocrates to Heart Transplants*. New York: St. Martin's Griffin; 1993.

Haubrich WS. *Medical Meanings: a Glossary of Word Origins*. Philadelphia: American College of Physicians; 1997.

Hendrickson R. *The Literary Life and Other Curiosities*. New York: Viking; 1981.

Holt AH. *Phrase and Word Origins: a Study of Familiar Expressions*. New York: Dover; 1961.

Huckleberry ER. *The Adventures of Dr. Huckleberry*. Portland, Oregon: Oregon Historical Society; 1970.

Huth EJ, Murray TJ. *Medicine in Quotations: View of Health and Disease Through the Ages*. Philadelphia: American College of Physicians; 2006.

Inglis B. *A History of Medicine*. New York: World; 1965.

Johnson WM. *The True Physician: the Modern "Doctor of the Old School"*. New York: Macmillan; 1936.

Lindsay JA. *Medical Axioms, Aphorisms and Clinical Memoranda*. London: H.K. Lewis Co.; 1923.

Lipkin M. *The Care of Patients*. New York: Oxford; 1974.

Magalini SI, Scrascia E. *Dictionary of Medical Syndromes*. 2nd ed. Philadelphia: Lippincott; 1981.

Maimonides M. In: Bos G, ed. *Medical Aphorisms: Treatises 1-5*. Provo UT: Brigham Young University Press; 2004.

Major RH. *Classic Descriptions of Disease*. 3rd ed. Springfield, IL: Charles C. Thomas; 1945.

Major RH. *Disease and Destiny*. New York: Appleton-Century; 1936.

Maleska ET. *A Pleasure in Words*. New York: Fireside Books; 1981.

Manning PR, DeBakey L. *Medicine: Preserving the Passion*. 2nd ed. New York: Springer; 2004.

Martí-Ibáñez F. *Men, Molds and History*. New York: MD Publications; 1958.

Martí-Ibáñez F. *A Prelude to Medical History*. New York: MD Publications; 1961.

Mayo CH, Mayo WJ. *Aphorisms of Dr. Charles Horace Mayo and Dr. William James Mayo*. Willius FA, editor. Rochester MN: Mayo Foundation for Medical Education and Research; 1988.

McDonald P. *Oxford Dictionary of Medical Quotations*. New York: Oxford University Press; 2004.

Meador CK. *A Little Book of Doctors' Rules II*. Philadelphia: Hanley & Belfus; 1999.

Oldstone MBA. *Viruses, Plagues and History*. New York: Oxford University Press; 1998.

Onions CT. *The Oxford Dictionary of English Etymology*. Oxford: Clarendon Press; 1979.

Osler W. *Aequanimitas with Other Addresses*. 3rd ed. Philadelphia: Blakiston; 1932.

Pellegrino ED. *Humanism and the Physician*. Knoxville, TN: University of Tennessee Press; 1979.

Penfield W. *The Torch*. Boston: Little, Brown and Co.; 1960.

Pepper OHP. *Medical Etymology*. Philadelphia: Saunders; 1949.

Post JM, Robins RS. *When Illness Strikes the Leader: the Dilemma of the Captive King*. New Haven, CT: Yale University Press; 1993.

Porter R. *The Greatest Benefit to Mankind*. New York: Norton; 1997.

Rapport S, Wright H. *Great Adventures in Medicine*. New York: Dial Press; 1952.

Reveno WS. *Medical Maxims*. Springfield, IL: Charles C. Thomas; 1951.

Reynolds R, Stone J, eds. *On Doctoring*. New York: Simon & Schuster; 1991.

Sebastian A. *The Dictionary of the History of Medicine*. New York: Parthenon; 1999.

Sherman IW. *The Power of Plagues*. Washington, DC: ASM Press; 2006.

Shipley JT. *Dictionary of Word Origins*. New York: Philosophical Library; 1945.

Shryock RH. *Medicine and Society in America: 1660-1860*. Ithaca New York: Cornell University Press; 1960.

Silverman ME, Murray TJ, Bryan CS. *The Quotable Osler*. Philadelphia: American College of Physicians; 2003.

Skinner HA. *The Origin of Medical Terms*. Baltimore: Williams & Wilkins; 1949.

Sosnik DB, Dowd MJ, Fournier R. *Applebee's America: How Successful Political, Business, and Religious Leaders Connect with the New American community*. New York: Simon & Schuster; 2006.

Starr P. *The Social Transformation of American medicine*. New York: Basic Books; 1982.

Strauss MB. *Familiar Medical Quotations*. Boston: Little, Brown; 1968.

Taylor RB. *Family Medicine: Principles and Practice*. 6th ed. New York: Springer; 2003.

Taylor RB. *White Coat Tales: Medicine' Heroes, Heritage and Misadventures*. New York: Springer; 2008.

Train J. *Remarkable Words with Astonishing Origins*. New York: Charles N. Potter; 1980.

Weiss AB. *Medical Odysseys: the Different and Sometimes Unexpected Pathways to 20th Century Medical Discoveries*. New Brunswick, NJ: Rutgers University Press; 1991.

Williamson P. *Office Diagnosis*. Philadelphia: Saunders; 1961.

Index